Notes of a Radiology Watcher

Stephen R. Baker

Notes of a Radiology Watcher

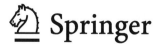 Springer

Stephen R. Baker, MD
Department of Radiology
UMDNJ-New Jersey Medical School
Newark, NJ
USA

ISBN 978-3-319-34707-3   ISBN 978-3-319-01677-1   (eBook)
DOI 10.1007/978-3-319-01677-1
Springer Cham Heidelberg Dordrecht London New York

Springer is part of Springer Science+Business Media (www.springer.com)

To the many medical students I have mentored, who by their enthusiasm and energy, make my work a pleasure.

Preface

This book, a compendium of many subjects all related to diagnostic imaging, is not the result of an organized, predetermined plan. Instead, it emerged in an organic fashion. The editorial style of each chapter grew out of an obligation to provide a monthly audio discussion in my capacity as coordinating editor of Practical Reviews in Radiology, a digest of contemporary radiology articles for CME content. I have edited and expanded on each of the topics I initially presented, and added many new ones, each similar in length to the other. Over the past decade, this exercise became a delightful habit for me. As I became aware of a potential or actual issue related to radiology, I researched it and consolidated my thoughts by putting them on paper.

The model for these remunerations was the column, "Notes of a Biology Watcher" by the late Lewis Thomas which appeared regularly in "The New England Journal of Medicine." I was impressed by the eclectic mix of his musings, his wide and deep erudition, and the trenchant comments that stick in one's mind years later.

I tried to bring the same characteristics to these collections of essays. They reflect my long experiences as an image interpreter, teacher of medical students and residents, program director, dean of Graduate Medical Education, member of the Radiology RRC, chairman, demographer, and geographer as well as my obsessive commitment to jargon-free reports and regular personal consultations between radiologists and referrers.

This format gives me a splendid opportunity to make known my opinions—some of which you may approve of and some of which you may not have thought about. If I pique your interest, I regard that as being a success, even though I may not necessarily persuade you by the force and content of my arguments.

I could not have organized this material alone. The coordination of various sections of the book and careful revision of the text required the dedicated efforts of six medical students—Shyam Patel, David Hansberry, Tekchand Ramchand, Hamid Bagce, Shivam Shah, and Jin Jung, all of whom I believe will become outstanding radiologists. They are all in my debt.

Newark, NJ, USA   Stephen R. Baker, MD

Contents

Part I

Early Residency: Preparation and Participation

The prospective resident must confront the issues of recruitment and selection and from there a choice of internships. Most trainees must reckon with the issue of a substantial debt burden. Also some need to be knowledgeable about imbalances in geographic opportunities during internship and beyond. A few may also have to confront adverse circumstances during their residency years. All these issues are addressed in Part I.

Centralized Interviews for Prospective Radiology Residents

Approximately 20 years ago, the match for radiology residency was imposed and became universally accepted. It has engendered a salutary effect for both the applicants and the training programs. Before then, program directors were free to interview candidates whenever they wished. Some often completed their first year rosters with beginning third year students or even with those still in the second year of medical school. Applicants had to guess when was the best time to seek interviews, a procedure which often interfered with participation in and completion of clinical clerkships. Some program directors demanded immediate confirmation of their decision to offer a residency, often leaving students in a quandary even before they could visit other places for which they had an interest. Moreover, potentially excellent residents who would likely eventually become superb practitioners and investigators in Radiology were denied opportunities to enter our specialty because they decided to pursue it too late. The need for the imposition of a match was acute to protect the interests of applicants who otherwise had no political means to protect themselves from the arbitrariness of recruitment. Programs gained as well from adherence to the requirements of the match. The interview season was specified to extend from the late Fall to the early Winter of the candidate's fourth year. Those who opted for Radiology after experiencing much of medical school were better able to articulate their reasons for seeking a career in our specialty. By then, for many, family situations had become more defined, allowing

candidates to look for programs that met their geographical predilections.

In the past 2 decades, advances in the technical virtuosity of Radiology as well as, frankly, augmented income expectations have made Radiology an increasingly popular career consideration, attractive especially to the most accomplished medical students. At least until recently when interest has declined somewhat, the competition for positions still is felt by the candidates to be keen indeed. Even though there are now 300 more first year slots than there were in 1999, prospective radiology residents initially apply on average to 20 or more programs in hopes of getting at least 15 interviews.

Moreover, there had been a consensus promulgated and maintained by program directors that interviews should not begin before the Dean's letter was received on or about the first of November. Yet today, some programs have now moved up their interviews to begin in September. Still, for the most part, interviews take place from mid-November through January. In that span, the typical candidate may visit 12–15 Radiology residency programs and also 5–6 internship sites.

However, there is no general consideration made by the program directors to make the interviewee's life easier during this two and a half month period by scheduling interviews in several programs in one city on consecutive days. Rather the prospective radiology resident must hope for the best as the luck of the draw determines the sequence of program visits. Most candidates are pleased if they are able to achieve their desired

S.R. Baker, *Notes of a Radiology Watcher*,
DOI 10.1007/978-3-319-01677-1_1, © Springer International Publishing Switzerland 2014

allotment of interviews including the programs they are most inclined to seek. Nonetheless, the proliferation of interviews often induces conflicts with the fulfillment of clinical responsibilities. For the most part, the consternation these scheduling difficulties may subject the applicant to, has not been the concern of program directors.

Thus, an unintended consequence of the otherwise beneficial reform afforded by the radiology match is now impinging on the prospective resident's undergraduate medical education as well as his or her pocketbook. Two to two and a half months of their fourth year is now devoted to interviews with little time remaining for coherent clinical education or research participation. If the average tuition at medical school is $35,000 then $7,000 is forsaken because of the length of the interview process. Approximately 85 % of medical students graduate with debt and the average debt is now between $130,000 and $200,000. Given the mean resident salary of $50,000 per annum, an indebted medical student cannot expect his or her financial obligations to be pared down before the end of specialty training. And added to that burden is the expense the candidate must bear by their odyssey within a region of the country or by crisscrossing the continent to appear at 15–20 separate places for interviews.

The costs of these trips includes (1) plane, train and car transportation, (2) accommodations and meals, sometimes shared with friends or relatives but more often taken in hotels (3) associated cab fares (4) incidental expenses such as dry cleaning, etc. As we all know commercial aviation in the US has become increasingly difficult for passengers. Frequent inconveniences are imposed by airport security, airway congestion, last minute cancelations and a host of other delays, all of which create anxiety and discomfort. December and January are particularly difficult months for flying with inclement weather too often an intrusion. And traffic impingements can be national in scope even if the weather is fine at the point of departure and at the destination. Similarly, the rising price of gas and bottlenecks on major roads makes car travel more bothersome and costly than ever before.

Procedures for interviews and admission to radiology residencies are not standardized. Some programs conduct their evaluation sessions on weekends, whereas other require an overnight stay to meet with the Director and other faculty at dinner interviews. Yet most interviews take place during the working day at which time a series of personal interviews is supplemented by a tour of the facility, a resident conference and a meal or two. Interview schedules vary, too, by the number of face to face exchanges with one or several faculty members and by separate evaluations by residents. Interview assessment protocols also are program-specific. Each has its particular way of doing things which program directors sometimes justify by the virtue of inclusiveness enhanced by multiple faculty involvement, the desire for resident participation and/or the maintenance of tradition.

Yet it is now time to take a new look at this process which like many other hiring practices are dictated by those in positions of leadership in the hierarchy of medicine. As such, they are defined by a tendency to address only the demands of the establishment not the needs of potential entrants. Is it not deemed crucial to consider in this process what is good for the applicant, who are young, often impoverished, at least temporarily, frequently anxious and fretful with their concerns underrepresented in the arena of popular opinion. At least in the spirit of fair play their voice should be heard and, in this matter, at least, heeded.

What I propose has been addressed to every applicant I have interviewed this season to date. They are unanimous in supporting a need to effect change as I will now outline. The opinions they express were extracted from a short questionnaire we give to each applicant as they start their interview day. At that time they have no knowledge of this proposal or our intent to bring it forward.

Why should interviews necessarily take place at the site of the facility the applicant seeks to join? Trainees are apt to apply to programs in cities where they would like to spend 4 years because they wish to reside there for a while or forever. Many of them have family or significant others they want to reside with or be near. For others, the residency itself is the draw irrespective of other geographical considerations. Whatever the impetus, the reasons for being favorably disposed to a program at a particular site, city or region are usually known to the applicant before a visit is undertaken. Even if a visit is not made in the context of a formal interview, revelations made in person about the hospital and its environment are seldom determinative in and of themselves. Moreover, much specific information can be gleaned before a visit by inspecting a web site, a CD, or a brochure provided by the program.

A tour of the facility is a ritual of all interview itineraries. Yet many tell me that in retrospect it is not memorable for them. Most say that upon reflection such excursions through the hospital and its clinics seem to run together in their minds with one place much like another. Furthermore, one might question how productive it really is to have four or five faculty members interview each applicant. In this era of increasing clinical responsibilities and higher RVU's expectations, multiple faculty participation in separate interviews and extended group evaluations sessions may be a luxury. Sure enough the applicant should spend time with residents and most properly be evaluated by them but a lean admissions committee may be just as effective as a fully-fledged one. Moreover, it may be efficient for at most, three or four rather than seven or eight individuals to conduct interviews of applicants both on site or off site.

So what might be done to reform the interview process? How could we decrease time away from school for applicants as well as reduce their expenses and discomfort, allowing them to pursue their medical education in November, December and January of their fourth year without obviating the opportunity for careful assessment by residency admission committees?

One answer is to focus the resident selection process in one or two central locations each over a 3 day to a 1 week period. Bringing interviewees and interviewers together can be accomplished in a short, concentrated interval thereby decreasing the dislocation and interruption of study and work that affects all prospective residents in their

quest for a residency position and impacts as well the faculty and residents who evaluate them. In a congenial, appropriately appointed environment, interviews can take place consecutively even at the rate of 10–15 each day. By convening in a central place, candidates and committee members need make only one or two weekend or one week trips to accomplish this task. To a great degree, the interviewees would not need to travel around the country on their own time and on their own dime, neither of which they have in abundance.

Of course, under such a scheme, an applicant would still be free to visit a facility if so interested, but not according to the structured context of a required formal interview protocol. And exempt from this schema of focused interviews would be the fourth year student who seeks admission to a residency position in the same institution where he or she is now enrolled or in a nearby, easily reached program in the same metropolitan area.

How could such a programmatic change be accomplished in Radiology? Currently there are 186 programs scattered throughout the nation, with total openings for nearly 1,200 applicants. A closer look at their dispersion reveals two interesting patterns of geographic distribution. Sixty-six programs accommodating approximately one third of all residency positions are all located within 30 miles of the I–95 corridor extending in a line Washington to Boston. The other two thirds are scattered in all other regions of the U.S. with a paucity only in the northern part of the Great Plains and the intermountain West. Hence the two assemblages of residencies can be considered like a chain and an archipelago. Outside the Northeast, only Chicago, Detroit, Los Angeles and San Francisco have more than three programs within their metropolitan area.

To ease the travel obligations currently borne by those seeking a position somewhere in the "archipelago", a likely place easily reached by plane from everywhere is Chicago. It could be the locus for a national interview weekend which would occur in December on the weekend after the RSNA. This time and location would also be least costly for interview committee members, many of whom would already be in Chicago for the RSNA meeting and thus would not need to make a separate trip there.

A separate weekend session for programs in the Northeast could take place also in December or January someplace along the Washington to Boston axis, preferably in a suburban hotel near New York so that parking would be free. The hotel site should be situated near major highways and also be with easy access to an Amtrak station.

If for no other reason we in the leadership of Radiology must consider the obligations we impose on our heirs in the specialty—those now in medical school and residency. To perhaps to a greater degree than we in our generation encountered, their experience is bound up with limitations of funds in the face of an extensive menu of mandated expenses for which they have few choices to reject.

They come from college to medical school in debt and leave medical school in much greater debt. By and large they cannot reduce the extent of their indebtedness during residency. Moreover, they are saddled with the costs of the ERAS application, the cost of the boards from their PGY 2 year onward, the costs of Steps 1, 2 and 3 of the USMLE exam, the costs of review courses, as well as the expense of licenses and fellowship interviews to name only some of their obligations consequent to training and progression to certification as a newly minted radiologist. Add to that the cost of traveling around the country at the convenience of stay at home evaluation committees. They deserve some consideration from us even though they may be too timid to express their disquiet and dismay at the exigent circumstances they have to confront, some of which are beyond our control to alter whereas others, like the locus of the interview process, are clearly within our capability to modify and improve.

To provide a perspective on the costs and obligations such a redirection of interview sites would encumber in time and expense, I provide the anticipated impact it could have on the conduct of our program, estimating costs and physician deployment on the one hand and reduction of obligations currently required on the other.

We accept five residents per year, placing us near the middle of programs in terms of resident complement. We receive about 400 applications and assign 90 slots for interviews. Usually 80 candidates accept the invitation and visit our department for a 5–6 h stay, including interviews with the two faculty members, assessment by our two chief residents, a tour, lunch and attendance at noon conference.

Of the 80 candidates, on average 10 are our fourth year students. Six come from our sister school, Robert Wood Johnson, 15 attend New York schools but currently live in nearby New Jersey or grew up there and have parents or other relatives still living in the area. Thus 50 other applicants must make a trip to see us. Of these, 25 reside within a 1–3 h drive from Southern Connecticut, Long Island, Westchester or Philadelphia. Twenty-five others come from further away, 7 or 8 from elsewhere in the Northeast and more distant locations, most commonly Florida, Chicago, Detroit, Texas and California.

Hence the introduction of off-site interviews to take place both in the center of the country and in a conveniently situated venue in the Northeast could accommodate 30 of our applicants from the Northeast and 18 to 20 from elsewhere in the U.S.

A distant location at a hotel in the country's middle for interviews requires a 2 1/2 day stay for two faculty and two residents (which incidentally encompasses our admission committee). Such an obligation would incur a cost of four airfares, 8 hotel day stays, meals for 2 1/2 days and transport to and from airports. This adds up to approximately $1,000 for airfare, $2,000 for hotels, $700 for food and $750 for airport transits for a total of $4,500. For the Northeast, the weekend costs would be about $3,000 if it included hotel stays and $1,500 if it did not.

The benefits to the department would be less disruption of regular work to interview approximately 50 applicants. Thus it would provide added daily capability to meet faculty and residents vacation requests in December and January, an opportunity currently restricted by the assignment of residents and faculty to be present to participate in the interview process. Overall, the costs a department must bear are not great, but the savings that a full implementation of this scheduling innovation will accrue to the applicant would be pronounced and profound, not only in time spent and fewer dollars expended on transportation, lodging and food but also on the restoration of time and focus to pursue tuition-supported, educational activities in this same time period.

A model already exists for the centralization of the interview process for prospective trainees in a post graduate medical discipline. For the past 9 years all applicants for podiatric residencies along with members of residency admission committees have convened at three locations in the country encompassing respectively an eastern, a central and a western site. The approximately 500 applicants and their evaluators spend a day and a half at these venues at which time between 15 and 18 interviews take place per program. This initiative has been a success. In 2010, the three sites changed to only one site consisting of a plenary interview session at a meeting facility in Dallas [1].

The number of interviews per program has not changed with the centralization process. Some but not all interested applicants still visit the home hospital and its clinics but they are able to see two or three facilities in one day, still more over consecutive days, on their own schedule and mostly on their own terms. As a result the time spent on the interview process has lessened for applicants and for committee members and travel expenses and travel interval have decreased for applicants. In the main all parties have been pleased with the process. There is no vocal minority of program directors seeking a return to the old paradigm of exclusive on site interviews in Podiatry.

Reference

1. American Association of Colleges of Podiatric Medicine—Centralized Residency Interview Program (CRIP). http://www.aacpm.org/html/about/index.asp.

A Critique of the Transitional Internship

Way, way, way back in 1968–1969 I pursued and completed a year of post graduate training which could be considered a prototype of the transitional year experience that approximately one third of prospective radiology residents opt for today. In many ways, my internship provided the perfect introduction for a career in radiology, exposing me to clinical encounters of such diversity and with many insightful interactions that I recall many of them vividly today. My training consisted of 8 months of medicine, including one ER month, and 4 months of surgery. The medical experience also encompassed 4 months of general medicine, 1 month on an oncology service at Montefiore Hospital—a full service academic medical center—and 2 months of medicine at Morrisania Hospital—a now defunct city hospital which served mostly indigent patients from the South and West Bronx. Morrisania was designed, can you believe it, into a series of open wards, 35 patients in one large room. The elevators often did not work and the lab was six flights up. Managing diabetic ketoacidosis patients was like marathon training.

My 4 months in surgery included 1 month in urology, 1 month in vascular surgery, and 2 months of general surgery.

It was rigorous—too rigorous because I was on every other night. There was nothing wonderful and everything wrong about that. My dad died unexpectedly in the sixth week of internship and 4 days later, I was hospitalized with infectious mononucleosis for which they kept me for 3 weeks as an in-patient. Imagine that also. But those particularities aside, the clinical experience that I received in breadth and depth, in variety and intensity involving adult patients, poor, middle class and very well off, was supported by some very excellent teachers and a few poor ones, too. It propelled me to take on responsibility for care although sometimes I was not prepared for it. I witnessed suffering and death engendered by the ravages of disease and, in truth, sometimes also occasioned by bad physician management. In most instances that care was ameliorated by compassion and competence exuded by physicians, nurses, and support staff. In sum, I learned about medical diseases and surgical diseases, I learned about the inevitability of physical decline and death as well as to appreciate the manifestations of effective treatment. We even saved a few lives too.

These are not ruminations activated by nostalgia. Rather, I want to create a counterpoise to the present day iteration of what was once called a rotating internship and is now labeled the transition year. I attempt here to examine and to critique how this 12 month period is organized and to relate how current radiologists view it. I also consider the economic advantages conveyed to hospitals that possess a TY program. In contradistinction to the relatively simple format of a rotating internship, the criteria for transitional internships are much more complex. Here are some of the interesting requirements as set forth by the transitional year residency review committee, an arm of the Accreditation Committee for Graduate Medical Educations. For each

S.R. Baker, *Notes of a Radiology Watcher*,
DOI 10.1007/978-3-319-01677-1_2, © Springer International Publishing Switzerland 2014

element I also offer some criticism as to the way it provides an experience for prospective radiologists.

Every transitional program, at least on paper, should have two coincident sponsoring residencies. At least one of those six sponsoring residencies must come from the following six disciplines; Emergency Medicine, Family Medicine, Internal Medicine, Obstetrics/Gynecology, Pediatrics and Surgery. A TY-program must have 24 weeks devoted to one or two of these disciplines. Each rotation should be a minimum of 4 weeks. The requirements also mandate 4 weeks of emergency medicine.

Well, what if a hospital with a transitional year program had core programs only in emergency medicine, and/or obstetrics and gynecology? It is likely that the 24 weeks of clinical experience that a prospective transitional intern must experience would be only in OB/GYN and ER. Of course, ER and OB/GYN provide patient experiences that would be helpful to a radiology resident. Yet, most of what a radiologist encounters aside from pediatric experience, as part of their residency for all but a few of the 48 months of training, are issues involving patients in medicine and surgery. Is enough clinical preparation engendered by such a meager requirement? Furthermore, only 24 weeks of the TY year requires actual clinical service i.e., taking care of patients. In a traditional internship devoted to a preliminary year in medicine or surgery or even in pediatrics no more than 2 months of electives are permitted on average. Add 1 month of vacation it means that the intern spends 40 weeks in clinical service, rather than only 24 weeks as in a transitional internship. And in a transitional program it is conceivable that one would have no experience in medicine or surgery.

On average, a transitional intern is able to take 5 months of electives. As part of the options of the educational program, a maximum of 8 weeks may be designated for nonclinical patient care experiences, such as research, administration and computer science. I know of several former transitional interns, now radiology residents, who took liberal arts courses during those 8 weeks. That is fine for one's general education, but during the

period of internship, the interval in which a radiologist can gain direct and sustained patient care experience, this often seems to me to be no more than a frill. Also transitional interns may take outside clinical electives providing that there is educational justification for the extraparietal rotation. No more than 8 weeks of transitional year rotations are permitted away from the primary institution or its affiliates. But it is permissible that those 8 weeks can take place at a community hospital that has no medical school affiliation whatsoever and the intern can be taught or not taught by physicians who have no relation to any medical school faculty nor have any direct participation in any residency aside from the fact that they are shepherding the individual who takes the rotation. Thus, there really is no oversight for such experiences. Opportunities for abuse are abound with such a circumstance.

Furthermore, most of these transitional programs do not take place in hospitals that are major affiliates of medical schools or academic medical centers. Rather, the bulk of them occur in community hospitals. Only those facilities that have one or two other residencies can assume the burden of a transitional year program. Well, for many hospitals it is not a burden but rather an advantage if looked upon in economical terms. It provides a financially favorable means to find the manpower needed to provide ward based clinical services. A community hospital could hire hospitalists but at a larger salary for each. Or they can hire other personnel supervised by attendings, bearing in mind that often private attendings make only short daily visits to inpatients, the rest of the day and night being covered by residents or physicians' assistants.

Let me consider more specifically the comparative finances that enable transitional internships to flourish. Inasmuch as transitional year interns can take up to 5 months of electives and have 1 month of vacation and have to provide only 24 weeks of labor on wards and 4 weeks in an emergency suite, two transitional interns equal the work of one full time care giver. I mean here not observerships on electives, but actual care of patients. An average intern's salary is $45,000 and with fringes approximately another $13,000, is required to compensate them. Two interns together, comprising one caregiver, would cost the institution about $115,000. Yet, if the same hospital would hire a full time equivalent PA that would mean 1.3 PA's because each must take a vacation and be off on some holidays. Hence, at $75,000–$80,000 annual salary the average physician's assistant starting salary with benefits of $18,000 equals about $100,000. However, transitional interns are expected for work for 70+ hours per week, whereas physician's assistants work no more than 40 h per week. Hence, to provide the same hours of care equivalent equal to one full-time equivalent transitional intern would require approximately 2.1 physician's assistants for which total salaries and fringes would equal $225,000 which is much more than the cost of the two interns. Furthermore, if that hospital was able to include those two interns within their Medicare cap allotment, then they would be reimbursed by Medicare for the work that is done by the residents through direct medical education transfer of funds and indirect medical education transfer of funds. And if that hospital was rich in elderly patients most of those costs would be covered by the Medicare payments. So it is conceivable in such hospitals that the cost of two interns would be zero considering the Medicare reimbursement vs. over $200,000 for a full time equivalent physician's assistant working the same number of hours as those two interns combined. Moreover, physician's assistants accumulate seniority in addition to raises, and over a few years, advances in rank by seniority increase their total compensation. On the other hand, new interns come every year at base salary. Thus, the transitional internship makes money for community hospitals, but does not make that much sense with respect to adequate clinical education.

One would assume that transitional interns enjoy their experience much better than conventional interns who go into radiology after completing training in medicine and surgery. We recently completed a survey of residents and fellows for the purpose of how they regarded their internship [1, 2]. We asked them if the internship was valuable for their development as a radiologist? Most of those who completed a surgical internship definitely said yes but only a minority of those who completed a transitional internship were affirmative. Among those who completed a preliminary year in medicine about half acknowledged its value and half did not. When we asked the respondents to submit written comments, approximately one quarter did. In this context, their opinions were even more defining of a difference. Nearly 75 % of the surgical interns who are now radiology residents or fellows acknowledged the value of their preliminary year whereas most of the written comments of transitional interns were distinctly negative.

Thus, the transitional internship is an economically viable source of cheap labor for hospitals. It is not in the main highly regarded by those who have completed such an internship. The oversight of such training opportunities is limited and in many ways ineffective. One has no direct way of knowing whether they are taught according to a curriculum in their elective months or whether those said to be their teachers are interested in education, and are good at it. The need for reform is clear. A reassertion of a structural rotating internship as I have it would be much better than many transitional programs which have liberal criteria that prevents the establishment and maintenance of rigor as it relates to clinical training.

Summary

Transitional internships are popular with prospective radiology residents. However, their curricula do not meet the clinical requirements for direct patient care because (1) they accord too much time to electives; (2) many programs cannot provide on-site clinical experiences in both internal medicine and general surgery; (3) the quality of program and faculty cannot be carefully judged as many programs take place in community hospitals with minimal or no relationship to medical schools; (4) electives at outlying facilities or departments without coexistent residency programs are even more problematic with respect to oversight; (5) assessment of the value of transitional internship by radiology trainees who have completed them is much less affirmative than assessment of straight medicine or surgery program by radiology residents and fellows who completed training in those traditional PGY (1) program.

A return to the more vigorous schedules of a rotating internship taking place in a bona fide academic medical center is likely to be a more pertinent way of spending the PGY (1) year than what is offered in many present-day transitional internships.

References

1. Baker SR, Tilak GS, Geannette C, Romero MJ, Patel A, Pan L. The value of the internship year for radiologists: a retrospective analysis as assessed by current residents and fellows. Acad Radiol. 2008;15(9):1205–10. doi:http://dx.doi.org/10.1016/j.acra.2008.04.015.
2. Baker SR, Tilak GS, Thakur U. Critique of the transitional year internship and its relationship to radiology residency. Acad Radiol. 2008;15(5):662–8. doi:http://dx.doi.org/10.1016/j.acra.2007.12.006.

Looking Back at the Value of the Internship

Several years ago, we explored residents and fellows perceptives of the internship. They were done at the same time that discussions about the organization of radiology trainee years were under fruitful analysis and eventual change to the new format currently being introduced at the time of this writing. This report and the one to follow explore the relationship of the preliminary year to the subsequent residency interval and beyond. Each considers the effect on the various types of internships and their remembrance of them by senior residents and fellows.

In Radiology, like all of medicine, nothing is constant. Continually, new techniques beseech our attention, some have become essential to our practice whereas others fade fast and are quickly forgotten, At the same time, threats from our colleagues, or should I say competitors, are a constant challenge differing in quantity and urgency so as to make for us each year a unique list of agenda items for problem resolution. Need I say much more about the intrusions of government regulators, insurance companies, malpractice providers and plaintiff's lawyers? And to top it off, the education of our residents, at least how that education is organized, has once more come under close inspection for possible alterations if not a complete metamorphosis.

Now some of you, many years beyond training, may look back fondly at your residency. Perhaps through rose colored glasses, you may recall that in those halcyon days the curriculum was predictable, stable and ordered. Or was it? Actually, abrupt change has been more profound than serene equanimity. In the early 1970s a 3 year residency encompassed education and training in diagnostic radiology, the emerging discipline of nuclear medicine and at least 10 months spent in clinical work and lectures in radiation oncology. Diagnostic radiology and radiation oncology split from each other in the time of the Carter administration. In Reagan's second term diagnostic radiology was lengthened to 4 years. A subsequent 1 or 2 year fellowship became de rigueur and the internship remained optional. But in the early 1990s the internship was made mandatory. Thus, what could have once been a 3 year course of post medical school graduate education for most has morphed into a 6 year obligation with internship and fellowship straddling a 4 year program. Yet by 2001 when the market for newly minted radiologists exploded, many decided to forego fellowship for immediate entry into practice. And today, there are opportunities for post post-graduate work in far flung places as teleradiology consultants. By the way, 35 years ago, offshore opportunity for young radiologists was limited to practice within the various services of Uncle Sam's armed forces.

So is it time once again to tinker with the terms and arrangement of a diagnostic radiology residency. Here are the possibilities, each sounding like the opening of a football play. 1-4-1, 1-3-2, 0-5-1 even 0-4-1. Hike. The choices will be debated this Spring by the program directors and the chief residents at the AUR, by SCARD also at the AUR and by the American Board of Radiology and the Residency Review Committee

S.R. Baker, *Notes of a Radiology Watcher*,
DOI 10.1007/978-3-319-01677-1_3, © Springer International Publishing Switzerland 2014

of the ACGME at a joint meeting in early June. The issues will revolve around two questions [1] do we need to train everybody in all branches of radiology over 4 years or can we aggregate the standard curriculum into an introductory period of 3 years and expand fellowship training to 2 years within a 5 year interval. What is the impetus for suggesting such a change? Well continuing the football analogy there are both offensive and defensive reasons for making this type of substitution. On the offense, we want the best trained or coached people to carry the ball for our specialty. Radiology knowledge is expanding rapidly, broadening and deepening the extent of our expertise as diagnosis in the main has in a sense been handed off to us while traditional methods like history and physical have retreated to the sideline. Yet, no one can be a triple threat, we need radiologists with specialized skills to move the team forward. It is maintained by some that 1 year of fellowship is not enough. The all purpose imaging physician went out with the single wing.

The defensive reasons are just as important. We cannot fumble and thereby lose possession of our hegemony to those in other specialties who are aggressive and hungry. That means we should play to our strength. Familiarity with the constraints of imaging, its appropriate utilization, its risks and uncertainties, our knowledge of the physics of the equipment we use, and our clinical acumen which extends over many medical disciplines are all in our favor in this enduring contest. Yet to first make and then continue to substantiate the claim to leadership we must work hard to be in the forefront of clinical practice and research as well as the application of translational investigations so we can maintain our lead as proprietors of innovation. But this can only happen, so say the quarterbacks of the three-two proposal, when everybody is truly a fully trained subspecialist.

The second question in the minds of the reformers is do we need the internship? Those wishing to do away with it argue that there really is no evidence that a clinical year makes us better doctors or better radiologists. And perhaps there could never be such evidence. How can one design it? What would be the criteria? If such a period of direct patient care can lead a radiologist to saving your life or the minimization of morbidity could it be shown? The prolonged debate persists, the conclusions remain elusive.

Moreover, the mandatory clinical *year* has spawned the transitional internship, a noble concept but honored in the breach by a few programs. For example in some of these internships the training can encompass up to 5 or 6 months of elective time enabling the trainee to do things both in medicine and out of it. In essence they enjoy part-time work and part-time vacation with months spent on soft subjects separate from patient care. Is this what such a year is about? Yet, others are steadfast in their belief that a good internship has meaningful, long-lasting results, incalculable perhaps in quantitative terms but nonetheless qualitatively evident for sure as such an experience necessarily enables a consideration for patients engendered by empathy and tempered by experience.

We have sought to explore this matter in detail by sending out a questionnaire to all radiology residents in the United States as well as those who are in their post residency year. We queried them about their perception of the benefits of the clinical year. The early results are somewhat surprising contrary at least, to my presumptions. Most of these trainees affirmed that the internship was helpful for their careers as radiologists. However, some opined that this 12 month period should be integrated into the four or five following years of training. An interesting speculation would then be what would those intercalary months encompass? More patient care or more radiology focused obligations? Would it make the point or be beside it? When all of the data in hand and analyzed, I will provide you an update in coming months [1].

Reference

1. Baker SR, Tialk G, Geannette C, Romero M. The value of the internship for radiologists. Acad Radiol. 2008;15:1210–5.

Radiology Residents: Internship Survey

Several years ago we undertook a study of the radiology residents' perception of value of their internship year. We were gratified by the response, surprised by the results and heartened by the fact that this study has already gained credence among leaders in radiology to the point where recommendations for modifications of some components of some types of internships will be made to national organizations. I believe the perceptions of residents today have changed little over the past 5 years and I present to you a reflection of continuing attitudes [1].

The questionnaire was sent out in 2007 to all residents in radiology and also those 1 year past training, most of whom were in fellowships. We were astonished by a 40 % response rate to the questionnaire. We asked the trainees six specific questions and called for additional data, including location of residency, the number of trainees and programs, current year of residency, internship type, and number of elective months during internship, expected subspecialty focus and other comments. The questions were. (1) Do you think the internship was *necessary* for your development as a radiologist? (2) Do you think the internship was *necessary* for your development as a physician? (3) Do you think the internship was necessary to provide perspective on the utilization of imaging resources? (4) Did the internship advance your capabilities and skills in specific procedures which have been helpful in your development as a radiologist? (5) Did the internship create further demands for your management of debt? And (6) did the internship further

affirm your decision to become a radiologist? For these six questions, there were five options on a Likert scale. 1—not at all, 2—hardly, 3—no influence, 4—mostly, and 5 absolutely. 5,500 questionnaires were sent out, 1,000 returned unopened, and nearly 2,000 completed and were returned to us.

Now for the specifics. Question one, (did you think the internship was necessary for your development as a radiologist). This was perhaps the most important question because the answer reflects what the residents feel about the pertinence of the first post graduate year. 52 % of those who responded indicated that the internship year was not at all necessary or hardly necessary or had no influence on the development as a radiologist whereas 48.8 % claimed that it did. If we eliminate the 12.3 % who claimed no influence, then our results indicate that 56 % thought the internship was vital for them and 44 % felt that it was not necessary.

These results could be compared with the results of question two i.e., do you think the internship was necessary for your development as a physician. For this question only 18 % registered an unfavorable opinion, 10 % had no opinion and 78 % thought that it was important or necessary. I will come back to some implications of questions 1 and 2 later.

For the third question—do you think the internship was necessary to provide perspective on utilization of imaging resources. While 32 % did not think that was important, more than 50 % agreed with the proposition. Regarding the next

S.R. Baker, *Notes of a Radiology Watcher*,
DOI 10.1007/978-3-319-01677-1_4, © Springer International Publishing Switzerland 2014

question, did the internship advance your capabilities and skills in procedures which have been helpful to your development as a radiologist, here only 32 % thought that it did whereas 31 % indicated not at all and 20 % said hardly. Thus the internship has value for the resident for humanistic concerns and diagnostic and therapeutic development, but not for mechanistic training. The fifth question—did the internship create further demands for your management of debt, 52 % claimed the internship year made demands on the management of debt, 22 % had no opinion, and only 24 % considered that it mattered not at all or hardly. And finally to the question did the internship year affirm your decision to become a radiologist? Well, a whopping 85 % thought yes. Many were relieved when it was over, the experience was long enough.

Returning to question one now disaggregating the results by resident year, the results here were interesting to us. I hope to you too. For PGY-2 and PGY-3 trainees about 50 % thought it was helpful. Similarly PGY-4 was favorably disposed to the internship as being necessary for their development as a radiologist. Yet in the fourth year of residency, the PGY-5 year the percent answering affirmatively was less than 50 %, whereas for those now in their post residency year which for many means within a fellowship, almost 60 % thought the internship was necessary for their development as a radiologist. Something happens in the fourth year engendering a dip in regard for the internship year as being necessary for their specialty development. Was it that preparation for the boards that colors everything? Was it some other factor? I suggest "board psychosis" but we cannot be sure.

We do not exactly know why, but it is gratifying for those who favor the internship to relate that immediately beyond residency, the internship year becomes more highly regarded with respect to a perception of the development of the individual as a radiologist.

We disaggregated the data once again in another fashion, this time by expectation of subspecialty choice? The results here were a little confusing. Whereas a slight plurality regarded it positively by those seeking a career in general

radiology, body imaging and women's imaging, those planning to concentrate in musculoskeletal radiology had a more negative opinion. On the other hand, interventional radiologists favored the notion by nearly 70 %, suggesting that some of the patient care skills and procedural developments learned in internship might be perceived to carry over as being valuable for preparation for interventional radiology.

One more time, question (1) was disaggregated now with respect to the type of internship that the residents pursued prior to beginning radiology training. Among internal medicine interns, who are now radiology residents, more than 50 % agreed with the proposition that the internship was necessary for their development. Yet among former transitional program interns, only 43 % thought so. Among former surgical interns, nearly 71 % affirmed the necessity of their internship for their career as a radiologist.

We then surveyed the extent of elective periods in the various internships, bearing in mind that a transitional internship was a choice of more than 50 % of the respondents, an internal medicine internship was completed by about 35 %, and surgical internship by about 14 %. The only other category that could fit the requirements is a pediatric internship of which there were only 5 respondents who followed this path. The number of elective months overall varied from 0 to more than 6. Most common were 2–3 months of elective which had a 27 % and 30 % response rate respectively, 4 months being the experience of 17 %, 5 months 9 % and 6 or more months 7 %. Yet in the transitional year, nearly 50 % of the interns had 5 or more months of electives. In internal medicine that number was only 11 % and in surgery only 2.5 %, in fact, nearly 80 % of surgical interns had no more than 2 elective months whereas in internal medicine nearly 65 % had 1–3 months.

Comments to our questionnaire were also requested and many were received. Among a group of 110 written responses, two-thirds favored the intern year with half of those in that group giving it a blanket endorsement. About one fourth felt the internship was necessary but should be shortened, and another one fourth believed the intern year was valuable but it should be more focused towards radiology, including more time in surgery, ortho, ER, ICU, and other specialties that emphasize the utilization of images. One third of the respondents who offered comments were negative about the time spent in an internship.

What inferences can be drawn from all of this information? There was a wide disparity of responses of course. Yet even though there is privation and stress in the internship year and even though many clinical issues in that year may be tangential to imaging, nonetheless, at least one half of those who responded overall felt that there was value to the internship year and that value was necessary for their development as a radiologist.

One issue brought to light by the data which was not generally known before the study was the great variation in elective time among the various internship categories. At a combined meeting of the Radiology Residency Review committee and the American Board of Radiology which was held on June 1, 2007 in Louisville, just prior to the board examination week, there was a consensus expressed that the internship year, as perceived by the residents and as recorded in our survey had value and should be retained. What also emerged from a discussion of the data were concerns about the utility and appropriateness of the transitional year given the great amount of elective time and the fact that many of these programs are conducted at community hospitals where opportunities for teaching are generally constrained.

A study published in JAMA in 1998 entitled Learning, Satisfaction And Mistreatment During Medical Internship A National Survey Of Working Conditions', provided corroboration of that notion. The investigation revealed that there was a moderate level of satisfaction by radiology residents with the first year of training. It is an exciting time in which they perceived enormous gain and knowledge in skills as well as the engendering of relationships with colleagues and attendings. Respondents to the JAMA survey which included other physicians besides radiologists, maintained that the greatest contribution of their learning came from resident colleagues, more even than by caring for patients. Interaction with attending physicians and reading followed closely in their collective esteem. Time with attending radiologists varied by specialty with residents in surgery having the most time with attendings and those in transitional internships having the least.

Reference

1. Baker SR, Tilak G, Geannette C, Romero M. The value of the internship for radiologists. Acad Radiol. 2008;14:1210–5.

Summary

The problem of debt repayment for entry level radiologist is not just one of financial challenge for the borrower. Rather it is an issue for all of Radiology as indebtedness directs career choices. And with the costs of college and medical school increasing coupled with relatively low salaries and mandated expenses throughout residency, average educational loan obligations of newly minted radiologist are well over $100,000. This has caused some trainees to consolidate their debt into a 30 year pay back agreement that allows the lender to alter the interest rate according to circumstance and opportunity.

An upshot of this phenomenon is the decision of some recent graduates of Radiology residencies to seek employment in private practice initially, even though their predilections might be for an academic position. The entry level differences between the two, average $50,000. Hence as behavior often follows the money, the lure of private practice is siren like. The issue of indebtedness affects the majority of residents. Perhaps to an even greater degree it is a constraint for minority residents because their debt load tends to be higher.

In this two part review, I will attempt to place resident debt in a socioeconomical context, offer data on the extent of the crisis for radiologists and for Radiology and also provide a few remedies.

The subject of this presentation is the debt crisis in education. What you might say, has this to do with Radiology practice and, on first glance perhaps for many of you who are outside academia, you might also say, what this has to do with me? Well, our specialty, like all others needs to maintain a modus vivendi among research, education and the provision of care. Ignore any of the three and the specialty would wither from lack of attention to new knowledge in a competitive environment among all specialties, lack of adequate training of those who will become our investigators and practitioners and lack of protection for practitioners as they seek opportunities to maintain and expand the fruits of their expertise. So we are all inextricably linked. A crisis in one should be an issue for all. And now there is indeed a crisis that bears upon the vitality of academic radiology although it also may appear to confer a Janus-faced benefit to private practice—a short term gain but a long term deficit.

What is the problem? The debt crisis is an infestation in the decision-making process of medical students, residents and young radiologists. It is a truism, with some exceptions, that behavior tends to follow the money. An emerging radiologist with an academic bent will likely choose private practice especially when a $150,000 loan must be paid even if the term extends to 30 years. Thus an investigative career is stillborn when one is in thrall to the exigencies of lenders. This is an issue particularly for minority residents possessing research interests. They are the ones probably most inclined to make discoveries with respect to diseases affecting members of their ethnic group. Yet, they may be particularly burdened by the weight of obligations they must bear to repay the costs of their education and training.

Debt repayment for education is an increasingly difficult problem for our country in general and is one borne most severely by the generation now being educated. Over the past 30 years income disparity between the more rich and the less rich has risen dramatically. The Gini coefficient is an economic index of inequality within a nation. It is displayed on a scale from 0 to 1 with 1.0 representing all of the income allocated to one wealthy person and none to the poor whereas a score of 0 indicates identical income for all. The Gini coefficient is highest in many Latin American countries—in Guatemala it is 0.59, in Brazil 0.57 and in Mexico 054. In Europe it is much lower. For example, it is 0.23 in Austria, 0.28 in Germany and 0.25 in Belgium. Among all industrialized countries, the United States has the highest Gini coefficient. It was 0.41 in 2000. And the trend towards income disparity in the past 3 decades has accelerated over the past 5 years with the Gini coefficient rising from 0.41 to 0.45.

You might not have experienced the ill effects of the yawning divide between the economic haves and have nots. No doubt we are all aware of the decline in manufacturing jobs and the rise in the number of poorly compensated service jobs with many of them created in retail business and hospitality enterprises. For example, in 1970 the largest employer in the U.S. was General Motors at which the median salary expressed in 2005 dollars was 17.50 an hour while today the largest employer is Wal-Mart at which the median hourly income is $8. In large measure, the disparity reflects educational attainments. A study of 5 year trends of mean real earnings by educational group reveals that high school drop-outs comprising 9.9 % of the population of all adults in the country experienced a real wage decline of 7.5 %. High school graduates comprising 30 % of the population saw a 0.5 % decline. Those with some college experience (28 % of the population) suffered a 3 % drop. College graduates, (21 % of all adults) had a 4.0 % diminution in income. Non-professionals with a master's degree representing 2.9 % of the population withstood a 2.5 % decline. The only real winners were PhD's

(1.5 % of the population) whose real earnings increased 3 % and MBA's, lawyers, and doctors together comprising 1.9 % of the population who collectively enjoyed a 10 % gain.

So income disparity has widened between the poor and the affluent and between the more educated and the less educated, but of the more educated, only those who had an MBA, PhD, LLB, or an MD prospered. And the disparity has widened also with respect to age, not because the young are earning less, although indeed they may be, but because the cost of their education beyond high school has increased so much. College tuition has grown faster than inflation for the past 30 years and faster than family income in the same time period. The trend has accelerated in the decade between 1994 and 2004. In that interval, median family income rose only 2 % while tuition at 4 *year* colleges have increased 59 %. The rate of rise of tuition at both public and private medical schools mirrors the upward trajectory of tuition in undergraduate schools. College has become more expensive because of the overall decline in public appropriations to institutions of higher learning, because of technology inputs into the learning process without coexistent productivity gains and because of increasing capital expenditures. I am sure your alma mater today has changed much from when you were a senior there. Athletic centers and student unions have become the new palaces. Part of that stems from competition with each university selling itself on amenities to prospective students, rather than the quality of education which is hard to discern amidst the hype, hoopla, and mystification. Food service in the cafeterias, new buildings, and excellent landscaping are easier to see and remember.

The two financial expedients that make it possible to complete college are loans and grants. And here also, the largest donor and lender, the federal government, has helped to worsen the cost squeeze. In 1981 of all federal dollars allocated for the support of individuals pursuing higher education, 41 % were in the form of loans and 59 % in grants whereas in 1999 there was nearly a mirror image reversal with 59 % of the pie in loans and 41 % in grants. Another relevant comparison regards Pell Grants, these monies designated for middle and lower income students, the awards of which have not been closely adjusted for inflation. Thirty years ago, grants paid 72 % of a 4 year public college education, but today only 36 % of the cost can be supported by a Pell Grants to those eligible. And over the years a much smaller percentage of students have been so eligible.

Although it has generally been assumed that with the passage and enforcement of civil rights legislation in the 1960s and 1970s and the imposition of affirmative action programs since then that less affluent minorities would become better enmeshed in the economic fabric of the nation. While it is true that African Americans are entering college in greater numbers, they are not completing their education in greater numbers because of the intrusion of debt repayments. In 1972, the gap between whites and blacks in college attendance was 5 % while in 2000 it increased to 11 %. Similarly for Hispanics the gap was 5 % for college attendance in 1972 and 13 % in 2000. If they cannot finish college, medical school is out of the question and radiology programs will never see them no matter how capable they could have been.

Debt should not be considered solely as an abstract number. Rather, it should be assessed as an expense in the totality of personal finance. Here, the concept of debt burden is important. Manageable rent should not exceed 33 % of income, and manageable debt should not exceed 8 % of income. Of student borrowers who graduated from college, 39 % live under the weight of unmanageable debt. In this group, 55 % of African American graduates and 58 % of Hispanic American graduates are so burdened. So even with affirmative action, the path to medical school and residency is open predominantly to more well off minority members and their parents, not everyone.

This background sets the stage for a more focused discussion of types of loans and grants and means of payment. I will also discuss the implications of the various repayment schemes as they affect medical students, radiology residents, and radiologists as they plan for a job. And, I will propose a few remedies to mitigate the situation for the sake of radiology in general and academic radiology in particular.

In the previous essay I provided some background about the education debt crisis. I discussed among other things, widening income disparities in this country by occupation, education and by age. In parallel, college tuition has increased much faster than family income. Furthermore, changes introduced by the federal government in support of funding through guaranteed loans rather than through grants have accentuated the debt management by college students, medical students, and physician trainees. In the discussion I delve into detail, especially in relation to medical education and the plight of residents. As measured in constant dollars, medical school costs have increased in the past 10 years by 50 % in private schools and 133 % in public schools. In the last 5 years the rate of increase has become steeper with each successive year. At public institutions, prices charged now are more than double the cost of education. To some degree, scholarships and grants can overcome part of the funding deficits in medical school education, and in fact, currently 27 % of the cost of tuition in both public and private institutions is covered by these grants.

If we use law students to illustrate the problem, remembering that they go to school for three rather than 4 years, and then enter practice rather than residency, their debt load has increased by 400 % in the last 15 years and 20 % of those with loans have defaulted on their obligations. At the same time, many law students moved their debt burden from public guaranteed loans to more private loans. Now in medical residencies, for most federal loans under the Stafford program, the

residents can opt for a period of deferment. There are two types of loans, one subsidized and the other unsubsidized. In subsidized loans the interest is not paid for the period of time spent in graduate school. When the interest resumes it is not capitalized. With unsubsidized loans, the interest accumulates over the several years of deferment and then is capitalized so the principal of the loan increases. Since 1983 it has been possible to consolidate loans, thus lowering the interest rate. In fact between 2001 and 2005 residents could consolidate their loans at very favorable interest rates, between 2 and 4 %. On the other hand, they must repay them over a 30 year term unless they accumulate the resources to pay it back sooner. And so it is conceivable that a resident will look to a 30 year period of loan repayment just for their education. For many they will finally complete that term after their children have completed college.

Well, how to pay for graduate school when one has additional obligations. Public loans are primarily supported by the federal government. They are more difficult to obtain for large amounts because of the extensive paperwork needed to secure the money. Seeking ease and convenience, many have opted for private loans, which is now a booming business. Unfortunately, the private loan business which has skyrocketed to 80 billion nationally will be facing perhaps the same problems that the subprime mortgage loan industry is facing today.

Yet for many residents, including about one fourth of those in my program, because of

S.R. Baker, *Notes of a Radiology Watcher*,
DOI 10.1007/978-3-319-01677-1_6, © Springer International Publishing Switzerland 2014

relatively meager resident salaries and other obligations, which I will touch upon in a minute, they cannot make ends meet just by repaying loans. So part of their education is repaid through credit cards. The trouble is, credit cards are ubiquitous, easy to get and the companies that issue them charge usurious rates. In essence, they are a bad bargain to bank on for repayment of education costs. But they are alluring because they allow ready access to credit so that trainees can pay back their loans in part, and pay for other things that they think they need or want. The average balance of students for credit cards in 1995 was $2,169. The average credit card debt in 1998 was $4,800 and in 2004, almost $8,000. So a resident for those few years of training may feel trapped. Private loans by the way require pay back immediately, they are not protected by bankruptcy laws and often they are sold through various medical schools. And increasingly they are marketed directly to consumers and can be purchased over the internet, a further attraction for these higher risk loans.

Let us now consider the cost of education borne by radiology residents. In a study that we did of the attendees to our review courses, we calculated that the expenses that are the obligation of residents, which include some or all of AFIP expenditures, an average of two board review courses, and the cost of the board examination itself calculated out to be $7,928 for trainees whose median salary was $50,000 [1]. Thus, 16 % of pre-taxed income was required to pay for education responsibilities they deem essential to their quest to become a full-fledged radiologist. Some departments give a book allowance, others pay all of the AFIP costs. Yet many do not, and most do not pay for more than one board review course. Furthermore, residents must travel for fellowship interviews and many take physics review courses away from their institution. They must pay for Step Three of the USMLE exam, and sometimes in the residency they must obtain a license. Hence, how is an indebted resident going to have enough money to pay for housing, automobiles, and food as well as some of the luxuries of life?

Well, do all of these things happen to have to occur? Can there be some other way of looking at this process? It is my opinion that many of the policies, which foist responsibility on the residents, have come from older individuals well beyond this age group, who are in a different economic status. They may have wistful memories of the past but that was back 20–30 years ago, when things were easier than they are at present. Therefore they cannot gauge the rigors and constraints that residents must go through.

One example of where changes can be made is in the cost of the board examination at all. The American Board of Radiology charges $2,800 to take the board examination series. Not counting travel to and from Louisville for the oral part, which is now replaced by a trip to Chicago or Phoenix to take the computer-based qualifying exam the board requires payment of $850 in the PGY-2 year, $500 in the PGY-3 year, $500 in the PGY-4 year and $950 in the last year of training. Why does the board demand beforehand payment from the residents when many of whom are hard put to scrape up the money? Was this arrangement set up to improve the boards' cash flow? It would be one thing if after the initial board certification the ABR's relationship with a radiologist would end. Well, that was the case up until 2002. Now with maintenance of certification, a radiologist is bound to the American Board of Radiology for life. Why not charge individuals more money when taking a MOC exam later in practice and reduce the price to the residents? Would this restructuring really be devastating to the ABR's cash flow, I think not. Once the change was made, they would not lose any money at all.

What is another response the residents can undertake to meet this debt burden? Well, they can moonlight. We have just completed a moonlighting survey, responded to by 65 chairmen representing 40 % of all radiology residents. We found that 86 % of programs allow moonlighting, either internal or external, or both. A minority of programs allows moonlighting internally by second year residents and a smaller minority allows second year residents to moonlight externally. Only some of the programs account for the time spent in external moonlighting and the time to travel to an external moonlighting source. Moonlighting has become a necessity for many residents to prevent them from defaulting on their loans. Incidentally, defaulting on a federal loan provides no bankruptcy protection and will disqualify individuals for receiving Medicare and Medicaid payment for services. That is a choice most do not want to undertake. Furthermore, moonlighting puts an additional strain on residents as they study for their qualifying exam. They need the money and they perceive they need to study extra hard. Consequently, time spent attending to their general residency duties are often either neglected or not given the attention they deserve. So the quandary continues; the end result for academic practice is that residents who have an interest in investigative activities and teaching are now confronted with the fact that finally they have come to the time to pay back their loans. No wonder private practice is attractive and academic practice is shunned by many who might enjoy a fruitful career there.

One proposal to address this issue takes note of the fact that starting salaries in academic practice are about $50,000 lower than starting salaries in private practice. Two medical schools have instituted a plan of a $50,000 signing bonus to those with an interest in academic radiology. If the radiologist leaves before 5 years, the bonus is forfeited. By that time, they should have settled into their career and no longer miss private practice as they are well enough compensated to meet their debt obligations. This is an idea that should be addressed by various institutions if they have the wherewithal to do it. And yet if they don't believe they have the resources to offer it, their success in recruiting will be compromised. With persisting if not widening income disparities between the academic and the private sector and with debt repayment remaining formidable, a bonus plan may not merely be an option but a necessity as long as young physicians have to accommodate to the mounting costs of at least 13 years of education and training beyond high school.

Reference

1. Baker SR, Sheen L, Varghese C. Debt and other expenses, the road gets harder for students and trainees. NJ J Med. 2011;2:26–8.

Radiology Resident Recruitment: Robustness in an Uncertain Environment

7

As most of you are now aware, these are parlous times for Radiology. The long run up in case volume has peaked. Although your practice may still be experiencing growth, for most of us we are now entering a period of retrenchment. The multi-decade expansion of our discipline has been accompanied by a 12 year interval of expansion of residency programs and now the former dearth in the number of newly minted specialists in our discipline has become a surplus [1].

Remember the managed care scare of the mid 1990s when it was predicted that volume would lessen with primary care doctors acting as gatekeepers. They would restrict utilization and then radiology practices should expect contraction. So some training programs decreased the size of their entering classes. But since then, even with the Medicare cap in place since 1997, nearly every program has become larger. So now we graduate approximately 1,100 residents annually up from 550, 15 years ago. And in the pipeline are even bigger classes. Thus with the specter of declining revenues and limitations of test-ordering just over the horizon (in essence a formula for decreased demand) coupled with increased supply, this uncertain future may be regarded with alarm by senior medical students. Since they are usually savvy consumers, we should see a declining interest by them in Radiology. Right? No wrong, or particularly wrong.

Judging by the record of the 2009 class and with no indication from preliminary results from the 2010 class of any change, radiology is still attracting in droves some of the best and highest achieving allopathic American medical students as well as a veritable flood of capable foreign medical graduates. But in the last 2 years, allopathic students are less inclined to seek radiology whereas foreign trained radiology seekers are still interested.

The following discussion will highlight details of the demographics of entrants to our unfavorable economic projections from seeking to join us.

In 2009, 1,095 positions were offered in the match. This represents nearly all available positions as far as can be determined. A few programs violated match by arranging with applicants for first year places separate from the match but that is done clandestinely and is probably distinctly uncommon and largely undetected. There were last year 1.4 applicants for every position. Of those, 931 who gained admittance were seniors from allopathic medical schools, 155 U.S. seniors from such schools applied but did not match. From the NRMP data 257 independent applicants, i.e., FMG's, osteopathic students and U.S. citizens who graduated from offshore schools, did not match whereas from this conglomerate group 134 did match. Yet I suspect that the number of so-called independent applicants was much larger. For example of the 600 applications we received for our program 300 were from foreign medical graduates. Of course the approximately 190 or SO American radiology residency programs under the aegis of the ACGME feel the effects occasioned by applicants, U.S. trained and others, who are applying to many more

S.R. Baker, *Notes of a Radiology Watcher*,
DOI 10.1007/978-3-319-01677-1_7, © Springer International Publishing Switzerland 2014

programs than in the past. That might account for the seeming throngs of FMG's knocking at Program Directors' doors which really may be a reflection of hyperactive churning of a relatively few and not the usual practice of a legion of place seekers. Yet I still suspect that a total of only 300 non-US medical school applicants to Radiology is too low a number.

Compared with other specialties, the figure of 1.4 applicants per position puts us right in the middle of the pack for this ratio among all specialties. Plastic Surgery at 1.9 and Dermatology at 1.7 are higher but their cadre of positions is much smaller. The notion of exclusivity, for larger specialty complements including Radiology, can be discerned by the ratio of matched positions gained by AMG vs. non AMG students and by the average Part I scores on the USMLE exam of applicants to these relatively large specialties. Let's take the first index first. Radiology competes well with anesthesiology, ER Medicine, Family Medicine, Internal Medicine, OB-GYN, Pediatrics, Psychiatry and General Surgery. Eighty six percent of all matched applicants in Radiology were AMGs which is the highest ratio amongst the nine most popular specialties. Second was Anesthesia at 83 %. Family Medicine at 41 % and Internal Medicine at 56 % were the lowest with respect to their popularity with graduates of allopathic American medical schools.

A discriminating factor often used by program directors to determine who should get an interview is their score on Step One of the tripartite USMLE exam. One may question whether the results of an exam testing basic science knowledge is in any way representative of how a radiology resident will perform or how he or she will function as a radiologist after residency. These doubts about the correspondence of the results of such a test with later achievement are legitimate. Nonetheless, in my experience, there seems to be a correlation at least between Part I scores and scores on the in-service exam given by the ACR during residency. But there the correlation ends. Yet with hundreds of applicants we need some objective measure to limit our interview season and the Step I test in the only objective

measure we have. Bear in mind that for foreign medical graduates Step 1 results tend to be higher because the applicants are often hindered by visa restrictions from prompt entry to the U.S. Hence, they tend to have enforced leisure, often enduring 1 or 2 years, with no work. Thus they can spend considerable time being prepped for the exam. Among all specialties only Dermatology, Plastic Surgery and Neurosurgery have admitted matched trainees with a higher Part I score range and for each it just barely exceeds that of Radiology. Most successful is Dermatology applicants who have scores that range from 232 to 251, Neurosurgery from 230 to 250 and Plastic Surgery from 238 to 251 whereas radiology applicants who gain a position in the match average between 230 and 248. In comparison ER's Part I range is 210–230, Family Medicine is 200–225, Internal Medicine is 210–230 and Psychiatry is 200–225 and General Surgery is 210–230 as is OB-GYN.

Hence, even today many excellent American allopathic medical students are seeking a career in Radiology and most are being accepted. Some of the matched applicants have Part I scores above 250 and, in fact, this year we have seen even more such highly accomplished test takers than last year. At the same time, we have interviewed some excellent applicants whose scores were lower than 230.

Now if you are a program director or an advisor to prospective residents what should you tell them about the frequency or multiplicity of interviews? Remember that primarily in December and January of their fourth year, they will need to be interviewed not only for Radiology but also for their preliminary year. Interviews are time consuming and travel to them can be expensive. Most students are still paying handsomely for their medical education even when they are on the interview trail and away from class and clinics so their education suffers from neglect during this period. Many advisors are telling them to apply to as many programs as they can to maximize their chance of getting an interview and then getting in. Is this good advice for highly competitive applicants, for average applicants or for those with relatively low Part I scores?

The data in this regard are revealing. The likelihood of matching for all candidates exceeds 90 % if just 9 programs are ranked, 98 % if 14 programs are ranked and 99 % if 20 programs are ranked. For the average to superior candidate the extra effort expended in proceeding with the eleventh through the twentieth interview, assuming all visited programs are placed on the match list affords little extra benefit. However, for those with poorer Part I scores, everything else being equal, more interviews may be necessary or the applicants' sights should be deflected away from the most prestigious programs where even if an interview is granted a match would be remote. The average Part I score of those that did not match in Radiology in 2009 was 220, in 2012 it was albeit the same. Undoubtedly many of the unmatched had too few interviews or had a match list that was way too meager. Yet for those with "better qualifications" a heightened fear of being shut out of the match engenders too much travail and traveling. Thus part of their interview season translates into a waste of time and money.

This discordance between current and expected near and medium term opportunity constriction on the one hand and avidity for radiology by superior students on the other is bound to lead to disappointment, misunderstanding and recrimination about promises unfulfilled. Not everybody who wants to go into Radiology is aware of this looming crisis at the other end of the pipeline. It is the responsibility of all of us to advise our potential junior colleagues to consider our specialty carefully before committing oneself to the rigors of the admission process on the front end and the uncertainty of the employment process when the training interval is over 5 or 6 years later.

Reference

1. Baker SR. Job prospects for radiologists in the United States. Imaging Manag. 2013;13(1):12–4.

Radiology Residencies: Disasters and Preparedness

8

For the past decade residency positions in radiology in America continue to be highly sought. The competition is fierce but when the match is published and the applicant has gained a place for training after internship, it is a cause for celebration as the stresses of the months long application process are finally relieved. However, entering a residency is no guarantee that it can be completed, independent of the enthusiasm and capabilities brought to the program by the trainee himself.

Externalities can affect the 4 year residency interval. There is no guarantee that the quality of the program will continue indefinitely as decline is as likely as improvement, although maintenance of the status quo is probably more frequent. In the United States today at times prized faculty members may be recruited away from the program, leaving the residents with fewer teachers of quality. The administration of the hospital may no longer be interested in maintaining a residency program, and might seek to end it after only a short transition period. This is not merely a theoretical concern as program closure has happened several times in the past few years and with financial constraints more burdensome such a consequence may become increasingly frequent. Worse, the program or the hospital may become bankrupt and then may no longer value the benefits of continuing to maintain a graduate medical education program. Under such a drastic scenario, trainees will then be compelled to seek other positions elsewhere and only get them if they are lucky. In these circumstances, there is little protection for the residents when the program declines or disintegrates.

Ad hoc procedures must be found to help residents in these unfortunate circumstances. Yet the record of the past several years is such that mechanisms are not always immediately successful in linking existing programs with displaced trainees even if the resident and his family has to relocate without delay. Moreover, the Radiology Residency Review Committee, an arm of the ACGME, meets only twice a year. When it convenes, it may conclude that a particular residency no longer passes muster and as a first warning, places it on probation. This is a good and bad thing at the same time. It is bad, because it tarnishes the reputation of the program. Perhaps such a report card will encourage the sponsoring agency to close the program or not make necessary investment to support it. Yet, it can also be good because it could be a wakeup call for the hospital or the medical school to now sustain the residency sufficiently after a period of decline and neglect. The Radiology Residency Review Committee could also opt to terminate the program immediately if the educational content is so wanting improvement that nothing can be done to fix it, an eventuality that is rare but not unheard of. Here, too, the resident now must find another place to complete his raining. However, a director of the disaccredited program may not be strongly motivated to help the displaced resident. So neglect, lack of investment, and economic vicissitudes can all contribute to a small but not negligible risk to any resident in any program.

S.R. Baker, *Notes of a Radiology Watcher*,
DOI 10.1007/978-3-319-01677-1_8, © Springer International Publishing Switzerland 2014

Hence, we have lessons to learn from the effect of Katrina on New Orleans programs. Also we can postulate rectifying responses, some of which have been instituted, and others as yet are not implemented or even not contemplated. The Centers for Medicare-Medicaid services, otherwise known as CMS, is the major paymaster for graduate medical education in the United States. It has recently recognized that when programs are disrupted there needs to be a policy to transfer personnel funding, either temporarily or permanently to a new host hospital from the old home hospital so that training can continue for that resident, even though the physical components of the damaged program have been placed in abeyance by adverse circumstances. The extent of change varied among the three programs. Ochsner Clinic, which stayed dry during the hurricane, nonetheless suffered considerably in the aftermath of Katrina. Its patient load went down and residency training was disrupted almost entirely for almost 6 weeks. Yet Ochsner was able to promptly reconstitute itself. The disruption of clinical training, its severity abbreviated, has not resulted in such a marked decrement in education that the quality of the program could not be restored.

Tulane Hospital which became non-operative after Katrina continued its radiology program after the transfer of residents to Houston. That necessitated the repositioning of the residents from New Orleans to another city hundreds of miles away with its associated difficulties in terms of maintenance of both quality of education and quality of life. In worse shape still was the LSU program which had been based for decades at the flooded and permanently closed Charity Hospital. The LSU residents were initially distributed to various clinical sites throughout Louisiana. Yet, that response was ineffectual from the standpoint of adherence to the standards of specialty training as prescribed in the Requirements for Graduate Medical Education in Radiology as well as by the General Requirements for all training programs under the aegis of the ACGME. Thus, the LSU program was terminated by the RRC, and later reconstituted as a markedly different program in personnel and structure. The trainees there had been made to search quickly for other places to provide education for them. Not all succeeded in finding a suitable program.

One other difficulty brought to light by the Katrina disaster was that while Medicare through CMS reimburses most residency positions in the United States, the Balanced Budget Act of 1997 requires there to be a cap of training slots at each facility, providing post-graduate medical education supported by federal funds. So, a hospital potentially willing to accept a resident in a program displaced by the disaster might then become reluctant to take on another trainee, because it would have to shoulder the entire burden of payment for that individual. CMS has responded to this predicament with the following proposed rules. It is a revision of existing regulations allowing home hospitals that have closed temporarily to transfer their full time equivalent residents who are paid for under Medicare to the new host hospitals, so that the receiving facility already training residents could obtain payment for the newly installed trainee who would join them either temporarily or permanently. Even though that means that such facilities would then exceed the level of the predetermined cap, further payment could be received by them in accordance with the number of new positions they would take from the New Orleans program. Under this arrangement, payment would be retroactive to the day of the disaster to incorporate new members at host hospitals, even if the host hospital is far away. This accommodation would be limited to no more than 3 years which creates a potential later issue for radiology with its 4 year residency requirement if a first year resident transfers particularly.

Under pre-existing conditions, it used to be that the hospital would be paid in its current year based upon a 3 year rolling average count of residents when they take on a new resident if the number of residents increased. Then the hospital would only get a portion of that increase based upon a prorated average. Under the new affiliation options related to Katrina and other anticipated disasters, as announced by CMS, payment for displaced residents occupying new positions will be excluded from the rolling average. The computation would instead simply be that the host hospitals will get the full amount of reimbursement for the resident and the home hospitals will get 2/3 of the reimbursement as well. Sounds great! However, remember reimbursement through Medicare in some institutions pays the full amount of the trainee salary and fringe benefits. Yet in others, especially those in which the Medicare component of the patient population is low, CMS only pays a fraction of such costs. It does not matter what the Medicare fraction was at the home hospitals, the new host hospital's increased payment would reflect indigenous Medicare rates for them, not the Medicare rate of the hospitals hit by the disaster. For example, in our institution, only 18 % of total salary for each line is received from CMS because the proportion of elderly patients in our institution is meager. Hence, if you wish to take on another resident, CMS will pay for it to the extent it has paid for other lines under the cap and no more.

So much for accommodating present residents in a disaster area and new residents who may be affected by future disasters. What should a program do in expectation that the next disaster may be knocking at its doorstep? Well, in this regard the lessons learned by the three Louisiana hospitals so far has been that a lesson has not actually been learned. Therefore, I make a suggestion. Either your institution with legal support, or your program itself, of course with legal support, should seek to develop a partnership arrangement with some other residency in radiology, located a distance away so that during the interval in which your hospital is disabled and cannot provide clinical and didactic experience for trainees, those residents could be transferred to the partner hospital under a preexisting agreement made before the cataclysmic event to allow for orderly transfer of trainees and enable the relatively uninterrupted continuance of education. Most likely a temporary accommodation consequent to such a partnership will gain the advantage afforded by the aforementioned rule of CMS which permits transfer payments to support displaced residents. Luck, as Branch Rickey once exclaimed, is "preparation meeting opportunity." We have insurance to protect us from untoward events related to injury or health. Similarly we should create our own insurance for residency training. A partnership agreements would be a good first step to give some measure of comfort so that for residents affected by the aftermath of the next disaster will be able to maintain a continuation of education even though everything else is disrupted or destroyed.

Another approach is to deny that these things will ever happen again, and for most of you, that will be sensible and require no effort. The odds are surely in your favor. However, we owe it to our residents to protect their education. They are innocents here; they enter a program not knowing whether its educational value will decline because of lack of money, lack of interest, lack of teachers, lack of clinical material, or lack of hospitals beds and clinic visits. It is our duty to protect them from these eventualities. Disaster preparedness is part of that responsibility.

Part II

Late Residency, Fellowship and Just Beyond

The reorientation of the board exams in radiology in content, context, and timing have allowed the introduction of curricular changes, especially with respect to the fourth year. Fellowships, too, must be reassessed to prepare better for challenges from other specialties and to maintain proper oversight of their educational content. The late residency period can be a time for experimentation. However newly graduated fellows and young practitioners must be aware that specific recertification obligations are being decided upon without representation by peers in their age group.

Reorganizing the Fourth Year: Curricular Organization—How Will the Fourth Year Be Redesigned?—Part I

9

At the time of this writing I have just finished interviewing prospective radiology residents who will begin their training. Soon I will submit my match list and I await the announcement of my roster in late March. I must say that despite the grumbling that Radiology may not be so attractive financially as it has been over the last decade, the quality of the applicants is outstanding. In fact it is the best I have ever encountered over the past 30 years which augurs well for the continuing vitality of our specialty. But this class is also special because it will be the first one to be trained under the new rules of the American Board of Radiology for first-time takers. As many of you may know the ABR has made radical changes in the content, context and timing of the board examinations. The former written examination will be transformed into a comprehensive qualifying exam to be taken at the end of the third year of residency. Among other modifications it will encompass physics in an integrative fashion and will include images to a greater extent than the current written test [1].

The end of the fourth year will not be the time of the certifying exam. That final test will occur 3 months into the year after the fellowship year (the present PGY-6). It will be computer-based like the aforementioned qualifying exam. No longer will the trainee have to endure the often stressful preparation for an oral exam and contemplate the lurking presence of an evaluator next to him or her for 10 half hour sessions. And no longer will getting right the first and second unknowns presented to him or her become the litmus test of equanimity during each session. Moreover, not only will the certifying test occur beyond residency and in a different format from the oral exam, it will be tailored to the practices, competencies and preferences of the individual test-taker. It will be intense in content but limited in scope. Thus one can be examined primarily in neuroradiology for example, and avoid having to answer a spectrum of questions across the range of the separate areas of imaging. For example, doing well in breast radiology will not be what could distinguish passing from failure for neuroradiologists.

The changed nature of the certifying exam and its removal to after the last year of residency and the following year of fellowship raises issues about the content of the curriculum of the final year of Radiology residency, now freed from the clutches of the dreaded oral exam experience.

What should the senior resident be assigned to do in this 12 month span now that it is open to opportunities for curricular reinvigoration? I have spoken about this with every one of the candidates who have come for interviews. They have been told by some program directors at their interviews that in this period they will have additional several months long rotations, usually three assignments in total, in the various sections of Radiology. Subspecialization training will remain confined to the subsequent fellowship year. At least that is how some programs envision it so my applicant scouts tell me. Other program directors are not sure about how to configure this year. After all they won't have to be definite about such assignments until 2014 when the present-day applicants enter their fourth year of residency. Those beginning the fourth year in July 2013 will be burdened by the qualifying exam which in that year alone takes place in late September or early October, 3 months into the final 12 months of residency.

The rationale for a "menu" if you will of additional months in various subspecialties is justified by the supposition that in practice, even if the junior radiologist is particularly trained in one thing, and most will be since more than 90 % of recent graduates pursue fellowship training, they will still need to know and perform as general radiologists because the needs of the group will require them to cross cover. A presumption informing that sentiment is that adequate training could not be achieved only through standard residency rotations in the first years and that the additional learning gained by a fourth year experience is crucial for work allocation after board passage. Moreover, it is even important for preparation for the certifying exam where evidence of competence will be vouchsafed by taking and passing during that exam questions in more than one subspecialty. At least that is the reason for what I would call the buffet table fourth year approach- put on your plate a little of this and a little of that and you will be nourished quite well.

We take a different approach. Instead of a buffet table, we are instituting a metaphoric training table. We will expect that in the fourth year, a resident will take 12 months in only one thing. That one thing could be basic research for one so inclined. But much more often, I suspect, the trainee will elect to concentrate on the same discipline he or she will follow in the ensuing fellowship year. Thus by the time of the certifying exam our resident will have completed 2 years as say a neuroradiologist making him or her likely to not worry that the certifying exam focused in neuroradiology primarily will be too challenging. Moreover, 2 years of in essence "post-graduate" subspecialty training makes that individual stand out compared with others who have followed the traditional 4 years of comprehensive education and then, in sequence, a single fellowship year.

Alternatively, a resident could spend the fourth year entirely in subspecialty one and the fellowship year in subspecialty two, making him or her marketable by a 12 month commitment to two disciplines of intense study in preparation for post-training employment. This 3-2 or 3-1-1 pattern has been followed successfully for 10 years at Duke University despite their contending with the oral boards situated in the fourth year. Furthermore, with the board exam delayed and refashioned, other programs including ours can adapt this model as well without the intrusion of a no holds barred "hyperintense" study interval. This could occur even if a program had no fellows with the Duke model modified to 3-1 and 1 instead of 3-2.

Which of these two approaches are more inline with appropriate preparation for a career in private practice? That will depend on evidence from three data sets; (1) the present arrangements of after hours work in academic practice (2) the present arrangements of after hours work in large private practices and (3) the penetration of U.S. based teleradiology services for after hours work for smaller practices.

We are currently in the midst of exploring the facts with respect to the first two uncertainties. Under the aegis of SCARD we have sent out a survey to all chairpersons requesting that they respond to a series of questions regarding the assignments of their subspecialists to after hours work. The responses indicate that mostly neuroradiologists and interventionalists are assigned only to their subspecialties both during the day and also off hours. Similarly, pediatric radiologists confine themselves to the radiology of children during the day, at night and on weekends and holidays and usually not to adult patients. Exclusive breast imagers often do not take call. Chest, Body and MSK radiologists, on the other hand, typically cover general and emergency radiology after hours. In fact, these three subspecialties might be considered the new general radiologists, even though they have limited fellowship training to the musculoskeletal, chest and GI and GU systems and their residency-only accumulated knowledge also of basic neuro CT and MR.

A division of labor strictly along subspecialty lines is seemingly more achievable in larger practices than in smaller practices. Yet if larger private assemblages of radiologists are relatively uncommon when compared with radiologists in smaller groups, then perhaps the particularities of after hours staffing would be a minor matter as cross coverage in the absence of teleradiology would be required. However, we all know that practices are getting larger. How prevalent has it become?

Evidence presented in a recent paper in JACR by Mythrei Bhargavan and Jonathan Sunshine of the ACR offers some answers. In their data from a 2007 survey with reference to earlier investigations in 1990, 1999, 2000 and 2003 revealed that the fraction of radiologists in very small practices (4 or less radiologists) decreased from 29 % in 1990 to 22 % 17 years later. Similarly over this interval in slightly larger practices (5–14 practitioners) the number of radiologists declined from 51 to 38 %. Groups of 15–29 F.T.E increased from 14 to 21 % and in practices of 30 or more radiologists the percentage change was from 5 to 19 % with most of the growth in very large groups of 60 or more radiologists. So the trend to larger and larger practices continues. Yet the median group size is still 11 radiologists.

The third trend, one that has occurred to the greatest degree since 2000, is the penetration of teleradiology. Actually with regard to after hour reading, teleradiology is really two distinct businesses (1) offshore readings which for Medicare regulations must be preliminary, not final and (2) onshore or intranational interpretations by board certified American radiologists licensed in the state that is the origin of the imaging studies. There the provenance of the radiological images are local but the definitive reading can be made by the remote teleradiologist.

One of the selling points of companies that provide U.S. based teleradiology is that their services are provided by subspecialists available for prompt reads both during the day and off hours. So those practicing in small groups may not have to be assigned for after hours interpretation of studies in their own hospital which are outside their particular subspecialty expertise as long as the subspecialty-trained teleradiologist is but a phone call away.

The evidence from these three sources of information are directly referable to the ascertainment of suitable curricular characteristics of the fourth year of radiology training. If exclusive subspecialty assignment will be the norm for the future and cross-covering outside of that discipline will be limited or absent from the roster of responsibilities of a newly-minted radiologist, then a fourth year curriculum consisting of buffet table reinforcement of all sections of radiology, (a few months of this followed by a few months of that) will be a mistake in comparison to the alternative of a fourth year of prolonged, focused education in one area to be followed by a fellowship which by design also focuses only on one area of radiology. This paradigm will be more in line with proper preparation for practice and will, in the aggregate, strengthen radiology by providing everywhere an adequate cadre of superbly trained subspecialists.

In contrast, if in many smaller practices the old model of cross-coverage without a definite final read teleradiology presence persists, then a well-rounded radiologist completing a range of rotation assignments in the fourth year to be followed by a fellowship in PGY5 will seem more appropriate.

My hunch is that neuroradiology, interventional radiology, pediatric radiology and breast imaging are now appropriately served by the dedicated single-focus fourth year model. And chest and body imaging may also gain from it because most of what they do they do during the night and on weekends is chest and body imaging. Perhaps for MSK radiologists who probably are often assigned to general radiology the buffet table approach, as opposed to the 1 year exclusive model, might still be more serviceable.

Summary

The recently enacted changes in the content and the timing of the Radiology board examination for first-time takers has called into question the curriculum of the fourth year of training. To many program directors, that year will be filled with a series of several months assignments in the various subspecialties of Radiology scheduled in a sense to round out the trainee's education. An alternative is a year-long intra-residency "fellowship" devoted only to one area, to be followed by further instruction in a similarly devoted fellowship in the same discipline in PGY-5, the traditional fellowship period. The strategic implication of both approaches is discussed in this essay.

Reference

1. Baker SR. Response to "my old Kentucky home, good night. Potential changes in radiology board certification process". AJR. 2008;1149–51.

Reorganizing the Fourth Year: The Fourth Year After the Boards Change—How Should It Be Constructed?—Part II

10

In July 1, 2004, the class of new residents in Radiology are the first group of trainees subject to the revision of the series of examinations leading to initial certification in your specialty. As you may know, the changes involve modification of the timing, content and context of these tests [1].

First of all, why were they changed? Many of you remember the challenge of the oral board examination which took place in late May or early June of the fourth year of residency. For those graybeards among us, you may remember that up until the early 1980s that momentous experience occurred as now 4 years after beginning residency, but which then lasted only 3 years.

You recall the positive and negative aspects of the test very well, I presume. At least everyone I have met has a store of stories about their preparation for it, about the test itself and about the anxious waiting for the results. Many of you also have not forgotten that the intensive studying for it was an excellent review of the entirety of diagnostic radiology. But at the same time you will acknowledge that to a greater or lesser degree you were infected with the virus causing "board psychosis". You were compelled by the worry over it, whether permitted or not, to neglect clinical duties during that fretful interval. Your previously assigned work was shunted to more junior residents so as not to bother you as you pursued your heroic journey leading to its climax in Louisville. And for this extended period of abject studying, you were paid in full or at least were able to maintain your resident's meager salary, no questions asked.

Also you might remember the dread of having to discuss cases in front of an examiner you could not see and could not charm. He or she expected you to be quick, glib and correct in every case set before you. The oral boards did not replicate normal viewing and interpreting in which a difficult case may be set aside for later deliberation. Rather the oral board was a performance, requiring extemporaneous and learned discussion of unknown images. No wonder it was scary in contemplation and stressful in realization.

Furthermore, the oral board exam tested one on nearly everything in diagnostic imaging. Since 1970 with the advent of multiple modalities Radiology has grown geometrically in both range of tests and in its corpus of knowledge. In the 1980s, to accommodate its broadening curriculum, Radiology residencies expanded to 4 years. In contrast our colleagues in Internal Medicine dealt with the problem of an ever expanding knowledge base by changing the term of the core residency to 3 years and by establishing and encouraging fellowships of 2–3 years in the 12 branches of Internal Medicine thereby engendering the establishment of subspecialists across the wide spectrum of the specialty. In Internal Medicine, then, subspecialization became early on a fact of life and the schedule of board examinations in the basic principles of internal medicine and in the various subspecialties were codified and subscribed to by their trainees.

S.R. Baker, *Notes of a Radiology Watcher*, DOI 10.1007/978-3-319-01677-1_10, © Springer International Publishing Switzerland 2014

In radiology, especially in the past 15 years, subspecialty training has been chosen by over 90 % of residents but more than half of them opt for programs for which there is not a test for added competence. They just have to finish the year and they can hold themselves out as a musculoskeletal or body imager, etc.

Yet all radiology residents have had to take the ten sections that comprise the comprehensive or more precisely perhaps the encyclopedic oral exam. For example, a resident who has decided to become a neuroradiologist still has to pass the Breast Imaging section of the oral board exam even if he or she will never again read a mammography study. All the preparation for each segment of the test will be with the intent of diagnosing correctly the eight to ten cases shown to him or her. And from then on, if he/she passes there will never be a need to see another breast case if Neuroradiology is what the individual will elect do exclusively.

To overcome the fear of the oral context, the exam will now be computer based. In order to avoid the over comprehensiveness of the certifying exam, one can limit that segment of test to one or two areas that conform to their expected areas of subspecialization interest. And to further the transformation of radiology training to the exigencies and impetus of subspecialization, the certifying exam will take place in the Fall after the fifth year or just after a fellowship is completed. Instead of the preliminary written exam a more comprehensive qualifying exam will also take place at the end of the third year or residency.

Where does this leave the fourth year of residency? It is no longer encumbered by the need to intensive and prolonged studying for an exam at the end of it. Fourth year residents are obviously more competent than junior house officers so they will undoubtedly be asked to take call at least equal proportion to their colleagues. Yet what will their curriculum be. There is wide latitude here for program directors. Presumably the two requirements for Nuclear Medicine and breast radiology will be largely satisfied by the beginning of the fourth year because the residents will need these rotations with their mandated time obligations completed before the qualifying test.

Many program directors have elected to break up the 12 months of the fourth year with several months of "mini fellowships" in order to give their trainees further experience in a range of subspecialty disciplines before proceeding to a true fellowship in the fifth year. In contrast we have chosen to require the trainee to pick one subspecialty for the entire 12 months; in essence a full fellowship within the temporal confines of the residency program. The resident could then take 2 years of de facto fellowship in the same discipline, one with us and one to follow or take two fellowships in different subspecialties, again one with us and one after their time in our residency.

Which is the better course? Let's divide the question into four parts. Is a 12 month "fellowship" in the fourth year better than successive mini fellowships for those entering academic practice and for those seeking a position in a private practice? And does the better choice depend on the specific fellowship? Is either choice an advantage for the budding neuroradiologist or body imager? To discover how these options will play out we surveyed the members of SCARD and the managers of the 25 largest private practices of Radiology to find out if their various subspecialty-trained faculty members or practicing radiologists cross cover other subspecialty disciplines for prescribed after hours coverage.

If generally they would not need to cross cover, then a fourth year of residency spent pursuing a full fellowship period of 12 months would be more advantageous for their career than a series of mini fellowships. But if they were required to regularly interpret studies apart from their subspecialty domain, then a fourth year of wider scope would be more appropriate.

More specifically in our survey we asked if a specialist in one area of Radiology regularly provided off hours coverage on duty or on call in body imaging, general ER Radiology, Interventional Radiology, Neuroradiology, Pediatric Radiology or none of the above. The specialists to whom those assignments may or may not occur were Neuroradiologists, Interventional Neuroradiologists, Interventionalists, Body Imagers, Chest Radiologists, Musculoskeletal Radiologists, Pediatric Radiologists, and Breast Radiologists.

The sizes of the attending staff of the 42 responding Academic Medical Center included five with fewer than 25 faculty, nine having 25–35 attending staff, 8 each for department with 35–45 and 45–55 attendings and 12 with more than 55 faculty who were practicing radiologists.

Among academic neuroradiologists more than three fourths had no responsibility off hours responsibility in other disciplines. For interventionists more than 90 % had no other film reading or procedure performance obligations. Among Interventional Neuroradiologstis only 22 % had no other on duty or on call assignments. Nearly 40 % of them cross-covered neuororadiology and surprisingly more than one quarter also covered pediatric radiology. 50 % of Body Imagers had no other scheduled after hours duties but half were responsible for general radiology and 15 % covered pediatric radiology as well. Chest radiologists were more likely to cover other disciplines than to be scheduled only for chest imaging. Two thirds of them were assigned to general radiology and one third to Body Imaging. Similarly more than two thirds of musculoskeletal radiologists were expected to interpret general radiology cases on nights and weekends. On the other hand three fourths of pediatric radiologists had no other responsibilities outside the regular work day aside from Pediatric Radiology call but only 50 % of breast imagers escaped being assigned to other subspecialties, mostly in general radiology.

Among the various private practices whose representatives answered our survey all had more than 55 radiologists. Three fourths of the neuroradiologists, 85 % of their interventionalists and 85 % of their interventional neuroradiologists had no other reading responsibility at night or on weekends. Surprisingly more than half of the body imagers at these facilities confined their work to body imaging only whereas nearly all musculoskeletal radiologists were assigned to general radiology. The overwhelming majority of pediatric radiologists and breast imagers confined themselves to their areas of primary responsibility after hours.

Hence, one tentative conclusion to be drawn from this data is if one is considering academic practice or practice in a large group a 12 months "fellowship" in the fourth year of residency followed by a fellowship in the fifth year would be a sensible decision for those seeking to be a neuroradiologist, an interventional radiologist, a neurointerventional radiologist, a pediatric radiologist or a breast imager. In this large professional aggregation, it would seem that having 2 years of fellowship in one subspecialty would make the newly-minted radiologist attractive to the group's admission committee. Moreover focusing on one's subspecialty alone would tend to make their prospective job more fulfilling at least in terms of focus on a restricted work experience congruent with their advanced training.

However, as a body imager, or a chest radiologist or a musculoskeletal radiologist you should expect to multitask at least in off hours assignments. And to be best prepared for that eventuality, before fellowship, in the fourth year of residency, you might be served better by completing a series of mini fellowships rather than spending that year doing one thing.

Reference

1. Amis ES, Baker SR, Becker GJ, et al. Panel discussions in radiology: changes in radiology training and new examination format. AJR. 2008;191:W217–30.

11

Reorganizing the Fourth Year: Reimagining the Fourth Year of Training in the of Training in the Era of Subspecialization— Part III

In Radiology, like all of medicine, nothing is constant. Continually, new techniques beseech our attention, some have become essential to our practice whereas others fade fast and are quickly forgotten. At the same time; threats from our colleagues, or should I say competitors, are a constant challenge differing in quantity and urgency so as to make for us each year a unique list of agenda items for problem resolution. Need I say much more about the intrusions of government regulators, insurance companies, malpractice providers and plaintiff's lawyers? And to top it off, the education of our residents, at least how that education is organized, has once more come under close inspection for possible alterations if not a complete metamorphosis.

Now some of you, many years beyond training, may look back fondly at your residency. Perhaps through rose-colored glasses, you may recall that in those halcyon days the curriculum was predictable, stable and ordered. Or was it? Actually, abrupt change has been more profound than serene equanimity. In the early 1970s a 3-year residency encompassed education and training in diagnostic radiology, the emerging discipline of nuclear medicine and at least 10 months spent in clinical work and lectures in radiation oncology. Diagnostic radiology and radiation oncology split from each other in the time of the Carter administration. In Reagan's second term diagnostic radiology was lengthened to 4 years. A subsequent 1 or 2 year fellowship became de rigueur and the internship remained optional. But in the early 1990s the internship was made mandatory. Thus, what could have once been a 3-year course of post medical school graduate education for most has morphed into a 6 year obligation with internship and fellowship straddling a 4 year program. Yet by 2001 when the market for newly minted radiologists exploded, many decided to forego fellowship for immediate entry into practice. And today, there are opportunities for post post-graduate work in far-flung places as teleradiology consultants. As a general comparison, offshore opportunities or young radiologists was limited to practice within the various services of Uncle Sam's armed forces.

So is it time once again to tinker with the terms and arrangement of a diagnostic radiology residency. Here are the possibilities, each sounding like the opening of a football play. 1-4-1, 1-3-2, 0-5-1 even 0-4-1. Hike. Those were the choices debated 6 years ago by the program directors and the chief residents at the AUR, by SCARD also at the AUR and by the American Board of Radiology and the Residency Review *Committee of* the ACGME at a joint meeting in early June. The issues will revolve around two questions (1) do we need to train everybody in all branches of radiology over 4 years or can we aggregate the standard curriculum into an introductory period of 3 years and expand fellowship training to 2 years within a 5 year interval. (2) What is the impetus for suggesting such a change? Well continuing the football analogy there are both offensive and defensive reasons for making this type of substitution. On the offense, we want the best trained or coached people to *carry* the ball for

S.R. Baker, *Notes of a Radiology Watcher*, DOI 10.1007/978-3-319-01677-1_11, © Springer International Publishing Switzerland 2014

our specialty. Radiology knowledge is expanding rapidly, broadening and deepening the extent of our expertise as diagnosis in the main has in a sense been handed off to us while traditional methods like history and physical have retreated to the sideline. Yet, no one can be a triple threat, we need radiologists with specialized skills to move the team forward. It is maintained by some that even 1 year of fellowship is not enough. The all-purpose imaging physician went out with the single wing.

The defensive reasons are just as important. We cannot fumble and thereby lose possession of our hegemony to those in other specialties who are aggressive and hungry. That means we should play to our strength. Familiarity with the constraints of imaging, its appropriate utilization, its risks and uncertainties, our knowledge of the physics of the equipment we use, and our clinical acumen which extends over many medical disciplines are all in our favor in this enduring contest. Yet to first make and then continue to substantiate the claim to leadership we must work hard *to* be *in* the forefront of clinical practice and research as well as the application of translational investigations so we can maintain our lead as proprietors of innovation. But this can only happen, so say the quarterbacks of *the* three-two proposal, when everybody is truly a fully trained subspecialist.

The second question in *the* minds of the reformers is do we need the internship? Those wishing to do away with it argue that there really is no evidence that a clinical year makes us better doctors or better radiologists. And perhaps there could never be such evidence. How can one design it? What would be the criteria? If such a period of direct patient care can lead a radiologist to saving your life or the minimization of morbidity could it be shown? The prolonged debate persists, the conclusions remain elusive.

Moreover, the mandatory clinical year has spawned the transitional internship, a noble concept but honored in the breach by a few programs. For example in some of these internships the training can encompass up to 5 or 6 months of elective time enabling the trainee to do things both in medicine and out it. In essence they enjoy part-time work and part-time vacation with months spent on soft subjects separate from patient care. Is this what such a year is about? Yet, others are steadfast in their belief that a good internship has meaningful, long-lasting results, incalculable perhaps in quantitative terms but nonetheless qualitatively evident for sure as such an experience necessarily enables a consideration for patients engendered by empathy and tempered by experience [1].

We have sought to explore this matter in detail by sending out a questionnaire to all radiology residents in the United States as well as those who are in their post residency year. We queried them about their perception of the benefits of the clinical year. The early results are somewhat surprisingly contrary at least, to my apprehensions. Most of these trainees affirmed that the internship was helpful for their careers as radiologists. However, some opined that this 12 month period should be integrated into the four or five following years of training. An interesting speculation would then be what would those intercalary months encompass? More patient care or more radiology focused obligations? Would it make the point or be beside it? When all of the data in hand and analyzed; I will provide you an update in coming months.

Reference

1. Baker SR, Luk L. After hours coverage of various radiologic subspecialties and its impact on the fourth year radiology residency curriculum. Acad Radiol. 2013;20:122–6.

Are We Losing the Certification Wars?   12

How do the various specialties and specialists in American medicine get along? Idealists might say that all differences and disputes are resolvable. For them the overall picture is one of collaboration and cooperation. Separation of responsibilities are agreed to in principle and have been authorized and validated by the formation of board certification from way back in the 1930s and by the creation of distinct curricula in the post war period which was strengthened by the increasingly specific regulations of the (ACGME) the Accreditation Council for Graduate Medical Education from the 1970s to today. Moreover, while state medical boards are concerned with licensure of physicians, a whole range of policies and regulations indicating criteria for insurance reimbursements, hospital payments, and malpractice case law, as well as focused accreditation programs have further defined the boundary conditions separating the work of each specialty.

Yet that splendid picture has a certain Currier and Ives quaintness quality to it, at least that is how the realists and skeptics might see it. Although there is perhaps a consensus regarding the separation of responsibilities among the treating specialists, such as between surgery and medicine (with the exception, perhaps of the face where oral surgeons, plastic surgeons, ophthalmologists, and otolaryngologists contend for turf) with regard to ancillary services, however, the situation is unsettled despite the perceived content and intent of its traditional practitioners in radiology, pathology and anesthesiology.

These various fields are considered fair game by medical imperialists wishing to expand into new territory.

Thus, we are all aware that more imaging is performed, interpreted and is the recipient of compensation by non-radiologists than by radiologists, at least in volume terms if not in dollars terms. Despite ostensibly congenial relationships, the imaging terrain is the locus for thrusts and parries by those who wish to compete with us. Until recently, the most promising ground for a non-radiologist was the imaging center. Many of our contending cardiologists or gastroenterologists function in these settings, some of them owning or at least leasing equipment there which indicates to all but the most naive that Stark regulations have a gap in it so wide that a tank could drive through them.

Recently the specter of the implementation of regulations under the Deficit Reduction Act coupled with an increasingly obtrusively active approach by Medicare with respect to their interpretation and enforcement of regulations has made new investments by non-radiologists in imaging facilities less attractive and perhaps current investments more burdensome than profitable. Nonetheless, the legitimacy mantra in the minds of non-radiologists, making justifiable their adventures in imaging, remains strong. They say I want to control imaging on my patient. That is a battle cry compelling our non-radiologist colleagues to venture into new areas where they think they can acquire imaging "gold". If not the imaging center, where they may seek the technical fee,

S.R. Baker, *Notes of a Radiology Watcher*,
DOI 10.1007/978-3-319-01677-1_12, © Springer International Publishing Switzerland 2014

they can at least collect the lower professional fee by gaining privileges at their local hospital to interpret studies. These examinations will be performed on hospital equipment whose volume they can stimulate and whose readings they can render. Perhaps it is small potatoes compared with the technical fee that they had or planned to capture at an imaging center. It is more work for less money but, nonetheless, promises to be a source of new income even if it means displacing the radiologist.

And in small hospitals where is the radiologist so displaced? Often he is only there part-time and sometimes not at all. If that small hospital is an ancillary part of a radiology group's multiple activities, the resident GI guy can make like the ER physician and say, because we are here, it is our business, not yours. Now ultrasound in the ER may be meager fare on the professional fee reimbursement menu but virtual colonoscopy promises bigger feasting. Projecting into the near future that small hospital's administrator might say, do we really need that limited commitment made by the multicentered radiology group in the neighborhood when we can contract with the well established American teleradiology company staffed by experts who will make themselves available to read day or night and do it well? Absence of commitment by those in person combined with excellence in reputation by those from afar is a superb recipe for outsourcing.

The key to the takeover within the hospital by local non-radiologists for high RVU reimbursement imaging procedures is accreditation and credentialing. Evidence of completing a course of study, interpretation of at least a minimum roster of images in a particular modality and successful passage of a board-type examination given by an "authoritative" organization is what most hospital administrators want to look at and approve as a requirement before allowing a physician to participate in an activity in their shop. For many administrators, it does not matter if that authoritative body is an upstart group lacking a track record of integrity in the pursuit of excellence or that the course of study is constricted compared with what radiologists do or if there is little attention paid to the curriculum to appreciate

utilization issues or radiation protection or physics instruction. What matters is the specificity and extent of definition with respect to the number of exams, and a mandatory certifying examination administered by a so called legitimate organization. These are what will determine what privileges will be granted.

The champion of this approach is cardiology. They currently have seven separate boards, each with a course of study, a number of interpretations as a minimum criterion especially in coronary CT, a board exam, which is time limited and recurring exams at a later date.

One might say, in Radiology we have ACGME fellowships which do the same thing. That is true, but how extensive are those fellowships in terms of encompassing all graduating residents. There are now seven ACGME accredited fellowships, each of them requires regular evaluations, each of them prescribes a course of study and each of them has a range of other specific requirements [1].

One fellowship, cardio-thoracic radiology, had only one participant in an ACGME fellowship the year before it was discontinued. All of the other fellowships are not at all fully subscribed. For example, in abdominal radiology, only 41 or 55 positions were filled recently. And in endovascular surgical neuroradiology there are only six residents in three ACGME programs; the rest are non-ACGME and occupied predominantly by Neurologists and Neurosurgeons, not Radiologists. Musculoskeletal radiology filled less than 100 % of its ACGME fellowship positions. In Neuroradiology 210 out of 274 positions were occupied, in Vascular and Interventional radiology 149 out of 268 were taken by trainees, in Pediatric radiology it was 65 out of 98 and in Nuclear radiology 14 out of 23 filled in 2008.

This does not mean that all of those in training were actually graduating residents. There are some, perhaps only a few individuals, who after several years in practice returned for fellowship training. And there are an untold number of non US graduated radiologists who have secured positions in ACGME-related radiology fellowships. Out of a total of 761 slots totaling all radiology ACGME fellowships only about half are occupied by individuals who will complete 4 years of training this year in an American Radiology residency. Hence, more than half of our residents will enter a fellowship program that consists of only a 1 year term of study. Such fellowships have no well-defined curriculum, no requirements for total number of studies and no certifying exam upon completion. On the other hand, Peds, Neuro and IR have CAQ's to further substantiate their credentials as a bona fide course of study for the acquisition of subspecialty expertise.

Now I have done a survey of individuals completing our recent review course. 147 individuals completed the survey, and to my great surprise, guess where they are going for fellowships? 1.5 % are entering to Military; only 10.3 % into practice; 4.1 % into cardiothoracic programs but none of them are ACGME; 10.8 % into Mammo and Women's imaging; 10.8 % into MR programs; 12.8 % are entering MSK fellowships but almost all of them are outside ACGME; 8.8 % are pursuing IR fellowships; 4.5 % Pediatric fellowships and 19 % have chosen Neuro fellowships. The largest number even exceeding Neuroradiology fellowships, is a body fellowship. As I mentioned, there are 41 individuals in ACGME body fellowships, but if I extrapolate the 29 out of my 147 who indicated they were going into body as the subject for post residency training, it comes out to 302 individuals in body fellowships nationally yet only 41 of them, slightly more than 10 % are in ACGME programs. So we have many individuals who are in the most popular of fellowships in programs for which there is no specific credentialing. The same is true for musculoskeletal radiology which prorates to 186 across the country who will go into fellowships but only 24 of them are in ACGME programs.

The point should be clear by now. If Radiology wants to compete for imaging turf, even within a hospital, it must reveal to those administrators in that hospital that the individuals who are board certified and have completed specialized training can be further demarcated by some standards beyond merely spending a term in a place for which they undergo more training. If our competitors are doing that in their fashion even though their training is less extensive and less adequate, they may take the business away from

us. At least, we have not protected the interests of more than half of our current residents who are now entering fellowships. If we fail in establishing at least competitive credentialing, than those junior residents can blame us for not thinking ahead to respond to what our contesting specialists are doing.

The prospect is stark. Excuse the pun. Yet it is up to us to secure a bright future for our graduates in face of the prospect that others are seeking our territory. They can claim to do it well because they perceive that imaging with 3D reconstruction has become so much easier. One may disagree with the notion that it has become much easier for them, but you cannot disagree with the obvious. At least with 3D many lesions are more readily observable even if the integration of findings remains a special capability which we alone possess.

A philosophy professor of mine once said "everything worth doing well is worth doing poorly." The conclusion of this message is the ambivalence associated with the word worth. Remember also behavior follows the money. And with credentialing, our nonradiology colleagues can now play for it. If we do not pay heed to what they are and will be doing, the game may be lost.

Summary

Radiology as a discipline must acknowledge the reality of competition from other specialties for control of imaging in hospitals. The rapid diffusion of 3D reconstruction has seemingly made abnormality recognition easier, thereby potentially emboldening the development of credentialing programs by competing physicians who are not radiologists. For them establishment of well-defined curricula of instruction, with a minimum number of interpreted studies, eventuating in a certifying exam and a "board" to oversee them are activities that can establish the "patina" of legitimacy.

Radiologists must meet these challenges by ensuring that their fellowship programs also involve credentialing structures. The ACGME fellowships in Radiology have requirements that address that objective, but the majority of graduating radiology residents are in programs with no codified credentials save the completion of a term of training. This will be insufficient in the inevitable struggle for dominance of hospital imaging. We must change our laissez-faire attitudes about it, pronto.

Reference

1. Accreditation Council for Graduate Medical Education; 2013. http://www.acgme.org/acgmeweb/. Accessed 11 July 2013.

The Trouble with Fellowships

13

One important element in the sustenance of Radiology as a vital specialty composed of physicians with special knowledge and expertise is the excellence of subspecialty training. It cannot be denied that the transformation of imaging as a discipline, which by dint of the incisiveness of newly introduced and continually improved imaging techniques, has transformed and increasingly dominated the diagnostic enterprise.

The fact that deployment and enhanced utilization of the core modalities of CT, MR, IR, and to a lesser extent ultrasonography has remained largely within the purview of Radiology is primarily because we have developed estimable fellowship programs to train our graduating residents so that they gain cognitive and procedural competence shared by no one else. But now our monopolies have come under challenge from other specialties who wish that imaging, too, could be in their grasp. The benefits of imaging to patients and to their practice are too enticing to be entrusted to us automatically especially when they have the wherewithal financially, administratively and even politically to claim a piece of the pie. The strength of our resolution to be the dominant player in the future depends in large measure on the vitality, the relevance, the specific qualities of education and the overall affirmative recognition of our fellowship programs.

And yet, today, among all the forums in which radiology education takes place undergraduate, GME, Public Medical Education, and CME, fellowship is the least assessed, the most unregulated, the least subject to quality control, and the most diverse in curriculum even within a particular discipline. To wit, programs outside the surveillance of the ACGME, by my estimate, direct the training for more than half of current fifth year learners. These fellows are like orphans. And those within the reach of RRC inspection are like the proverbial step-child getting less attention and consideration than other siblings in the house. It is time then to look at the fellowship experience closely, noting deficiencies in order to search for ways to better organize and superintend the education received by young radiologists during this year of training and to bolster the credentials a graduating fellow can present to his or her next employer.

As a first step in this critique, it may be helpful to look back to the seminal stage of fellowship development in the 1970s and early 1980s.

Discipline-based fellowships as situated within a post-residency year of further training in many branches of Radiology was uncommon at the beginning of the modern era of Radiology, i.e., the time of the introduction of cross-sectional imaging modalities in the 1970s. And in comparison with Internal Medicine around 1980, the two specialties went their separate ways in their approach to subspecialty education beyond residency. Internal Medicine fixed the period of residency at 3 years allowing for the introduction of 2 and 3 year subsequent fellowships in the maturing subspecialties of cardiology, gastroenterology, etc. The most vigorous of these subspecialties have been those most procedurally oriented in part because reimbursement policy in the U.S. favors procedural over cognitive work.

Radiology leaders at that time realized also that the corpus of knowledge had grown so vast that a 3 year term of specialty training was not long enough, so in the late 1980s the residency term lengthened to 4 years. Nonetheless, it became apparent soon after that further training focused in one area was needed even beyond a 4 year residency. Thus, fellowships gained in importance and in number, even though in the 1990s and until very recently many questioned whether the additional seasoning occasioned by a fellowship was really necessary for those entering the private practice of Radiology. So the alternative of direct entry into practice positions was still an option some thought to be a valid and economically secure career move.

Yet surprisingly most graduating residents thought otherwise as they perceived the value of subspecialty training within a fellowship to be an enhancement of their prospects even though it meant another year of low salary. And the prominence of this view surprisingly is not a very recent one. In fact, in a study from 1999, a survey directed to senior residents in Radiology, encompassing 402 fourth year and 395 third year residents, revealed that 80.1 % and 84 % respectively had accepted fellowship offers. In a questionnaire filled out in the spring of 2008 by residents at our annual review course, 93 % of registrants were planning to begin fellowship training 2 months later. The same survey given again in 2009 to senior residents indicated that 95 % of trainees in their fourth year were planning to enter a fellowship upon completion of their residency. So fellowship has become nearly ubiquitous as residents have endorsed by their intent its immediate value as a learning experience and also its enduring, enriching value as a prerequisite for special competence, recognized and supported by radiology groups, hospital administrations and third party payers. Further acknowledgement was signaled when the American Board of Radiology in 2007 decided to change the content and timing of their certifying examination. The modification in schedule and allowance for choice in subjects to be taken during this examination were both clear validation of the prominence if not the essentiality of fellowship training.

Comparing the fellowship choices of residents in 1999–2000 with those 9 and 10 years later reveals some significant changes. Body imaging and interventional radiology were the two most frequently chosen subspecialties but both later decreased in popularity. Interventional Radiology which was opted for by approximately 28 % of those surveyed at the earlier time, 5 years ago, was the choice of only 9.5 %. Body Imaging has decreased from 30 % to an average of 18 %. However, in the 2 years of surveys, in 2008 and 2009, there was a wide variance in this fellowship with 23.4 % pursuing it in 2008 and only 14.5 % in 2009. Recent growth has occurred in MR fellowships or MR fellowships combined with options like women's imaging or informatics. These fellowships were picked by less than 1 % 10 years ago and 5 years ago encompassed approximately 13 % of all fellowships. Cardiothoracic Radiology which is no longer an ACGME survey program, increased from 0 to 3.6 %. Neuroradiology continues to be a moderately popular choice and on average has not claimed more or less of a percentage of fourth year residents than before. In contrast, MSK has also risen from 3.3 to 13 %. Thus there has been a significant change in the mix of fellowship choices over the last 10 years.

But taste in fellowships is apt to change quickly. Among those residents finishing in 2013 and among rising fourth year trainees, women's imaging fellowships are now widely sought because of the apparent security of breast radiology—entirely a monopoly under our purview. Also Interventional Radiology is now considered by many a vital discipline with an optimistic future. Correspondingly other fellowships in Body and MSK are less popular because volume and reimbursement in these fields will continue to be constrained.

In essence there are three categories of fellowships. There are those post-residency programs for which a CAQ examination is available for individuals after the completion of their training. In fact, the CAQ has made ACGME surveillance necessary. Consequently there are no fellowships in Pediatric Radiology, Interventional Radiology and Neuroradiology outside the ACGME umbrella. In the most recent surveys approximately one third of individuals in fellowships are in programs in these three disciplines. The secondary category is fellowships in which ACGME surveillance is a possibility but non-ACGME fellowships are also an option. For the most part this includes the fellowships of musculoskeletal radiology and body radiology. In our last two surveys again, approximately one third of those in fellowships concentrated on the Abdomen and MSK. As an aside ACGME oversight had been available in cardiothoracic radiology but because so few programs elected for this type of surveillance, the ACGME discontinued their relationship with them. ACGME surveillance also extends to nuclear medicine. Again it has very few programs and very few registrants. In these programs, the Radiology RRC will conduct reviews if a connection with the ACGME is made. Yet by far most of these programs are outside the surveillance of this accrediting body. For example, in the last 2 years, 54 slots were offered in abdominal radiology in the U.S. in ACGME programs. Only, 41 were occupied. However, there are additionally 250 other positions in programs outside the ACGME oversight in Abdominal Radiology. Similarly, for musculoskeletal radiology, there are 27 positions offered, 24 are occupied in ACGME programs but there are approximately 150 other positions in a range of programs that are beyond the ACGME's surveillance. Of the approximately 1,100 positions available to graduating residents only 500 (or 47 %) are in programs subject to RRC inspection. Strictly non-ACGME fellowships include MR and women's imaging. Together these make up a third of all fellowships. A recent article estimated the number of breast imaging programs at between 84 and 130 positions each year and a guess at MR fellowship slots is between 130 and 160.

However, the total number of fellowship offerings is not known precisely and really has never been known. Fellowship positions may be available in some programs for 1 year and unavailable the next. Outside the ACGME tent such programs have the option of starting and stopping whenever they wish. Thus, one of the issues we must contend with in fellowships is their quality. We do not know about many because we do not know where they are, how many positions are offered, what is the curriculum of such programs and how are they evaluated. This is one of the major hurdles to improving fellowships. An issue particularly acute for non-ACGME fellowships is criteria definition. Competing specialties seeking opportunities for imaging such as gastroenterology and especially cardiology have devised well-defined criteria with clearly specified levels of competence backed by a requisite number of cases in various categories. For non-ACGME fellowships in Radiology in which there is no regulation or control, those completing such training may become competent radiologists but they leave the program with no credentials to demonstrate that competence to imaging groups, third-party payers or hospitals. Thus, they are at least at an administrative disadvantage compared with others seeking our imaging turf.

The decision to set up a non-ACGME fellowship is chosen by many programs to avoid the hassle of RRC surveillance which indeed confers a spectrum of obligations on the program and its director. Moreover, non-ACGME fellowships allow a wide range of programmatic flexibility to modify requirements to meet current needs, wants and limitations. Furthermore, it provides the trainee with an opportunity to pursue moonlighting and to bill for his or her services outside the area of the fellowship. In Radiology programs within ACGME oversight, fellows cannot bill.

ACGME regulations, as I mentioned before, are time consuming, expensive, somewhat mysterious and require statistical measures and preparation for an RRC review every several years.

What about the ACGME programs themselves? Here as well there is need for improvement. The record of CAQ-fellowship regulation compliance is disturbing. Consider only ACGME programs in Radiology both fellowship and core. There are 186 core residencies, 93 vascular interventional programs, 85 neuroradiology programs and 45 pediatric radiology programs, encompassing 4,500 radiology residents and 436 fellows. Thus, one would expect that the number of citations in the fellowship programs, given their smaller faculty and fewer number of trainees, would be much less than in the core programs. Yet the record is otherwise. In neuroradiology on average there are 4.7 positions per program, in interventional radiology 3.0 and pediatric radiology 3.2. The average core Radiology program consists of 24 trainees.

Looking at citations per program in both the core and subspecialty areas from 2003 to 2007 one finds a disproportionate number of citations in fellowships. In scholarly activities the core programs had 19 citations and IR had 16. In duty hours work environment the core program had five citations, IR had four and neuro had three. In the important area of procedural experience, the core programs had 13 citations, IR 16 and neuro 13. Regarding the meeting of didactic components the core programs and neuro each had 8 citations but IR had 21. In education programs in relation to patient care the core programs overall had three citations and IR had 11. In the evaluation of residents the core programs had 14 citations, IR had 11 and neuro had 9. This recitation of citations is a special concern with IR. And in a further review of nine IR programs five had credentialing issues, seven had faculty lacking ABR certification, 13 faculty lacked the CAQ, which is a requirement for the program director but not necessarily for the faculty, and three program directors had no CAQ. IR and to a lesser extent neuroradiology, even with surveillance by the Radiology Residency Review committee of the ACGME, has significant compliance problems. Who is responsible for this? Well, one could fault the RRC for not emphasizing to program directors the crucial importance of following regulations. One could also fault the APDR, the Association of Program Directors in Radiology for no heeding this problem and of course one could fault the chairman for not given it full attention. Moreover, a survey of 69 chairmen illustrated that fellowships were not a major concern for them.

Thus, I have set the stage for considerations of improvement. In the next essay I will delve a little deeper and present as well remedies and proposals to bring these fellowships into the fold, making them more part of the family, so to speak.

And here is where the metaphor of step-child and orphan apply. Because there are two types of fellowships available to Radiology residents, those under the watchful eye of the Radiology Review Committee, an arm of the Accreditation Council for Graduate Medical Education (ACGME) and those that are entirely bereft of any official oversight. The RRC conducts regular surveys of programs within its purview. It has the power to issue citations, place programs on probation or terminate them altogether. It demands that program directors maintain records of procedures performed, conduct evaluations under specified rules and it further demands that the institution at which the program is based conduct formal scheduled reviews. Also, it requires that the programs provide the equipment and support to enable a fellow to meet the clinical opportunities he or she needs to gain competence. Furthermore it restricts the fellow by his or her designation as a "student". And he or she is unable to bill for services when functioning in his or her capacity as a learner in the subject of the fellowship. One who is a neuroradiology fellow, for example, must have all neuroradiology studies reviewed by an attending and the reimbursement for professional services will be received by the faculty member, not the "student".

Summary

The recently enacted changes in the content and the timing of the Radiology board examination for first-time takers has called into question the curriculum of the fourth year of training. To many program directors, that year will be filled with a series of several months assignments in the various subspecialties of Radiology scheduled in a sense to round out the trainee's education. An alternative is a year-long intraresidency "fellowship" devoted only to one area, to be followed by further instruction in a similarly devoted fellowship in the same discipline in PGY-5, the traditional fellowship period. The strategic implication of both approaches is discussed in this essay [1].

Reference

1.   Baker SR, Luk L, Clarkin K. The trouble with fellowships. JACR. 2010;7:446–57.

The Changing Board Exam Schedule in the U.S.: Will General Radiologists and Emergency Radiologists Become Synonymous?

14

Change is a constant in radiology. Yet the visibility of that change depends upon the thing altered. The introduction of a new modality or an advanced technique is readily manifest as it is demonstrated in the production of novel images. Modifications of reimbursement or the announcement of new regulations are usually publicized before their imposition so that while they may be startling, they are not unexpected, at least in the immediate term. In contradistinction, there are profound changes that do not broadcast their arrival as they are the result of gradual alterations of attitude or slowly developing realignments of opportunities or even sometimes the subliminal redirection of perspectives held by regulators policy planners, or competitors. Such new realities are generally perceptible in both their evolution and inevitability by those attuned to look for trends. Yet for most radiologists, they are apt to burst on the scene assertively, belatedly and unheralded.

Just such a metamorphosis will soon occur in the U.S. 30 years ago, with the advent of cross-sectional displays accorded by CT and ultrasonography, we took on the roles of interpreter and explainer to referring physicians about 3D phenomena as depicted in stacks of 2D slices of information, encompassing the span of a body region. We became the keystone of the diagnostic process for most conditions as advances in CT, provided with each quantum improvement in pictorial rendering, more incisive and comprehensive images whose diagnostic import could only be discerned by the application of our distinctive knowledge and specific training.

Yet, today, further advances in imaging are reorienting the paradigm, leaving those who profess general capabilities in radiology in the uncomfortable position of not being that essential after all. Anatomy and gross pathology can now be observed readily in 3D arrays, revealed in multiplanar reformations rendering composite images, which are relatively easy to interpret. Thus, our once exclusive proprietorship of the intellectual manipulation of the 2D to 3D transformation has been challenged. Such a change threatens to engulf the claims of expertise formerly and until recently held by general radiologists. Because of the already vast and continually accumulating expanse of newly available information instituted by technical advances, they can now no longer lay claim to the possession of recondite knowledge and know how. Other specialists who care for patients directly can now have at their disposal detailed static depictions of disease height, width, and depth, as well as video clips and with exciting functional data. Hence, with such newly-acquired accessibility to this enhanced diagnostic armamentarium, reliance will only be placed on those radiologists who are specialized in accord within the referrer's discipline. The neurosurgeon will still benefit from the insights of the neuroradiologist and the thoracic surgeon will continue to seek advice from the chest radiologist. But the general radiologist increasingly will have little to offer to treating physicians who possess specialist credentials. After all our clinical colleagues' residency education and practice are suffused now with sophisticated image instruction. Many have gained technical facility with image-guided procedures. From now on, the radiologist must be a specialist to other specialists or face obsolescence.

Whither the general radiologist? Of course, this job category will not disappear overnight. In small and outlying facilities, the general radiologist will stay vital but in a narrowing, reduced role servicing primary physicians and other caregivers who have had relatively little training in imaging interpretation. Yet in hospitals of at least medium size, larger radiology groups must become more differentiated along subspecialty lines if they want to keep their turf.

Radiology education must adapt to this impertinent and insistent actuality. Radiologists in the U.S. can no longer be measured by 4 years of residency education which, incidentally, is now the longest interval between internship and fellowship of any non-surgical specialty. The timing, content and context of the written and oral boards now nearly fully implemented were motivated by a desire to redirect residency education to emphasize subspecialty options.

And these calls have been heard. Despite strident urgings by those resistant to and reluctant for change, the American Board of Radiology has taken the bold step of fundamentally reorienting residency training. The traditional oral board examination with the candidate and reviewer in close communication has been replaced by computer directed tests which will go a long way to diminish the fear which, in anticipation at least, such verbal byplay has induced. The schedule of examinations has been altered. The former written examination taken in the fourth year has been superseded by an image-rich, comprehensive test occurring after 36 months of residency. And in the place of the oral exam will be a subspecialty-oriented certifying exam taken 15 months after the completion of the fourth year of residency.

The purpose of the intrusion of those innovations is more than to diminish anxiety for the test taker. Rather they are meant, among other things, to stimulate subspecialty training which will likely commence after the initial exam, allowing for much of the concluding 12 months of residency to focus on the intensive development of

expertise in one or two realms of subspecialty knowledge in preparation to the continuance of focused training in a fellowship, which would follow as before in the fifth year of radiology training.

But what about the person who does not want to specialize? What would that fifth year be? What would the opportunities be for practice as well? The generalist of today will be no more. Perhaps the generalist of tomorrow will be, lo and behold, the emergency radiologist. Just as subspecialty practice is an imperative, so too will be the need for around-the-clock radiology coverage. Where is the predominant locus of after-hours practice? It is in the emergency suite, of course. Teleradiology may suffice for ER coverage in small hospitals. However, for larger, more busy facilities the radiologist on site will be a necessity if imaging by radiologists is to exist at all. And such an individual will have to demonstrate by education and confidence, advanced knowledge of a range of modalities adapted to emergency patients and trauma patients. Thus, emergency radiology will not be confined to one technology or one organ system or one body region but to one realm of conditions affecting the acutely ill or injured.

Over the years, emergency radiologists have been in many ways the odd men out. They have not had a separate section of the oral board exam even though they have created a curriculum entailing their distinctive corpus of knowledge. They have very few fellowship slots. In various radiology organization schema they have often been an afterthought despite the fact that in some hospitals up to 50 % or even more imaging studies take place in the ER. With the expected transformation of radiology training from a 4-1 to a 3-2 or a 3-1-1 continuum of general and specialty training, it is time now for emergency radiology to claim that it too can provide meaningful educational experiences so that those who wish not to be bound by an organ system or an age group or a single technique can find a place and thrive. We must provide the needed guidance and expertise to enable newly minted radiologists to function not as a replica of the old fashioned general radiologist but rather to perform as its vibrant successor, as a superspecialist serving the emergently ill and injured and the highly trained physicians and surgeons who care for them.

To me, the path ahead is clear. In the new environment having 3D imaging ubiquitously available, the emergency radiologist must step up. His or her commitment has always been to enable the establishment of diagnoses according to rapid assessment according to protocols which allow prompt institution of therapy. Emergency radiology has as its own hallmark, the willingness of its practitioners to be available at any time and with teleradiology, anywhere. Emergency radiologists are conversant with new imaging techniques and they are comfortable with establishing and maintaining a continuing and coherent dialog with emergency physicians and trauma surgeons, even under the stress of the moment.

But what they lack are enough fellowships to create an enlarging cadre of experts. It is time now before it is too late to press for more subspecialty training lines. They need not be ACGME authorized because if such were to be created, the trainee could not bill for his or her diagnostic services. Rather, non-ACGME fellowships would be the way to go because as a graduate of a 4-year residency program, the fellow would be permitted to be compensated for his interpretations even as he gains experience under the tutelage of his instructors.

But as one prescient observer once said, opportunities are like flies coming at you and elephants going away. Soon, maybe, the general radiologist will be the emergency radiologist if we deem it and make it so or else imaging of the urgently distressed will be a subsection of some other specialty [1].

Reference

1. Baker SR. The oral boards: why radiology has it wrong and why it must be changed now. JACR. 2008;5:5–9.

Bubble Trouble

15

One of the most infectious maladies humans as social animals are at risk of suffering is excessive, misplaced optimism. An exuberantly affirming view of the near and medium term is exploited by the cunning and enthusiastic to excite the naïve. And no matter how sophisticated we might appear to be the lure of the prize is an ever present susceptibility ready to snare us when our guard is down.

Just think of how irrational we become when a national lottery revs up to provide an award of $100 million or more. Nearly everyone wants to buy a ticket- Hey, you never know-even when the odds of winning are infinitesimally low.

And it is not just games of chance that intrigue us. Excessive speculation can intrude into commerce and investing. Remember the dot.com bubble that broke in 2000? Can you forget the housing bubble that burst in 2007 and 2008? Currently we are in a global commodity bubble with the price of copper, for example, never higher because of the unreasonable assumption that the Chinese economy will continue to grow fast and indefinitely or at least until it surpasses the U.S. in total wealth and later in GNP per individual. But the early dotcoms generated no profits, houses were overvalued and the Chinese economy is now slowing so we should expect commodity prices to fall soon as demand recedes.

Well, radiology is not bubble proof either. We are now just starting to experience the effects of one we initiated back in 1999. The adverse consequences of the unrealistic estimations and actions that informed it are now being felt in many ways.

We enlarged our residencies beginning 13 years ago in anticipation of unremitting expansion of imaging under Radiology's purview, led by the heightened capabilities and expanding utilization of CT and MR. Yet now, for the past several years imaging volume has fallen, putting the lie to the notion that because of increasing population, especially of the elderly, and a permissive reimbursement system, unfettered growth will remain a thing of the present and a certainty for the future.

Well, it isn't any longer. The job market for newly minted radiologists is drying up; the number of senior students interested in our specialty is decreasing year by year. In the last match, vacancies increased to about 8 % of offered slots, Medicare continues to attempt to ratchet down payments per case and insurance companies are insisting on more denials. And yet, despite these worrying signals, the cadre of radiology residents keeps expanding [1].

Let's look at the record. In December 1996, Medicare capped the number of residency positions for which it offered payment. The cap, unaltered, is still in place today. In order for a particular residency program to increase its complement of trainees and still be reimbursed by Medicare it would have to take them from another residency program in the same institution. A very unlikely scenario, to be sure. To enlarge its residency it is much more likely that it would have to generate the money for salary and fringe benefits from its clinical revenue. In the mid-1990s, the specter of managed care influenced manpower

S.R. Baker, *Notes of a Radiology Watcher*,
DOI 10.1007/978-3-319-01677-1_15, © Springer International Publishing Switzerland 2014

decisions. There were about 4,000 radiology residents in 1992 in the U.S.A. But a compelling notion back then was that the advent of capitation and other money-saving innovations would constrict demand for imaging by about one fourth. So many residencies followed suit. In 1999, there were only 3,591 residents in allopathic radiology residencies in the U.S.

But the unexpected happened. Advances in CT with respect to speed of image generation and incisiveness of pictorial definition made it possible to routinely scan children and uncooperative adults. New uses were found for computed tomography like the demonstration of pulmonary emboli. Significant improvement in MR also took place. The result was that the growth of these two modalities was astounding, generating a need for more radiologists in both academic and private practice and cheaper professional labor i.e., residents and fellows so that CTs could be performed and interpreted around the clock.

The agency responsible for approving accreditation of residencies is the Accreditation Council for Graduate Medical Education (ACGME). Through its Radiology Residency Committee it is called upon to evaluate requests for program expansion solely on the basis of the educational capabilities possessed by that program. If both volume and teaching staff were adequate in number and qualifications, then the RRC would almost assuredly approve a request for more. National demographic implications were deemed irrelevant for decision-making. I was on the Radiology Review Committee during much of the last decade and I am therefore very aware of the approval process and the policies that underlie it.

So it was a period of resplendent expansion. Imaging volume was continually going up, reimbursement was relatively unencumbered and money became available to find more residency lines. Each year from 1999 to 2010, the number of training positions increased by more than 115 annually from 2001 to 2004 and by no less than 30 each successive year. So by 2010, there were 4,531 slots filled by residents which over the decade encompassed a 20.03 % rise. Compared with many other residencies radiology leads the pack. For example, pediatrics grew by 7 %,

internal medicine by 3 %, OB-Gyn and Urology stayed constant while surgery, pathology, family medicine and ophthalmology declined. Orthopedics has grown rapidly recently as have ENT and Plastic Surgery. These three residencies are considerably smaller than Radiology so that the actual number of additional positions is likewise smaller than it has been for Radiology.

Along the way over this decade there have been years when demand and supply were slightly out of sync but the corresponding rises in supply and demand kept residency allotments overall in lockstep with utilization.

And in fact, imaging had been growing for a long time- for 40 years or so with the continued broadening of the spectrum of imaging tests finding widespread acceptance by referring physicians, insurance companies, the federal government and the public at large. It seemed that the steady upward progress of imaging utilization would go on forever. This presumption in fact set the stage for the manpower bubble now in progress.

Why is the bubble now bursting? Could it be that volume is actually decreasing? And it is. Traditionally the most reliable source of data on imaging utilization in the U.S. has been derived from Medicare files. Information about the specifics of healthcare diagnostic choices and their costs applied to the care of the elderly serves as a reasonably reliable proxy of U.S. health care indices for the population as a whole.

And the Medicare data reveals that even as the number of radiology residents has gone up, the utilization of imaging has now started to go down after first leveling off. A study from the Moran Company of Imaging Services billed to Part B Medicare Carrier and paid under the Medicare Physicians fee schedule from 1999 to 2009 revealed growth exceeding 5 % per annum from 1999 to 2005, then a decrease in the rate of expansion from 2005 to 2008 averaging 1.1 % each year. But in the 2008–2009 year, there was a 7.1 % drop in volume and 2.1 % decline in spending. Even earlier from 2006 to 2007, expenditures per beneficiary decreased from $419 to $375. Advanced imaging tests as a percentage of all imaging tests continue to rise and the number of CTs has grown albeit more slowly until 2010 but now it has too begun to decline while MR volume has remained flat. Furthermore, in an analysis of utilization of all insured patients, not in Medicare, the 2010 year revealed a 5.4 % drop in radiology procedures following a 0.2 % decline in 2008 and a 1.0 % reduction in 2009.

Radiology positions increased progressively in this decade of growth. But at its tail end and presumably also for the medium term ahead volume and reimbursement will be in decline. Yet the radiology trainees who were brought on stream to service the growth spurt are not commodities to be disposed of when economic conditions turn unfavorable. Instead they are young physicians about to begin a career. Have we made a Faustian bargain with our junior colleagues, enticing them to join our illustrious specialty just at the time when our 40-year span of nearly uninterrupted technological advance and enhanced prosperity is coming to an end or at best entering a prolonged period of retrenchment?

And has that technology itself become another kind of Faustian bargain to be redeemed to our detriment? Have we made imaging interpretation compatible with advances in computer investigation so that the diagnostic interpretation itself will become the province of algorithms instead of our expertise? The possibility of inroads by computerization is inevitable and I think imminent. Radiologists must adapt and redeploy the application of their expertise to preserve their favored position as practitioners today. And at the same time they must provide new opportunities for our residents and newly-installed diplomats, who despite these countervailing unfavorable trends that I have outlined, are still bubbling with enthusiasm for our specialty.

Summary

We are now entering an uncomfortable time requiring adjusting to unfavorable manpower conditions in Radiology. Since 1999 we have been increasing the complement of residents in our programs, the number rising from about 3,500 then to more than 4,500 now. This advance in the extent of the trainee roster was deemed acceptable when volume was increasing as it had been until 2008. But now after plateauing CT and MR utilization has decreased and probably will continue to decrease. So the problem is too much supply and diminishing demand with both going their contrary ways for the foreseeable future. Now the job market is tight and will get tighter even as Radiology has lost its cachet with many medical students as witnessed by an 8 % vacancy rate in matched positions this Spring.

Reference

1. Luk L, Baker SR. After-hours coverage of various radiologic subspecialties and its impact on the fourth-year radiology residency curriculum. Acad Radiol. 2013;20(1):122–7. doi:http://dx.doi.org/10.1016/j.acra.2012.05.021.

Regulation Without Representation

16

A few weeks ago, the quadrennial exercise in collective bargaining began in earnest at my home institution. At the table sat housestaff members and paid officials of the Residents Union on one side and labor negotiators and the Deans for Graduate Medical Education of the three medical schools in our university system on the other. The setting has a particular piquancy for me because as the Associate Dean for Graduate Medical Education of New Jersey Medical School, my job is to represent management. Yet I recollect very well when as a senior resident I was also the President of the Committee of Interns and Residents. Then I represented my trainee constituents in the turbulent 1970s in New York City where collective bargaining was more of a free for all than it is today.

Although many of the issues which we are discussing in this ongoing deliberation are different from what they were more than 30 years ago, some are nearly the same. Salaries are of the utmost concern, yet movement on them is much constrained given the economic stringencies impinging upon house officers and medical institutions, especially medical institutions like ours, supported to a significant degree by our state whose leaders in turn are wrestling with unprecedented budget deficits.

In preparation for the bargaining process, I contacted the Association of American Medical Colleges (AAMC) to get some data regarding the economic conditions of residents in general. The results, while expected, were nonetheless startling. In constant dollars, resident salaries are essentially unchanged from what they were 40 years ago. But what has changed is the extent of indebtedness in both actual and constant dollars from even 10 years ago. The average amount owed by a beginning intern is $175,000 whereas in equivalent currency it was less than $100,000 even 8 years ago. Moreover, the cost of living measured again with consideration of inflation is greater today than ever before. Two years ago we published a paper indicating that approximately 15 % of a third and fourth year radiology resident's salary, pretax, on average has to be allocated for mandated educational expenses to be borne by him or her. Included in this roster of expenses are AFIP-related costs for housing, travel and enrollment, the costs of Step 3 of the USMLE examination, a trip to Louisville for the oral board exam, and the costs of review courses in preparation for the exam. In our survey of those taking at least one review course, the mean number of such courses actually attended was two such extraparietal exercises. Add to that the cost of travel for fellowship interviews and further impingements by adverse changes in loan repayment requirements and it is clear to see that the cost squeeze on many recent medical graduates is profound.

Now, eventually, if present trends continue, most radiologists after several years in practice will begin to get out of the hole. But the effect of a period of penury may have a lasting influence on the job choices of recent graduates as well as on their attitudes towards income accumulation and location considerations. Hence any initiative

S.R. Baker, *Notes of a Radiology Watcher*,
DOI 10.1007/978-3-319-01677-1_16, © Springer International Publishing Switzerland 2014

that can serve to lengthen the period of recompense or defer expenses until the debtor is able to pay may have a salutary effect not only on cash flow but also on how one might view the world without the incubus of financial obligation on one's back. Put another way, any abrupt expense imposed on residents that can be meted out in a more prolonged fashion rather than all at once deserves consideration for its benevolence and its practicality.

So one might ask why are PGY(1)'s encouraged to pay upfront the costs of the board examination to be taken several years later. The American Board of Radiology so advises them to pay for the boards well-before taking them thus giving the ABR the use of the money thereby depriving the newly-minted residents from use of sources of money from savings or debt.

Why is this so? Does the ABR need to capture the dollars from these junior physicians promptly because if not they will lose revenue? Hardly! The certificates earned by diplomates of the ABR are time-limited, valid for only 10 years. More likely than not a radiologist will be better off financially a decade after entering training which is 5 years after gaining board certification. Then why not lower the charges to a beginning resident and raise them for the costs of subsequent certification when the candidate, now already established in his specialty most likely will be able to afford it?

These days, a radiologist has no choice but to the pass the tests the American Board of Radiology sets before him. After all the ABR is a monopoly. It clearly meets the definition of that model of economic power. It is the only seller of its product with certification a consequence of passage of an examination the ABR constructs and administers. Eligibility criteria of candidates trained in the U.S. deemed suitable to obtain its products is severely limited, open to only those who are now or have completed training in an ACGME approved Radiology residency. One cannot take the boards as can some law students who may be allowed to sit for the Bar Exam in some states without having attended law school. Barriers to competition by alternative certifying agents are practically insurmountable because an imprimatur by this board, the ABR is honored by tradition and by the respect held for it by all interested parties who have a stake in the maintenance of high standards for a practicing specialist. These parties include patients, state and local governments, hospitals, clinics, other physicians, the radiologists themselves and insurance companies. Therefore, upstart boards have little chance to break into the business.

Hence if there is such a consensus about the value of ABR certification and a lack of alternatives to it, the board bears a special responsibility to the individuals it represents. While many actors are dependent on the role the ABR plays as a protector of patients, in effect the owners of that board, if you will "are the community of radiologists" for the standards it imposes for the common good are directed in particular to vouchsafe the quality of radiologists and hence the quality of radiology. And therefore even though it sits in judgment it too can be judged.

Paramount among any board's responsibility is to be accountable to its owners, i.e., all radiologists. Hence in the words of John Carver, a leading theorist of board function, "the board must be in a position to understand the various views held in the community".

In fact, the ABR is very careful who it chooses to be its members. The quality of these individuals is high. The ABR respectively takes into account diversity, too. The present day complement of diagnostic radiologists on it includes representative from all regions of the country, from all subspecialties of radiology and from both genders.

Yet what the board is not representative of is the age range of its members. The average age of first time takers of the test for initial certification is roughly 30 yet the mean age of its members is 59.4 years. Only one member is below 50. In this regard, the ABR is not alone although its mean age is nearly the highest among all specialty boards. In OBGYN it is 58.4, in Pediatrics it is 59.2, in Surgery 55.1, in Internal Medicine 56.7, in Anesthesiology 55.0, in Pathology 57.0, ER Medicine 59.1, Dermatology 56.4 and Neurosurgery 53.5. Only Psychiatry and Neurology, a combined board, has an older member complement on average with a mean age of 60.4 years.

Moreover, none of these boards has a young diplomate on its membership roster. Perhaps it is presumed that junior diplomates lack the experience, expertise or wisdom to participate in board deliberations and decisions. Yet what they may lack in years in the profession, they could make up for in awareness of the problems and attitudes of junior "owners" of the specialty.

The avoidance of young colleagues, while a near unanimous position of specialty boards, is not subscribed to by the ACGME and its 24 RRC's. All of them have at least one resident member and internal medicine has two. In fact among the 251 RRC members in all specialties 27 or 10.76 % of them are residents and each resident is a voting member of his or her respective RRC. Bear in mind that residents have not yet completed their period of training and yet are entrusted with a policy-making role in all specialties. On the other hand, junior board certified specialists are given no equivalent opportunity by the ABR and like board organizations.

The AMA has a student board member with full voting rights as does the AAMC. Among the specialty colleges such as the ACR more than half have resident members on their respective boards. In a survey of the board constituents of the largest universities in each of the 50 states, some public and others private, 70 % have a student member and in nearly all of these, the students so chosen have voting rights [1].

Thus with respect to board certification in Radiology, the generation gap is alive and well whereas with program accreditation the gap has been closed. A monopolistic organization lacking representation by one of its constituencies, i.e., its junior members, will make policies like accelerated payment in part or in full for initial certification giving little heed to the constraints it places on residents who are a class of individuals with no bargaining power. This policy is ultimately harmful to radiology by impinging further on the weak. It is time now for the board to change its membership personality by admitting at least one junior member. By so doing it will be compelled to look more closely at how it is imposing costs on those who cannot afford to meet them without enduring further privation.

Reference

1. Williams KJ. Improving the NRMP board: why not direct representation? Acad Med. 1998;73(6):623–4.

Part III

Radiology Elsewhere in the World

In this part, American healthcare and particularly American radiology is discussed in reference to O.E.C.D data encompassing 34 countries. American radiology residency education is compared with the characteristics of training in Europe. Also two countries with markedly different scales of wealth, Japan and Cuba, are evaluated. Both in their particular context have been successful in the delivery of healthcare and the provision of radiology resources.

O.E.C.D. Health Data: Where Does the U.S. Stack Up?

17

The national health debate, centered for the past several years on the efficacy and later the constitutionality of the Affordable Care Act, has been characterized by passionate discussions and diatribes focused on the controversy regarding the obligations of government to manage the health of its citizens even to the extent to which it intrudes on individual freedom of action. What an affluent society-one that can provide the wherewithal to improve healthcare-should be most concerned with ought to frame the content of the conversation about what kind of system do we need and what and how are we to pay for it. The means and mechanisms by which we should promote health, prevent disease, cure or at least treat illness and provide rehabilitation is by contemporary rhetoric often lost in the shuffle, at least in my view.

So if you will allow me, I would like to acquaint you with the health indices of other countries, most of which are similar to ours with respect to per capita income. Extensive information about the components of their health care is readily available from the files of the Organization for Economic Co-operation and Development (O.E.C.D.). Two years ago it had made available statistics for each of its member countries, providing an opportunity to scan a scorecard, if you will, comparing the American experience with others. It allows us to redirect our attention towards the transcendent concern of long term trends with enduringly relevant data focusing beyond immediate political issues and certainly beyond radiology and even organized medicine as a whole. This information offers an assessment over a 50 year span. In this two part evaluation, I will compare all 34 nations first and then in the second part concentrate on Japan as a counterpoise to the US.

The O.E.C.D. currently consists of 34 member countries. It includes Switzerland, Norway, Iceland and nearly all nations in the European Union, excluding Malta, Cyprus, Latvia, Lithuania, Bulgaria and Romania. Also not on its roster are all the countries resulting from the dismembering of Yugoslavia, except Slovenia, and the 15 nations who once constituted the Soviet Union. The ten other members include two from North America, the U.S. and Canada, two from Latin America, Mexico and Chile, two from Oceania, Australia and New Zealand, two from East Asia, Japan and South Korea and two from West Asia, Turkey and Israel. Other noteworthy non-members include Brazil, Argentina, Indonesia, Taiwan, Singapore, India, Pakistan and China. The population of its constituent countries varies from 300,000 in Iceland to more than 300 million in the U.S.

Since 1960, the O.E.C.D. has accumulated annual national health statistics. Not every country is represented by an uninterrupted skein of contributions to all of these indices. Not everyone has contributed yearly data, but by and large, especially in the last 15 years, the data are extensive even if not exhaustive. For most of the categories and for most of the countries the long term, and particularly, the recent records are robust.

The health-related information amassed by the O.E.C.D. includes overall expenditures in

S.R. Baker, *Notes of a Radiology Watcher*,
DOI 10.1007/978-3-319-01677-1_17, © Springer International Publishing Switzerland 2014

this economic sector as a percentage of gross domestic products, the annual growth rate of these expenditures, the fraction of health care costs expended through public resources and for each annual record, the percentage of costs paid out of pocket. Health Care Activities and Resources charted by O.E.C.D. include average length of stay overall in hospitals, total hospital beds per 1,000 population as well as acute care length of stay data.

Health statistics measures are provided including life expectancy at birth, overall, and for men and women; life expectancy by gender at age 65; causal mortality in two areas, suicide and infant mortality; the number of physicians and nurses each for 1,000 population. Physician activities as assessed by per capita annual consultations with patients. Also, physicians and nursing graduates per 100,000 population are given for each nation. Risk factors, too, are the subject of annual data including tobacco consumption, both for all citizens and by gender, alcohol consumption per annum and obesity as a percentage of all men and all women as derived from self-reporting and also by measurement of weight by health care workers. Finally there are multinational per annum ratios of CT examinations by 1,000 population overall and further delimited by those obtained in ambulatory care facilities and those done in hospitals. The number of CTs per million population from country to country is listed as well. Similarly MR use overall and disaggregated by ambulatory care facilities and hospitals, are part of the data set as are the number of MR units per million. Mammography studies per year per country per million population and radiation therapy equipment per million, round out the information directly pertinent to Radiology.

Before proceeding with an evaluation of inferences to be drawn from this trove of data certain limitations and caveats should be acknowledge. Anyone who assesses these data from the O.E.C.D. website cannot promptly check the accuracy or completeness of the information, at least not on a first inspection of them without seeking recourse to more detailed explanations of data quality. Secondly, the age structure of the national populations varies from country to country and over time. Although there appears to be a coming together, a closing of the differences in wealth and health say between very rich Luxembourg and still developing Mexico, a yawning gap between them yet exists. The issues of income distribution wide in Latin America and narrow in Scandinavia may be obscured by national statistics which veil differences by per capita income and region. These disclaimers notwithstanding, I believe meaningful comparisons can be made of distinctive approaches to health and perhaps differing effectiveness of these approaches country by country through examination of the data. I provide for you some highlights.

As of 2009 the percentage of the growth domestic product devoted to health care in the United States was 17.4 %. The next country in its devotion of resources for this purpose was Finland at 11.8 %, followed by France 11.6 %, Sweden 11.4 %, Belgium 11.3 %, Switzerland 10.8 % and Germany 9.6 %. Japan is ranked 20th at 8.6 %. Mexico is at 12 % but its total GDP is much lower than average and Luxembourg is at 6.1 % but its GDP is much higher than all other O.E.C.D. members. The annual growth rate in real dollars in the U.S. was 5 % in 2000–2001 and 6.7 % in 2001–2002 but since then it has averaged 2.2 % per annum. Over the past 50 years the growth of the percentage of health care in the U.S. as a component of GDP has had an uninterrupted rise from 5.1 % in 1960 to 7.4 % in 1972 to 10.6 % in 1988 and to 13.9 % in 2000. The fastest rate of increase was in the early 70s just before President Nixon sought to impose price controls on hospital charges.

With respect to the percentage of public expenditures for health as a fraction of total health expenditures only three of the 34 countries are below 50 %-Chile, Mexico and the U.S. all at 47 %. Hence, while the shibboleth of socialized medicine enters into disputes in the political arena about American health care, 31 of the 34 O.E.C.D. members have more of it than the U.S. and in all of them it costs less of their national treasure than in the USA. For example, public related health costs in the U.K. are 84 % of their health dollar, in Canada 70 %, Japan 77 % and

Switzerland 59 %. Yet the rate of increase in the percentage of public expenditure is increasing in our country. Since 2000 it has grown more than twice as fast as the rise in the percent of GDP spent on health overall.

Since 1965, on the other hand, out of pocket payment as a percentage of all health care expenditures has declined from 45.1 to 14.4 % in 1995 and leveled off since then being only 12.3 % now. This is the result of the penetration of Medicare, Medicaid and other insurance plans. The percentages vary greatly elsewhere- 49 % in Mexico to 14 % in Canada.

With respect to health status, the U.S. trails most other nations in the O.E.C.D. In the U.S. in 2009, life expectancy at birth was 78.9 years ranking us 26th of 34. For females here it is 80.6 years. For that we are in 25th place and for males at 75.7 years—27th place. For life expectancy at age 65 for women it is 19.9 years 24th place, and for men at age 65 we live on average 17.3 years placing us higher on the scale but only in 21st place. Hence, by these important indices, one might claim that we are not getting a bang for our buck in health care—no matter how it is allocated.

Part of the long gain in life expectancy showed by all O.E.C.D. members is related to the decline in infant mortality. In the U.S. it is now 6/1,000 which is not bad relative to the past but it is exceeded by many other O.E.C.D. countries. Moreover, all 34 countries have decreased their infant mortality steadily. Since 1960 the U.S. rate has declined from 26 to 6 per 1,000 births. But this percentage decline is the worst among all O.E.C.D. members. We are now still far behind last year's rate in Iceland of 1 per 1,000. And our childhood immunization rates are nothing to be proud of either. Only 90 % of children in the U.S. are immunized against measles while in several other countries the rate exceeds 98 %. The U.S. performance with respect to DPT immunizations last year was only 83.9 %. In some countries all children have been immunized against these diseases.

The density of physicians in the U.S. including those both American and foreign trained was 2.4. per 1,000 which puts us 26th of 34 and nurses per 1,000 averages 33.7, situating us in the bottom half of countries. The shortage of doctors here is reflected too in medical graduates per 100,000 where we rank in the bottom third, Also in consultations by physicians per capita per year we are similarly below the mean of OECD members.

But now let's look at Radiology. For CT examinations per capita, for the last year for which there is a record in the U.S. we did 227.9 exams per 1,000 populations, far ahead of Luxembourg and Belgium, each the next closest at 180 per 1,000. In the U.S. approximately 80 % are done in hospitals, presumably reflecting the contribution of E.R. requests among other indications to the total mix of CT studies. We have 34.3 scanners per one million residents, a percentage exceeded slightly by 5 other countries. We just use them more intensively. Incidentally, well ahead of us in CT availability is Australia. With MR the situation is about the same. We do more magnetic resonance imaging than every other country except Japan-where use exceeds America's record by 20 %. Remember their %GDP devoted to health care is half of ours.

At this juncture, we should all agree that the U.S. is an outlier with respect to many of these health indices. I will continue this analysis in part two addressing further the habits of Americans and their relation to health. We are markedly different in this regard from most other O.E.C.D. member nations. I will focus specific attention on Japan which is as distinct from other OECD countries as we are but for different reasons.

The O.E.C.D, a so-called "rich country's club" of 34 nations, 22 in Europe and including also Japan, Korea, the U.S., Canada and Australia has provided annual statistics for each national member including health expenditures, health activities and personnel data. Inspection of these data reveal that the U.S., despite assigning the greatest percentage by far of GNP toward health, performs poorly in many pertinent categories. Life expectancy is worse than in most other O.E.C.D. countries, the number of physicians and nurses per capita is relatively low and so are measurements of infant mortality and immunization rate. In contrast, we are near the top in number per population of CT and MR machines and we use them more extensively than is the practice in most other O.E.C.D. countries. Also, the obese person percentage of the population is much higher in the U.S. than that found in other nations. In essence, we are unique, generally, in the high cost of care and a laggard in measurements of the effectiveness of our health care enterprise to ensure prolongation of a healthful life for our citizens, at least in reference to similarly "advanced" countries on all continents [1].

Reference

1. Mattke S, Epstein AM, Leatherman S. The OECD health care quality indicators project: history and background. Int J Qual Health Care. 2006;18 Suppl 1:1–4.

Characteristics of Radiology Training Programs in Europe in Comparison with Those in The United States

Often in matters of comparison of health care between the U.S. and elsewhere I take a critical view of the American product. Not this time. I want to say straight out that after a visit to participate in the annual meeting of an organization called Management in Radiology, which is an association of European radiologists akin in purpose and purview to the Society of Chairman of Academic Radiology Departments (SCARD) in the US, I came away with the conviction that in our country we prepare our residents much better than they do in every country in Europe. Our training paradigms are evidently more extensive in scope, more uniform in content and more committed to the education of radiologists of the future than is the case in most European countries. We have incorporated into them standardized instruments and policies for review and surveillance that are mostly lacking on the other side of the North Atlantic.

This comparison is based upon two major distinctions between here and there. In the US, our capacity for organization and our zeal in providing structure in medical education is built on a long-standing tradition beginning with the Flexner Report for medical school education in the early 1900s progressing to the establishment of specialty boards and board examinations in the 1930s and afterward to the development and maturation of the Accreditation Committee for Graduate Medical Education in the 1970s and 1980s and with its mandate for specific regulations which are constantly in evolution.

In comparison, Europe is a collection of 50 plus countries, some very large, and others mere statelets. They have differing organizations and systems of healthcare of medicine, and differing perceptions of the balance between the profit motive and the need for universally available social services. Recent efforts at integration of care across national borders have followed in the wake of the expansion of the European Union but they are not in lockstep with it. Moreover, to a much greater extent than in the US the number of radiologists in relation to population varies widely from place to place, and especially from country to country. Thus, it should not be expected that there would be homogeneity in Radiology training programs across Europe.

Recent attempts at integration are well-meaning, but they are limited in scope and halting in implementation. Two important developments stand out; both of which have occurred in the last 5 years. In 2004, in order to assess the existing differences in radiology graduate medical education, a survey was conducted by the European Association of Radiology (EAR), an organization which has since 2005 been known as the European Society of Radiology (ESR). In any event, in 2004 the survey was addressed to the various national radiology societies to gain an overview of the nature of residency training in each. The results of the survey demonstrated the existence then and now, of a wide spectrum of permutations with respect to entry requirements, training schemes, curricular manifestations and resident evaluations. Responses were collected from 24 of those countries including most of the large nations and a range of smaller ones. Notable omissions included Finland, Turkey, Bulgaria, Serbia, Belarus, and the Ukraine.

Here are some specifics which I hope you find interesting. Overall, in relation to US programs and among European countries, I found disparities to be much greater than resemblances. For example, residencies in 12 countries mandate passing a national examination before beginning residency, and 6 countries require passing a local exam. Therefore, six countries have *no such* requirement for entrance. In Ireland, Netherlands and Russia, a national exam before beginning residency is the only pre-requisite besides an MD degree. In some ways, this is analogous to the US where passage of parts 1 and 2 of the USLME test is necessary. Seventeen countries require an interview prior to entry. In most programs in the US an interview is also part of the application process. However, in Austria, Denmark and Greece, there are no specified entry criteria beyond the holding of an MD degree. Furthermore, unlike the US, there is no computer based match program anywhere in Europe. Now, we might regard that as a fundamental difference yet it should be remembered that the match for radiology residencies only began about 20 years ago. Two countries do not require an MD degree before beginning training; France and Switzerland. In France, final certification occurs at the end of training whereas in Switzerland—which has a 6 year program analogous to the US with an internship often in the first year of training and then a 5 year residency, features analogous to our 4 years of residency plus 1 year of fellowship—the MD degree is issued later than just before entry, sometime early on in the 6 year training interval.

An internship is required by program directors in only 8 of 24 countries before beginning a radiology residency. In the US the value of the internship is subject to continuing controversy and debate. In a study that we published a few years ago in Academic Radiology, after assessing current trainees in residency and fellowship we reported that a slight majority favored the internship. When disaggregated by internship type, 70 % of those who completed a surgical residency viewed it as valuable; and those having done a medical internship were mildly supportive of it based on their experience. In contrast only 40 % of those who completed a transitional internship regarded their preliminary year as a necessary and worthwhile experience of time and effort.

Internship length varies among these European countries but in most, it is 1 year long. However, in the UK and in Ireland it is 2 years. On the other hand, in Poland it is only 3 months, in France, Germany and Hungary, clinical experience occurs during training, not before it.

Several countries take a distinctly idiosyncratic approach to radiology training which merit separate mention. In Russia, there are no national exams and no local exam before or after the period of training. Also there is no internship requirement and no national curriculum. Furthermore, there is no obligatory formal teaching and until 2004 training length was only 2 years. It may have been extended to 4 years recently, but it is not clear at this time, from the data I was able to review whether that change has occurred there. On the other hand, there is fellowship training beyond residency in Russia.

No other national program is less than 4 years, except in the Ukraine which incidentally has no radiologists per se. That is right, none! Education is only in the techniques of radiology to be performed by doctors who possess system-specific designations such as gastroenterology. Thus, in that country, Radiology is not vocation specific. Hence there are no training programs in radiology nor are there fellowships nor certifying exams. A typical person doing radiology is a GI doctor who does GI procedures, including those involving diagnostic imaging.

In Italy, there is no national curriculum, no on call responsibilities, no log books or procedures, requirements and attendance. Attendance at Radiology meetings off-site is not required. There are no fellowships and there is no recognized subspecialty training. There is a final examination, but it is advisory to the applicant, not determinative of competence as regarded by future employers. Moreover, Radiology training is limited to 46 h per week, which makes the absence of night call understandable.

Most of these 24 countries have a national curriculum except for Italy, Slovakia and Norway. The assumption of on call responsibility occurs in a majority of programs but starting time is very variable. Most European residents begin on call in the second year, but in Norway, it occurs after 2 months of training, in Switzerland after 3 months and in Greece after 6 months. This is a major departure from the US in which all cases are reviewed by attendings. In Europe supervision by attending radiologists diminishes as training advances. Trainees perform and report procedures *always* under the supervision of a senior radiologist in only five European countries of the 24 in the survey. In all others, independent unreviewed interpretations occur by the third year and in four countries it begins before the end of the first year [1].

Like in the US, most training schedules involve successive rotations in the various subspecialties. In 19 of the 24 countries, training intervals are both organ specific and modality specific rotations. In three it is modality-based only and in two it is organ specific only. Formal teaching is mandatory in 18 but not obligatory in six.

Here is another fundamental difference with the US. Subspecialty training occurs in only half of the 24 countries. Even more astounding, at least to me, only 7 countries include nuclear medicine in their curricula and none provides instruction in PET. Moreover, Denmark, France, Netherlands, Norway and Spain have no board examinations.

Now, given these marked dissimilarities, the European Society of Radiology, newly named as such in 2005, announced in that year a plan to introduce a detailed, continent-wide curriculum, at least among the nations in the European Union. It was stated that resident radiologists at the end of 3 years should be fully conversant with the basic aspects of the corpus of common knowledge for general radiology. This will be achieved by a mixture of didactic and practical training. Furthermore, the duration of training in

radiology would be 5 years. The content of the first 3 years is a structured program including radiological anatomy, disease manifestations and core radiological skills. The fourth and fifth years would be structured more flexibly to develop sufficient competence enabling the trainee to function autonomously as a *general* radiologist. Please note the emphasis on general radiology. In the US, the ABR by moving the certifying board exam to 3 months after the fifth year, made a clear commitment to mandate subspecialty training for residents. The fifth year will consist of a formal fellowship format and the fourth year in most residencies would focus on training in one or two areas. In many programs this would be in effect a second fellowship.

The emphasis in Europe is a 5 year educational experience to create a general radiologist. It was also declared by the ESR that the curriculum should include education in cell function physiology, anatomy, physics, medical legal issues and administration and management. At present, while there is a consensus to move towards a general curriculum for Europe, it has not been implemented and in many respects it is honored in the breach instead of in its details. Note that that despite the rhetoric, the teaching of interpretive skills in, for example, ethics and management, does not occur in the UK or in Italy or in Greece and in fact it is only a feature of radiology residencies in Germany and Switzerland.

Sub-specialty training is limited in Europe. Fifteen of the 24 countries offer fellowships, but they are not as comprehensive in variety as in the US where fellowships abound in Body, Neuro, Peds, MSK, Women's Imaging, MR, etc. For example, Austria has recognized subspecialty training only in Interventional, Neuroradiology and Pediatrics, in Germany it is Neuroradiology and Pediatrics and in other countries only Ultrasound. In fact, only two countries offer more than three fellowships—Ireland and the UK. Moreover, the percentage of residents doing fellowships is very low in almost every country, except for Ireland and Germany. In France, for instance only 10–15 % of graduating trainees go on to fellowships. In the UK, it is 5–10 %. And when they have completed fellowships most individuals practice in that subspecialty only a fraction of the time per week, not like in the US where many subspecialty trained radiologists practice in their subspecialty nearly 100 % of the time.

What are the implications for US radiology resident and fellowship programs when their directors seek to hire foreign radiologists with training so-called "equivalent to board certification" as stated in the ACGME requirements for Radiology fellowships? Are European radiologists as fully trained as are radiologists who go through the American system? Well, many European trainees do not take a board examination, their national curricula vary and most residencies are not as extensive or intensive as in the US, in the pursuance of such requirements. In many programs, in most countries, the evaluation mechanisms and supervisory polices are either not in place nor they are not formalized and consistent.

Are European radiologists as fully trained as subspecialists as the US? Not at all. Overall, there are only a few fellowships offered, there is only fractional participation by them in subspecialties as a practitioner. Furthermore, teaching competence is not formally assessed in many fellowships there.

This analysis does not mean to imply that there are not excellent radiologists in Europe. There are many. Nor does it mean to suggest that radiologists are merely generalists and none obtain subspecialty training or gain subspecialty expertise. That probably is not true either but the mechanisms of education are limited when compared with the US. Thus, the number of subspecialists is less, their quality in the aggregate is probably much less, and the quality of education from place to place varies.

Can there be achievement of a unified curriculum? Probably not. Here are two reasons. The percentage of radiologists working in the private sector after training varies considerably. It is 60 % in Greece and 0 % in UK. In fact, in most places in Europe, private practice is limited or non-existent. Furthermore, the ratio of radiologists to population differs markedly. Thus the concerns of radiologist will also differ markedly from country to country. In Greece, there is one radiologist for every 4,500 people whereas in the UK there is one radiologist for every 28,000 residents. In the US there is one per 10,000. The training programs of Greece and the UK have to differ given that Britain has 7 times fewer radiologists than Greece where the majority of radiologists are in private practice and MR utilization is very strong. In contradistinction, in Britain it appears that a major consideration for training and practice is meeting a backlog of ultrasound examinations. Incidentally, most of those sonographic studies are done by the radiologist, not by a technologist.

I come away from this analysis being reassured that in the US we are doing the right things in terms of supervised education. I am assured that we are forward thinking especially with increasing emphasis in the later part of training on learning a subspecialty. Such comprehensiveness may be just a side benefit of the fact that the expanse of our country is continental in reach but is organized under one polity whereas Europe is a collection of states with a long history of rivalry among them. Whatever the antecedents, Radiology resident education in the US is in my opinion, qualitatively superior to what currently occurs to the East of us across the North Atlantic Ocean.

Reference

1. Baker SR. The training of radiology residents in the United States and Europe, major differences and some similarities. In: Second international society of radiology, virtual congress; April 2009.

Japan: A Country with a Currently Successful Radiology Model of Health Care

19

In a previous essay I presented data derived from the Organization of Economic Cooperation and Development (the OECD). These statistics encompass information from each of the 34 members of the OECD, popularly known as a rich country's club. Forty eight annual health-care related indices accumulated over 50 years from 1960 comprise the data base. It makes for fascinating reading and analysis.

Two countries for which many of the health-related categories stand out as outliers are the United States and Japan. The former is notable for its extravagant use of its national treasure as 17.5 % of its Gross Domestic Product is devoted to health care in the U.S. A distant second is Finland at 11.8 %. Yet despite this largesse, we fare poorly. For instance, we rank near the bottom in life expectancy. Similarly we are ranked 31st of 34 in deaths per live births under age of 1 today when we were 12th of 34 in 1960. We are 32nd of 34 in medical graduates per 100,000, 29th of 34 in the number of hospital beds because we have found hospitalization to be too expensive. Moreover, with respect to the number of doctor consultations per year we are in 30th place. There are things to be proud of course in the US including access to care-assuming you have insurance-and innovations in technology. But overall it is fair to claim that our health care system needs major reforms.

Japan's health care has a radically different statistical profile. Life-expectancy at birth both genders, is 83.0 years—in the US, it is 78.2. Life expectancy at age 65 for women is 24 versus 20.0 years in the U.S. Infant mortality in Japan is 2.4 deaths per 1,000 births in infants up to 1 year of age. In the U.S. it is nearly 3 times higher. The U.S. and Japan have about the same number of physicians and annual medical graduates proportionate to the population but in Japan, doctor consultation per capita per year is 23.2-nearly 4 times the American average. Japan has more than 3 times the number of acute care beds than we do and average length of stay is an unbelievable three and a half times higher at 18.5 days-yes that is 18.5 days.

With respect to imaging equipment, the differences are also astounding! The U.S. is ranked fifth in the number of CT scanners per million people at 34.3 putting us closely behind, Greece, Iceland and Australia in ascending order. Australia has 42.5 scanners per million while Japan has 97.3 per million, 3 time per capita as many as the U.S. What is not known from this data collecting is the utilization of these machines in Japan. Remarkably in Greece one CT study is performed on average per year in 320 of every 1,000 persons. In the US it is 228 but in Australia only 94 of 1,000.

With regard to MR units, Japan still leads by a lot but less dramatically than with CT. There are 43.1 MR units per million inhabitants in Japan. The US is second, far behind, with 28.9 per one million. Again utilization is not known from Japan whereas in Greece it is nearly one MR per 10 persons, slightly ahead of the United States in MR use intensity.

Hence in Japan, people live longer than in any other large country, they have a lot of hospital beds and patients spend a long time there with each admission on average. They have few

S.R. Baker, *Notes of a Radiology Watcher*,
DOI 10.1007/978-3-319-01677-1_19, © Springer International Publishing Switzerland 2014

doctors but many doctor visits and they have disproportionately more CT and MR units. Yet Japan devotes only 8.6 % of GNP to health exactly one half as much per capita as the United States. How it that possible?

Moreover, despite having nearly one quarter of its population over age 60, long term care insurance is provided to each aged Japanese citizen and noncontributory care by patients is also afforded its children. Despite providing more physician visits, perhaps the Japanese by virtue of diet, life style, wealth distribution are seemingly healthier? Here the evidence is mixed. Today one third of Americans are obese, a percentage exceeded perhaps only by Tonga in the South Pacific, whereas in Japan the percent of obese in the population has nearly doubled but from only 2 to 3.9 % over the past 30 years. On the other hand 39 % of Japanese smoke while in the US it is now only 14 % who do so. The Japanese pressure to work life-style may not be as healthy as it would be in a more relaxed society. Yet hypertension, a precursor to stroke, which has long been a major cause of death, is now more controlled with better drugs and a national consensus to seek measures for protection from the ravages of high blood pressure has helped as well.

Is there a single explanation for the Japanese success? No, but here are a few clues. A collectivist ethos informs all the institutions in Japan whereas the initiative of the individual is at least a conceit if not a philosophical directive of the American character. Adoption of preventive testing supported by employers is more accepted and utilized in Japan than in the U.S. or Europe. Perhaps that explains in part why they are healthier. Yet why despite their prolific investments in CT, MR, and Hospital beds-typically with people in them-are costs relatively low there?

For one thing, physician compensation is lower. In a study from 2005 comparing the salaries of generalist physicians as measured by purchasing power per person converted into dollars the average monthly income for such American doctors was $8,170 whereas in Japan comparable physicians earned only $4,600 or about $55,000 annually. Assume that unlike the United States where radiologists' salaries are about 4 times that of general practitioners, in Japan it is rather most likely just twice as much. Hence lower physician income brings costs down.

Inasmuch as the government participates in the purchase of high-tech imaging machines they can command a lower price from manufacturers, making CT and MR more affordable and ubiquitous. Comparable costs of an average MR illustrate other differences strikingly. In Japan an MR costs about $200, $100 for the professional charge and $100 for the technical side. In the US the average bill for the same procedure could be $1,050 one $100 for the physicians' interpretation and $950 for the facility as the technical charge. Here is another reason why health care is more affordable for residents of that nation.

Of course, there are countless other reasons for the cost differential but each probably refers to the overriding collectivist mentality in Japan which imposes discipline on the allocation of resources and profits.

Yet is such a system of high tech investment in imaging and hospital-based care for both immediate medical needs as well as for a center for recuperation, sustainable as the population continues to age and as immigration is limited and the economy remains sluggish? By 2030 it is estimated that a combination of good health for the elderly and a less than replacement level birth rate will result in 40 % of the population being over age 60. That will be an unprecedented demographic phenomenon. With such an increase in the dependency ratio could Japan continue to satisfy the needs of those who are near the end of life who are also apt to utilize more health-related resources extensively than those who are younger? Or will rationing come to Japan despite the relatively low percent of national income devoted to the health care sector of the economy. While we strive in some ways to improve our overall health, the Japanese will undoubtedly struggle to maintain their exemplary record. But the burden may be too much for any society to bear given that as time progresses fewer and fewer of its citizens will be wage earners and more will be health care consumers [1].

Reference

1. Fahs MC. Japan's Universal and Affordable Health Care: Lessons for the United States? Japan's Universal and Affordable Health Care: Lessons for the United States? N.p., n.d. Web. 11 July 2013. http://www.nyu.edu/projects/rodwin/lessons.html.

Radiology in Cuba: A Different Path with Fewer Resources and More Compulsion

20

American radiologists have good reason to be self-congratulatory about the current state and bright prospects of their specialty. Imaging is now, more than ever, in the ascendancy as an essential component of diagnosis and therapy for a lengthening array of pathologic conditions. Every month new developments are highlighted by feature articles emphasizing the vitality of our specialty and the expanding range of techniques and machines under our purview. The boast that American Radiology is the best in the world is not without some foundation.

Yet, such a comparison between us and others is open to clarification and question. Radiology is but one item on the health care ledger. Also included are matters of cost, access and proper utilization of resources. The issue of ultimate value must therefore be looked at in the context of socioeconomic considerations. One of the essential responsibilities of any polity to its citizens is the provision of health care. This obligation includes not only the detection and treatment of illness and injury, but also its prevention. And disease prevention involves not only public health measures per se, but the availability of food and shelter and the necessary infrastructure to sustain wellness and to tend to the sick.

Consequently, the two most fundamental indices of the success of a nation in meeting its health care priorities are life expectancy and access of the population to medical care. Life expectancy in the U.S. is near the highest in the world, but universal access has not been achieved and probably will not be in the near future. In most European countries where the mix of imaging modalities is directed less to CT and MR and more to ultrasound than in the U.S., life expectancy is similar to ours and in most countries care is more widely accessible. One might assume that wealth is necessary for health; the lesser issue of the specifics of the distribution of resources depends on organizational arrangements and political will.

Yet, is affluence a necessary prerequisite? In other nations less lavishly endowed with resources and capital than ours, great accomplishments have been made in securing both an average long life and universal coverage for illness. For example, in Kerala, a province in southwestern India with a per capita income of less than $1,000 per annum, life expectancy exceeds 70 years and care is available to all residents via a mix of state run and private facilities. The key to this accomplishment was not the availability of abundant funds but a consensus reached among all segments of society that health is a priority even if few are able to get rich from it.

Perhaps even more surprising, a similar success has been achieved in Cuba, where private enterprise of any kind is prohibited, political dissent is muted, freedom to travel is restricted and access to the free exchange of information has been limited, at least before the advent of the Internet. Before proceeding with a specific discussion of radiology in this island nation, some background on the transformation of healthcare in Cuba is necessary. By any measure, advances made in the past 40 years have been phenomenal. I restrict my comments here to the measures of improvement rather

S.R. Baker, *Notes of a Radiology Watcher*,
DOI 10.1007/978-3-319-01677-1_20, © Springer International Publishing Switzerland 2014

than the means, coercive and otherwise, by which that improvement has occurred. By no account do I proffer an endorsement of the existing government, even though through its agency, the metamorphosis has been made to happen. Thus, I will concentrate on results.

One of the main features of the Cuban health system is that every individual and family in the community, whether relatively well-off or poor, urban or rural, black or white, is completely covered by comprehensive services. Use of the healthcare system is free of charge to all citizens. That relates not only to primary and secondary care but also to specialized facilities at referral sites where radiology is available. Each individual is guaranteed access to a clinic nurse, doctor or other health care worker 24 h a day. Physicians, including radiologists, are required to live in the community in which they practice. Their incomes are similar to other workers. Healthcare comprises between 10 and 15 % of the gross national product in Cuba, a percentage allocation which is at or close to the highest in the world. Obviously, the provision of free care must be subsidized by income from other sectors.

Currently, Cuba ranks second in the world in infant mortality. Life expectancy for men and women is approximately 74 years of age. The common diseases in Cuba, cancer, heart disease and diabetes are similar in incidence to current experience in the United States. Only 30 years ago infectious disease and parasitic infestation were rife throughout the country. That does not mean that Cuba is now unaffected by diseases caused by microorganisms. A resurgence of an epidemic of dengue fever recently occurred. Eradication of the infection has been achieved as a result of coordinated efforts from the central government on down and from local governments upward.

An area where especially notable achievements have been made is in perinatal care. Every maternal death is evaluated at both provincial and national levels and all births must occur in a hospital. Incidentally, men are not allowed in the birthing room, a policy perhaps not related to healthcare but to the continuance of machismo in this society. Women average 23.6 prenatal visits per pregnancy and all receive free ultrasound tests throughout the pregnancy.

Mammography, until 1990, was provided for all women 35 and older. Now that frequency has decreased because of a worsening shortage of mammography film. For all patients, sonography is universally available and most radiologists have gained expertise with this technique. Of the limited funds available for modern equipment, most are directed to the purchase and maintenance of ultrasound machines. A dependence of sonography can be gauged from the fact that at the major referral center in the country, the Hermanos Almeirjias hospital in downtown Havana, approximately 500,000 imaging examinations are performed per year of which 200,000 are sonography studies. This hospital also has two CTs and one MR machine, each of which do no more than 15 studies per day and they are frequently down. In fact, throughout Cuba there is limited access to computed tomography and in the present period of economic austerity it is not likely that CT will grow in number of studies or number of machines. Moreover, there is a debate among health care policy as whether to proceed to a greater reliance on high-tech modalities in central sites or seek a more widespread diffusion of conventional imaging.

There are 60,000 physicians in a country of 11,000,000 people, by far, the highest ration of physicians to population in the world. That is why Cuba has, for the last 30 years, exported physicians to other countries in the world, especially to Africa, Latin American and parts of the former Soviet Union. In the United States, about 4 % of all physicians are radiologists. In Cuba, the 200 radiologists comprise only 4 in 1,000 of the physician work force.

Cuban medicine suffers from a lack of supplies and equipment. Nonetheless, its advances have been astounding as measured by life expectancy, fetal mortality and the ratio of physicians to population. Cuban radiology also is hindered by the lack of access to advanced imaging but its accomplishments are nonetheless noteworthy.

Despite reductions and privations, diagnostic imaging appears to be meeting much of the population's needs, not so much for some specific diseases, for which the absence of nationwide dissemination of multidetector CT or high field MR might confer a benefit, but for most of the illnesses for which imaging can play a part. As measured by the results of health care initiatives over the past 20 years, the Cuban example indicates that health and wealth need not be considered an inseparable pair if success is to be gained [1, 2].

References

1. Baker SR. Pneumoperitoneum something Pneu under the diaphragm. Diagnostic imaging in Cuba, an international of congress (syllabus). Havana, Cuba; 2002.
2. Baker SR. Technology, shifting tides and uncertain tidings, Editorial. Emerg Radiol. 2002;9:247–8.

Geography and Radiology: Perfect Together

21

In addition to my duties as a Radiology Chairman, Program Director and Graduate Medical Education Dean, I have a second career or rather a hobby in overdrive. I am a card-carrying geographer. I earned two master's degrees at Columbia University, attending class in my afternoon off and in the evening away from my radiology day job. Part of the tuition was paid for by the G.I. Bill as a benefit I received from serving as a radiologist with the 101st Airborne Division at the tail end of the Vietnam era.

As I gained some facility in geography I suggested to the department head that I could teach a course in Medical Geography bringing together my knowledge in both disciplines. He accepted and for 15 years I taught the course to a heterogeneous assemblage of undergraduates, MPH students, matriculates in the School of General Studies and students from the Schools of Journalism and Architecture. It was an enriching experience which only ended when my duties here at New Jersey Medical School got too hectic.

But along the way my involvement in geography as a student, teacher and researcher profoundly aided my capabilities as a radiologist in some ways immediately obvious but in others initially ineffable and which are only now slowly gaining clarity. It was not that geography imparted a methodological advance in thinking through a problem or capitalizing on an insight. Instead it gave me a new way of contemplating disease in an individual, considering its antecedents, its likelihood and its susceptibility to occur in particular sets of people. It is not that social,

occupational and travel history were not novel or recondite subjects. But geography made the acquisition of those pertinences crucial for me, not footnotes to the medical history but often part of the heart of the matter. As such neglecting to have that knowledge became an irritant for me- my geographical predilection made having it essential. And reducing the announcement of a patient's race or ethnicity to a meaningless overgeneralization sticks in my craw as an example of deficient history taking.

Today, for example a 44 year old man was presented to me as being "Spanish". I asked the intern was he from Spain-raising the question but already knowing the answer. No she said. He is Hispanic. I said that term is forbidden to be used in our department because while it may have value in political discussions and projections- even though it mixes many disparate groups- for medical purposes it has no value because a Mayan from the highlands of Guatemala and Porteno from Buenos Aires, the son of Italian immigrants, have nothing else in common except that they speak different dialects of Spanish. The term Hispanic, by the way, was invented by the old Department of Health Education and Welfare in 1973 as a wastebasket term to account for those who were deemed neither to be black nor white.

Yet requiring that the country of origin be provided in imaging requests often too might not even be enough. We have a lot of immigrants here from Ecuador. There are two main population centers in that country-one clustered at the seaport of Guayaquil and the other in Quito and surroundings in the Andes-most of them living at altitudes above 9,000 feet. In Guayaquil, a hematocrit of 40 is normal, in Quito it reflects anemia.

Not only stated country of origin and specific time of departure from there to the U.S. are important when immediately sensed by language and appearance. Outmoded approximations can be made by not digging deeper into relevant geographical considerations. Many of the so-called African-Americans that we see as patients or work as hospital staff including many in my department are actually not Americans but they are Africans. The recent increases in legal migration from Africa especially to the East Coast is a little appreciated phenomenon but it encompasses a major percentage of recent immigrants. They do not share the specific-history of oppression which have hardened African-Americans for many generations. They do not carry the same legacy as those whose ancestry suffered as slaves, yet in our nation in which discrimination still exists they may be exposed to the same slights that are still part of the national scene even though less overt than formerly. And they have different diseases suffered in Africa that are not to be found in Americans of similar racial category.

One way of discerning origin- either birthplace or ancestry is by employing the geography of names. Now with a computer nearby almost any name can be mapped promptly. So some surnames most likely to be the moniker of an American black female are Tyree, Alleyne, Jeter or Hairston even though generations ago their forefathers came from islands to the South. Nearly everyone whose last name is Rolle came from Florida because most of their ancestors were from the Bahamas. Beckles is a Jamaican name. Alleyne is Barbadian whom then immigrated to Panama to build the canal. Honeychurch is likely to be from Dominica. On the other hand most Ravenales are White and from South Carolina and Childress and Hickman are almost exclusively Caucasians from the Southeast U.S. More people named Garza are from Mexico than from Cuba, Puerto Rico or the Dominican Republic.

Among Africans in Ghana and the Ivory Coast, but not in Nigeria, for some ethnic groups, those apt to emigrate-each gender has only seven first names representing respectively the days of the week. Hence, if one is Kwame-Saturday or Kofi-Friday you are a male of the Ashanti tribe from Ghana most likely born and raised in the second city of Kumasi. The experiences of these now known to be from a specific place can be gained or at least anticipated if you bring these facts and the predilection to know more in a focused way to the analysis of a clinical presentation.

On the other hand, denial of geographical facts can limit one's capabilities. Several years ago I was invited by my good friend, an Italian radiologist from Naples, to address the Italian Emergency Radiology Society. He recently took on the position of Chief of Radiology at a hospital in Castel Volturno, a small coastal city about 30 miles from Naples. My research indicated that Castel Volturno is the entry port for both legal and illegal immigrants from West Africa, with most coming from Nigeria and most of them from Southern Nigeria so they were likely to be Christian, at least nominally. Knowing beforehand that the majority of the residents of the town are black, I prepared a talk on emergency radiology findings in patients with sickle cell disease and trait, figuring that the local radiology department would see such cases. Driving into Castel Volturno, my preliminary research affirmed nearly every person was black. But my audience, nearly all white Southern Italian radiologists asked why did I bother to talk on such a topic-it had little relevance to them, even though the patients and these African diseases would likely be part of their daily work.

On the whole, the influx of Africans into Italy while not vast in numbers is a source of consternation. There has been little impetus to engage or embrace these immigrants who still stand outside of Italian society. The radiologists in my audience took a distinctly antigeographic view of the special medical susceptibilities of the population they had to serve, I am sure to the immigrants' detriment.

These are just a sample of the insights I have gleaned from thinking geographically as well of one instance where such inferences were shunned. I feel strongly that the more you know about the place a person hails from or where his ancestors came from both, spatially and ethnically, the better you can practice the craft of diagnostician.

Part IV

Radiologist Inclusiveness: Minority Features

Demographic considerations should be a source of continued interest as taste and economics change with respect to specialty choice. In this regard, radiology is in a state of flux. Increasing still are the absolute number and percentages of individuals, now mostly American, of South Asian ancestry, while the percentage of women trainees stays stubbornly constant.

22

Who Will Be the New Radiologists?: A 2012 Assessment

I believe we are deep into a period of uncertainty in Radiology. That uncertainty has manifold dimensions. Will the downturn in overall imaging use continue at its present rate of decline? For those of you who may not appreciate the reality of this national trend because you are still doing OK with respect to volume of high tech studies such as CT and MR countrywide the yearly decrease in MR utilization is now 6 years old and the decline in CT has begun more recently. The optimists or perhaps the fantasists out there may not worry because when the Affordable Care Act a.k.a Obamacare comes fully on stream in 2014, then all those uninsured will now get imaged and presumably the decline will reverse. Maybe so but the results from Massachusetts indicate no imaging volume flood from the institution of the more comprehensive inclusion of all its citizens in reimbursable health care coverage.

Hence, with no new imaging devices in the offering, we should expect to see nothing like the expansionary period from 1998 to 2006 which upon reflection might be fondly remembered as the Golden Age of Imaging. In response to that time of rapid growth and perhaps unfettered optimism buttressed by the rapid and steady increase in average income of radiologists, residency programs expanded all over the country. The justification for hiring more trainees had to be presented to the Residency Review Committee for Radiology, an arm of the Accreditation Committee for Graduate Education. Only two criteria are deemed relevant to grant such requests, considering of course, that the petitioning program was otherwise in good standing. Those criteria were and are (1) there are enough cases in all modalities to accommodate the additional residents and (2) there was adequate attending staff in all modalities to teach them.

I was a member of the Radiology Residency Committee for much of this expansionary period with my term recently. Although some of us pondered the ultimate demographic consequences of the aggregate effect of frequent justified approval of requests for program enlargement, such speculations were outside the boundaries of decision-making.

So now the number of residents is 25 % greater than it was in 1999 and requests for further accretions to trainee complement have kept coming in through 2012. Only two medical disciplines have expanded their trainee complement more in this interval, Anesthesiology and, even to a greater extent, Emergency Medicine. All other major specialties have limited growth and some like Family Medicine have seen their cadre of residents decrease. Inasmuch as since 1997 the number of trainees reimbursed through Medicare has been capped, expansion of one program often must coincide with a decrement in some other program in institutions having a common sponsor. Thus, much of the increase in E.R. trainees has occurred at the expense of other residencies like Family Medicine.

But for Radiology such horse trading has been less frequent, especially when hospital administrators and medical school deans must pay obeisance to the chorus of observers who seek the

S.R. Baker, *Notes of a Radiology Watcher*,
DOI 10.1007/978-3-319-01677-1_22, © Springer International Publishing Switzerland 2014

primacy of primary care. Radiology programs for the most part have funded these additional positions from the revenue they have gained from their expanding volume of work. At least until recently. Now we are at an inflection point as each of these newly minted radiologists have found it increasingly difficult to find jobs. And if present trends continue, those who will finish fellowship each coming year, with each year there will be more of them. The job market will be tighter (forget Obamacare for the moment) and tighter. Now, senior medical students, while callow in some respects, are often avid and accomplished readers of tea leaves. They are quick to react to perceptions of opportunities enlarged and opportunities constricted. After all, choice of a specialty is one of any young physician's major life decisions, less important perhaps than choice of a spouse but for many even more important than choice of where to live.

In view of a perceived turning away from growth in Radiology studies in the past 2 years indicate that allopathic medical graduates are turning away from Radiology.

In the 2011 match for Radiology positions commencing on July 1, 2013, for the first time in several years not all programs filled completely. Of more than 1,100 positions offered 3.4 % positions were unfilled on match day, a phenomenon affecting at least one slot for 10.4 % of Radiology residencies. This past year, the trend continued and the results were worse. Now 7.7 % of positions-more than 80 slots-did not fill, creating an immediate problem for 23.8 % of programs.

At my institution where I serve as Chair and Program Director of Radiology, a great emphasis is placed on stimulating medical students (who first possess a nascent interest in Radiology) to seek it as their career. We had been very successful in convincing between 12 and 20 students out of a class of 185 to apply for a Radiology residency each year from 2000 to 2010. But this past year only seven applied and this new year it will only be three. And for the following class as of yet I have only two who have expressed interest. So I expect that the unfilled rate at the next match will be still higher and more programs will have to deal with the problem.

Yet, despite the weakening of interest, the aggregate applicants that I talk with generally feel that the competition is strong. So abetted by the concerns of deans of students, some of whom are frankly behind the times, they encourage their students to apply to 30, 50 even 60 programs. Yet, the data are clear, the marginal utility of the eleventh interview or beyond is very small. On the other side of the divide, program directors must interview many applicants. In fact, a good rule of thumb is to interview at least 12 times the number of available positions because mostly you are assessing the same cadre of students everyone else is chasing, at least if they will be allopathic graduates. But most programs start the process with applications from several 100 eligible students. In programs situated in the Northeast along the corridor from Boston to Virginia which encompasses the training sites of 55 % of all Radiology residents, these non-allopathic applicants come from five other sources-osteopathic schools, Caribbean schools, graduates of medical schools in India, graduates of medical schools in Iran, and graduates of medical schools in other countries. Some training programs still consider only Americans who are graduates of the 120 plus medical colleges that are members of the American Association of Medical Schools, whereas most programs now will grant interviews to some applicants who come from medical schools in those other categories.

What criteria or criterion has been used to rank these non-allopathic residency seekers? Well, there is only one objective measure-one that only tangentially relates to the prospect of the capability of a candidate as a radiology resident. And by the way, that metric relates even less to his or her ultimate performance as a fully-fledged radiologist. I refer here to the Part (1) score of the U.S.M.L.E. exams, which every applicant must take by the time they are to be considered for acceptance. Of course, Part (1) is designed to test for knowledge acquired in the first 2 years of the standard curriculum in American medical schools. It is a test of basic medical knowledge not clinical knowledge.

Last year, we compared the results of the applicants from the six groups of medical schools. I listed above reviewing the scores for all but the miscellaneous group of graduates of medical schools from various countries. Some qualifications-Iranians and Indian graduates have usually completed medical school several years before applying and thus could have used this additional time to prep for the exam. But I have found that the few residents who have come from these two sources perform just as well as U.S. based, American graduates. As for the offshore or Caribbean students, most of whom are American citizens in examining the curriculum and performance indices of one typical school, I noted that the MCAT average score of entrants to the school is 25, well below the allopathic school average. Nonetheless, I have also found that those I have chosen and these are, admittedly just a few, they too, function no worse than their colleagues who were educated stateside.

So I expect that Radiology will be more and more populated by graduates of these other types of institutions. That may be a partial solution to Radiology's emerging lack of popularity among graduates of American non-osteopathic medical schools. But it will lead to further questions, not to be pursued in this essay, about the professional braindrain or about the insufficient number of physicians in the U.S. with radiology now perhaps becoming a glaring exception. As the need for other physicians increase, we will now see a dearth of prospects for residents in the pipeline and a lessening of interest among those once likely to enthusiastically choose us and now fearful about doing so [1].

Reference

1. Fink J. Staffing companies: how to profit from Obamacare's job outsourcing. Invest Daily. N.p., 23 July 2013. Web. 11 July 2013. http://www.investing-daily.com/15482/staffing-companies-how-to-profit-from-obamacares-job-outsourcing/.

Women in Radiology

23

The responsibilities of any medical specialty that has earned and continues to merit the public's trust are to maintain quality, to expand the application of its expertise and to assess and later to employ new technologies that enhance its capability to provide care. But in our society we must add another consideration—i.e., the demography of any specialty should be in general accord with the various constituencies of the national population so that all those who aspire to enter the profession sense that the opportunity to do so is available to them.

Over the past 40 years the overwhelming sentiment of the electorate has been to foster diversity among the capable and interested. This does not necessarily mean the imposition of quotas but rather it encompasses both vigilance and provisions for encouragement with the goal that the specifics of the distribution of minorities and women in a specialty reflect the population at large to as great a degree as possible. This entails creating opportunities instead of obligations. Yet, such a policy of opening of possibilities to all runs the risk of allowing the less qualified candidate to be admitted to residency training at the expense of the more accomplished. So it is with surprise and chagrin that the leadership of Radiology is confronted with the disturbing fact that whereas 45 % of all medical students are women and 40 % of all residents are women, only 25 % of Radiology residents are of that gender. Moreover, the percentage of women in Radiology residencies has not grown in the past 10 years. It was 26.9 % in 1994 and 25.7 % in

2003. If we exclude the six military radiology residency programs, which naturally are more likely to have a higher percentage of male trainees, then the percentage rate increases only to 27.3 %. Even in 2012 it remains at 27 %, a peculiar constant when all other demographic indices with respect to female participation, are growing. My program here at New Jersey Medical School is representative of the national average. In 2002, 24 % of applicants to our program were female and in 2003 it was 27 %. We are near the middle among all programs by having 26 % of the residents as females as current trainees. Among the 186 Radiology residency programs the standard deviation for the percentage of women was 12.2 % surrounding a mean of 25.7 %. Twenty programs are more than one standard deviation below the mean in terms of percent of women. Perhaps discrimination exists yet it appears to have no relation to program size, to urban, suburban or rural location or to region of the country except that five of the seven university programs having less than 11 % of women trainees are in the South. In fact, there is one university program there that has a roster of 25 men and one woman and another with 22 men and three women. However, these are distinct outliers. On the other hand, there are female preponderant programs-one with 66 % of residents being women and a few with more than 50 %. One might ask if these differences relate to the fact that some male program directors have a bias against female residents. Yet, this is probably not the case. In 2006 22 % of programs directors are women and in the programs with a low percentage of female residents approximately one fifth of those programs have directors who are also women. There is no consistent pattern here.

Is the apparent underrepresentation of women a situation that occurs only in the United States? Well, in Canada there are 16 medical schools, 59 % of the medical students are women. Yet, only 37 % of radiology residents there are women. This is a situation analogous to what is present in the United States where there is a 20 % difference between the percentage of women as medical students and the percentage of women as radiology residents. In many competing specialties in the United States over the past 10 years the percentage of women has grown. The number of women in so-called ancillary services analogous to ours in terms of lifestyle choices reflects the general trend which is at variance from the Radiology experience. In Anesthesiology there has been a slight increase from 1995 to 2003 in the percentage of women trainees, rising from 24 to 27 %. In Pathology the acceleration is even greater, advancing from 41 % to nearly 50 % female trainees and in Pediatrics, which is a customary haven for women seeking specialty training, the percentage has increased from 60 to 66 %. Even in Urology, an unlikely specialty, perhaps, for women to seek a residency position, the percentage of females has increased from 6.5 to 10.9 %, while it has remained constant at about 19 % in Surgery.

Another question that might be asked is, is it likely that the reason why women are not going into Radiology because they do not think they can advance in academic or private practice? In 2007 among the ACR membership in 2000 of a total of more than 30,000 radiologists, 13.1 % are women. Yet, they are not underrepresented in that organization inasmuch as 20 % of ACR officers are women and the percentages on the board of chancellors, the steering committee and specialty commissions is 15 %, which mirrors the total percentage of women in practice in all types of Radiology. There is also very little difference among ACR percentages of women regionally. Of all the regions in the U.S. there appears to be a greater number of women in relation to all radiologists only in the Middle Atlantic States. Even when we look at state chapter officers we find out that the percentage of women approximates their general percentage. So, at least among the ACR, there are apparently no barriers preventing women from assuming positions of leadership.

In the RSNA the demography of leadership is similar. Overall 15.8 % of RSNA members are women. Among refresher course committee members 12 % are women, in the scientific program 19 % are women and among its subcommittee chairs, a role which is often a stepping stone to further advancement, 4 of the 16 chairs are women. The regional distribution of women among members of the RSNA is more or less homogeneous with an increased percentage in the Middle Atlantic States. In the Society of Chairman of Academic Radiology Departments (SCARD), the number of women has consistently been low but it is increasing. It is now 13 % a rise from about 2 % a few years ago. And if we look at the masthead of the two leading journals in our specialty, Radiology and AJR, in 2002 approximately 11 % of radiologists appearing as editors or assistant editors in Radiology were women, a number that has not varied much in the past decade. In AJR, the percentage of women increased from 7 %, where it had been from 1990 to 1997, to 15 % in 1998. It has grown little since. Thus, from these data, there appears to be no widespread institutional discrimination against women entering Radiology, although there are some suspicious outliers. Moreover, there appears to be no apparent institutional barriers preventing the advancement of women into positions of leadership. Hence, other considerations including lifestyle, career balancing and the nature of the work should be considered to explain the relative unattractiveness of Radiology as a specialty choice for American female medical school graduates.

What are some of those issues that might make Radiology less enticing for women? Even without sufficient data for full substantiation, the following possibilities should be considered. First, fear of physics. We have a tendency to conclude that women do not do science as well as men nor with as much interest. Perhaps there is a fear of physics out there that prevents women from going into Radiology despite the attractiveness of the specialty in terms of income, opportunities and lifestyle. This factor needs further assessment. Although I think it is really a red herring.

Another possibility is fear of radiation. This is probably an emotional concern only yet it is one that may inform individuals considering a career in our specialty. We now know that for many generations, except for interventional radiology, the chance of radiologists receiving excessive exposure has been very limited. Yet, perception of radiation danger may be a notion held strongly by female medical students preventing them from seeking a career in Radiology.

The fact of underrepresentation in our specialty by females should not be ignored. Further study is needed to help investigate this problem and come up with possible correction in action and policy. Most importantly, the education of medical students should take place with radiology integral to the curriculum from the first year on. This is desirable if only to dispel false notions about radiation risk and to acquaint students about the specialty's allure. If we want Radiology to be diversely represented we cannot sit back and just bemoan these statistics. Rather we should get out there as medical educators to influence female medical students early in their careers about how fantastic our specialty is and how we need them to join us in greater numbers.

I have another explanation derived from the context of comments of women who have entered radiology and those who were interested but turned away from it. Among American female medical students, there is a widely felt notion that friends, peers, and family want them to enter a field in which they will provide direct patient care, connected with the expectation that their capability as nurturers will be utilized. In contradistinction, many Pathology residents are women occupying positions in another non-nurturing specialty. But most female pathology residents are South and East Asian by birth or background where the nurturing connection is apparently not as strong [1].

Reference

1. Baker SR, Barry M, Chaudry H, Hubbi B. Women as radiologists: are there barriers to entry and advancements. JACR. 2006;3:131–5.

Radiologists of South Asian nativity or ancestry are increasing in number, especially among trainees in our specialty. Although there are no overt barriers to their advancement through the hierarchy of national radiology organization, their representation in positions of leadership is surprisingly meager. The issue of participation of South Asian radiologists needs to be addressed for the sake of substantiating inclusiveness, so that the contributions of radiologists of all ethnicities can confidently aspire to reach fulfillment as fully-fledged contributors to our specialty.

The previous essay focused on women. It emphasized the notion that women are not entering the field in proportion to their percentage as medical students. We concluded that there appears to be no institutional barrier, either to entry or advancement and that the reasons to why our specialty is not as popular to them as expected must relate to psychological and/or lifestyle factors that need to be further explored. When we come to the issue of Indian radiologists i.e., both those born in India or the children of those born in India who have been raised in the United States who seek to enter Radiology training, the situation is a little bit different. Here, we do not see a lack of interest in Radiology but rather an intensification of interest. Yet, there is also evidence, perhaps of a glass ceiling preventing Indian radiologists, designated either by nativity or ancestry, from advancing up the rungs of organized Radiology. The explanations for this phenomenon, to be described herein, are still a matter of speculation.

It is important that the more we know about the distribution in space of any group the better we can understand how we are accommodating their aspirations, proclivities and particular needs. To learn about their distribution is the first step in perceiving the barriers that limit opportunities.

South Asians were few and far between in the U.S. until the adoption of the Immigration and National Amendment of 1965, otherwise known as the Hart-Celler Act, the landmark legislation passed during the Johnson Administration. This law enabled large scale immigration from places outside of Europe, based upon specific needs and talents. In the past 3 decades Indian immigration has increased every year. In 1997 for example, there were nearly 750,000 Indian immigrants in the United States, which represent 2.9 % of all legally documented foreign born. There are also 489,000 permanent residents from there in the U.S. as of 2005.

In 1997, India ranked sixth in frequency among all countries supplying immigrants to the U.S. after Mexico, the Philippines, China, Vietnam and Cuba. Yet, among physicians, Indian immigrants are by far the most common of all non-American nationalities comprising 21 % of all FMG who practice in the United States. Natives of India in the U.S. have shown a predilection for a wide but distinctive range of occupations including motel owners and retail clerks on one hand, and software engineers, university professors and physicians on the other. South Asian immigrants are now widespread in the United States but focal areas of high concentration remain in the Middle

Atlantic and Mid Western states. Yet, there has been in recent decades a centrifugal movement of Indian physicians, including those either immigrating directly from India or those who, after initially residing in the Northeast and Midwest, have relocated to the South and West.

There are now approximately 800,000 physicians in the United States and 40,000 of these are ethnic South Asians. Compare that with only 1,500 Taiwanese physicians in our country. Today, radiologists of Indian nativity or ancestry comprise the largest non-indigenous, non-European ethnic group among radiologists. In 1982 there were 300 Indian-educated, board-certified radiologists in the United States and in 1996 there were 600 representing 2 % of all radiologists. As of 2004 they comprised about 3.5 % of all practitioners in our specialty.

India is a country of one billion plus people distributed within 27 provinces. Each of those provinces differ from each other to a greater extent perhaps than European countries do because of significant variance in history, caste, religion, language and political organization. In fact, most Indian radiologists come only from two states and the lead of these two states continues to advance over all others. They are respectively Gujarat in the Western part of the country and Andhra Pradesh in the southeast. In the U.S. there also is a smattering of radiologists from the Indian diaspora who have migrated here principally from the U.K., Uganda, Tanzania, Zambia, Guyana, Surinam and FIJI. But today, the largest group of ethnic South Asian radiologists are not foreigners educated elsewhere but American medical graduates. From 1965 to 1985 the predominant segment of the U.S. based Indian radiology community were those who received degrees abroad. Today, it is their children, born and raised here, who make up the majority of this group.

In some medical schools, the preponderance of students of Indian or Pakistani ancestry is very significant. For example, here at New Jersey Medical School, 35 % of the student body is of South Asian origin. Last year we had 500 applicants to our radiology residency program. South Asian applicants comprised 121 of those. Of that number 70 were American medical graduates and 51 received their MD degrees outside the U.S. One quarter of those on our rank list were South Asian by ancestry and approximately 35 % of our residents are ethnically Indian.

Now, if we look at the listing of membership in the RSNA and the ACR, the findings are, at the very least, interesting. In 2002 among the 25,000 members of the RSNA, individuals of South Asian ancestry, as identified by surname, comprised 5.5 % of the membership. A more detailed examination of last names was undertaken to get an idea of the rate of change of Indian membership in the RSNA. The two commonest last names in Gujarat are Patel and Shah, and the two commonest last names in Andhra Pradesh, are Rao and Reddy. We assessed their frequency on membership lists over time. From 1994 to 2003 the number of individuals named Patel increased from 58 to 89. Even more significantly, the number of Patels who are trainees increased from 12 to 28.

A slightly lesser degree of increase was noted among Raos and Reddys but among the Shahs, the other Gujarati surname, from 2000 to 2003 there was a doubling, rising from 11 to 22. Gujarati immigrants and their descendents have increased by 67 % in the membership of the RSNA recently.

Note the changes between 2003 and 2004. In this year the number of Patels increased yet again from 89 to 113. In 2003, 141 members of the RSNA had the last name of Smith and in 2004 it was 147. So if we project forward, considering no slowing or quickening of rate of change, in 3 years Patel will be the most common last name among RSNA members. And in fact, among trainees in all programs, 13.3 % are South Asian. I repeat, only 3.3 % of all radiologists are South Asian but 13.3 % of all trainees are of Indian or Pakistani ethnicity. In many residency programs more than 25 % of the residents are South Asian. So, unlike women medical graduates who are not seeking our specialty as much as one would expect, the South Asians are becoming an enlarging cadre of radiologists now and increasingly in the years to come.

The distribution of ethnic Indian trainees varies widely across the United States. In those states with more than 50 radiology residents, Michigan leads with 30.9 %, while North Carolina has only 1.6 %. Other states vary between these extremes.

If we now look at the leadership of the RSNA in 2003, consulting the lists of members who are Board of Directors officers, R & E Foundation Trustees, R&E Foundation Honors Council, Audit Committee, Bylaws Committee, CME Advisory committee, Corporate Relations, Educational Council and Ethics Committee, surprisingly we found no South Asian representatives, either FMGs or AMGs. On the important refresher course committee there are 9 % South Asian and in the scientific committee only 1.7 % are South Asian but there are no subcommittee chairs with this pedigree.

Consider now the ACR. If we look at the American College of Radiology membership list, in 1999, the last year for which these figures were available, among the roster of ACR officers, Board of Chancellor members, Council Steering Committee members, and all Free Standing Committee members and Task Forces, the number of South Asians is zero. In the operation committee 2 of 329 are South Asian and on specialty committees of all stripes, 9 of 579 were South Asians. Hence, I have endeavored to outline the particularities and peculiarities of a minority group of radiologists who have been in the U.S. for nearly two generations are now growing rapidly in number. Specifically, second generation South Asians, those who are Indian by ancestry, not by nativity, are now populating residency programs is proportionately. Yet, still today, South Asians are not represented in leadership of the two major organizations. Furthermore, if we take aspy the mastheads at the two leading radiology journals, AJR and Radiology, lack of representation exists there as well. In Radiology,

the number of South Asians among editors and assistant editors, as listed in the masthead, has risen in the past 10 years from 0 to 2 %. In AJR there has been a corresponding decline from 5 % in 1994 to 2 % currently. Moreover, only 2.5 % of all residency program directors are South Asian. Consequently, there are few role models for young South Asian ethnic radiologists despite the fact that the cultural identity of South Asian ancestry remains strong. Incidentally, proof of that fact is illustrated by the retention of Indian first names and Indian surnames even among those who are second and third generations in the U.S.

Ethnic groups first define themselves culturally through associational activity. Such cultural consciousness provides legitimacy and cohesiveness to pursue further advocacy both clinically and professionally. The lessons of incorporation of other groups into hierarchical participation in medicine and in the larger American society should be applied to the rapidly increasing segment of our specialty consisting of individuals of South Asian background. At the very least, the exclusion of South Asians from positions of prestige and power in Radiology is anomalous, if not discriminatory. This issue should be addressed by radiologists both among the rank and file and by the leaders in our specialty in the expectation that all radiologists should become confident that matters of place of birth or ethnicity are irrelevant and that advancement should be based exclusively on merit [1].

Reference

1. Baker SR, Broe DM, Kumar V. Characteristics of the distribution of emigrant Indian radiologists, pathologists and anesthesiologists in the United States. Soc Sci Med. 1984;19(8):885–91.

South Asians in Radiology in the United States, Part II

25

This essay is an update from the preceding one, written 8 years before. Incorporation of radiologists of Indian ancestry into all segments of American radiology has occurred despite the united reserve previously cited. The number and percentage of South Asians continues to grow remarkably. In short another example of the typical American success story.

Immigration, integration and assimilation are three salient features of the American experience from the founding of St. Augustine, Jamestown and Plymouth to today. At times, barriers to these processes have been raised and at other times lowered. And today at least for legal immigration they soon may be readjusted through legislation. The vagaries of politics aside, we as a nation are in great measure the products of the efforts of migrants to our shores. For most of us, if we are not newly arrived here ourselves, we are also their descendents. So the study of migration can be fascinating not just as for the knowledge it imparts but also for the relevance of that knowledge to our understanding of what we are and appear to be.

Medicine in the U.S., over the past 50 years, is informed by the opportunities, complications and vicissitudes related to the incorporation into its workforce of foreign-trained and foreign-born/ foreign-trained physicians. After all, we graduate 18,000 allopathic medical doctors each year and we must find approximately 25,000 physicians to fill existing residency slots per annum. Moreover, most of those foreign physicians stay here after training, becoming citizens and raising children some of whom go on to gain the M.D. degree also. These sons and daughters of immigrants even though thoroughly Americanized nonetheless often manifest the cultural traits and inclinations inherited from their immigrant parents and forebears.

The physician workforce in turn tends to reflect the broader American distribution of newcomers and those with a longstanding American pedigree. Yet it does not perfectly replicate the population at large, as some migrant groups have become proportionately more highly represented than their general numbers. One of these groups is the South Asians- ethnically Indians primarily but also those of Pakistani, Sri Lankan, and Bangladeshi lineage-both immigrants and their offspring.

In Radiology, the penetration of South Asians has been profound over the last 40 years. The purpose of this essay is to provide data on this progressing phenomenon including a charting of their increasing numbers both relatively and absolutely and the varying collective penetrance by those who immigrated from certain parts of India and not others.

Before providing that information, a few notes on data acquisition. Indians (at least the majority who are Hindu) both resident and itinerant can be recognized by their distinctive surnames. Unlike other arrivals, they tend not to change their cognomens to make them sound more "American", so to speak. Moreover they generally do not adopt traditional Anglo-Saxon or trendy first names common in the general population and they! at least

S.R. Baker, *Notes of a Radiology Watcher*,
DOI 10.1007/978-3-319-01677-1_25, © Springer International Publishing Switzerland 2014

maintain Indian style given names into and beyond the second generation. So when examining a list of radiologists it is usually easy to pick out those characteristic of South Asian ethnicity.

Yet India too has a diaspora which extends beyond the United States including Canada, many European countries, South and East Africa, Australia, Fiji, and Guyana. The latter is a small country not very far away from the U.S. relatively, in which descendants of immigrants from India comprise about 50 % of the population. South Asians residing there have been Guyanese for three generations at least. Hence many have loosened ties with India as evidenced by their forsaking Indian-style first names for more American sounding ones. This naming tendency makes it possible to cull them from lists of South Asian descendants in which connections with the subcontinent remain close because of the likelihood of continuing linkage afforded by ease of communication and transportation.

Therefore one can gain a pretty good grasp of the size of the community of radiologists who are South Asian descendants by scanning the names of all members at large and finding them within the group. Furthermore, if we consider that in many ways each Indian province is more unique and largely more populous than the various European countries, surname analysis can allow us to discern intra-Indian trends because even today last names to a considerable extent are tied to specific provinces.

I have been studying the issue of Indian radiologists in American practice for more than 30 years now. During that time I have observed this cohort enlarge in number and national penetration. I have also recognized the persisting trend of selective-out migration in certain Indian provinces and their absence in others.

As I have indicated in my previous reports, I also am the credentialing officer for radiologists who are or who wish to become enrolled in One-Call Medical, a PPO provider that engages radiologists to interpret workmen's compensation imaging examinations. The company has enjoyed unabated growth over the years. Past and present enrollees now comprise a group of over 19,000 radiologists i.e., more than half of active radiologists in the U.S. This large list constitutes the rolls from which we have been able to determine the percentage of Indian-associated radiologists among all radiologists as well as the likely ancestral home of those that left there including both immigrant physicians and native-born Americans of Indian parentage. This set of names also enables us to distinguish those regions in the U.S. that have been attractive to migrant radiologists to our shores and those that have not.

I have published three previous studies on this subject published in 1984, 2000, and 2008, using RSNA and ACR rosters as my source. While differing in number now when compared to those earlier investigations, the present list reveals increasing, actually accelerating, growth and a persistent pattern of relocation predilections for those undertaking a unilateral move from India to the U.S [1].

Reference

1. Baker SR, Mann S, Hill H. The distribution of emigrant radiologists, revisited: characteristics of cohort arriving after 1980. Asia Oceanian J Radiol. 2002;7(2): 104–10.

Part V

The Appearances and Implications of the Radiology Report

We are evaluated by our referees primarily by the language of our reports. Do we communicate and consult effectively? Are our phrases and explanatory descriptions too jargon-laden? Is our use of metaphors effective communication or unwanted obfuscation? What will be the effect of the electronic medical record on our communicative capabilities. All these topics are considered here.

Towards More Literate Reports: Avoiding Words and Phrases You Should Not Say

26

The emerging categorization of quality assessment, utilized now by most accrediting agencies in medical education divides the roster of evaluation into six distinct areas of inquiry and measurement, They are medical knowledge, professionalism, system based practice, practice-based learning, patient care and interpersonal and communication skills. All of these competencies are important for physicians, both those in training and those beyond residency. For radiologists, despite our distance from direct contact with patients as an essential component of most of our daily work, they are still no less important.

We must be knowledgeable and concerned with our patients even as we are mostly at a remove from them. Also we must be aware of and participate in the management of care locally in the context of national regulations. And, of course, we have to be good communicators. sharing and receiving expertise in our conversations with referrers. Perhaps more than other specialists, our communication skills relate to the written word as manifest in our dictated reports. So this competency must be in the forefront of our commitment to quality [1].

Now more than ever to maintain the excellence of the enduring statements we render, we have to skillfully recognize imaging findings and the implication of those findings through written expressions that must be clear, succinct and apt. Why now more than ever before? Because our reports will likely be read not only by the doctors and other caregivers we know and see and talk with on a daily or regular basis, but also our reports must be unambiguous and comprehended by clinicians we do not know but with whom we will be linked through the widening availability of the electronic medical record. When a patient is treated elsewhere at some distance from you and at some time in the future, the message of your report will be essential by itself inasmuch as clarification may be more difficult to render to supplement what you have proffered in the first place. And the individual, remote in place and time who reads it may not be a physician. So what you relate must be intelligible to everyone qualified to provide care. Hence, the language of the report must be pitched to the level of medical sophistication enjoyed by a physician assistant or nurse practitioner.

Under this potentially extended distribution of the fruits of your expertise, highly specialized vocabularies become an impediment to understanding. Jargon does have its psychological benefits for those who profess and comprehend it. It reinforces exclusivity, sometimes affording a comforting smugness to know that you are one of the cognoscenti who can converse with a special word roster to others as informed as you are even though outsiders are excluded. It lets you share confidence through the use of coded phrases and terms. But jargon and its coconspirator, abbreviation, are in themselves potentially dangerous because they inhibit widespread communication and consultation. They do not promote comprehension but serve to restrict it. The pertinent slogan should be: if you want to be understood by a few, use jargon but if you want to be not misunderstood by many, use English. In the context of a radiologist's written reports, the level of medical English to strive for is intelligibility by primary care physicians or their surrogates (PAs and their like).

With that as a background, we should look with a discerning eye at some patterns of expression that have infiltrated the customary parlance found in many radiology reports. The purpose is to expose and root out habitual misuses we have become comfortable with but which can engender confusion leading to mistaken conclusions and sometimes, to the uninitiated, bewilderment and befuddlement-all of which by the way serves to weaken our ethos as experts.

I have compiled a list of 64 things you should not say or write, each of which has frequently appeared in radiology reports from everywhere. But their frequency and commonness should not be a justification for their continued use because misinformation, ambiguousness and obfuscation should not be our stock in trade. We can do better, we are expected to do better in this objective category, and the recognition and removal of errors and foibles of expressions will lead to better care. I have disaggregated these pesky problem terms into distinct groupings, each with a common theme within the rubrics of figures of speech. With regard to precision, our dictation must be as specific as possible about what is being observed and commented upon. Everything that is extraneous to the satisfaction of this principle should be avoided even though such words and phrases have become encrusted through habit and custom. Those that perpetuate less than a rigorous literal exposition that can be immediately and unequivocally comprehended should be deleted from your lexicon.

In this category are various examples of incompleteness that have become inappropriately commonplace in reports. Because we are anatomists we should provide exact anatomic references. Therefore, by itself "vascular" is imprecise because most of the time you know if it is a vein or an artery Moreover, you know, of course, only certain arteries calcify and outside of phleboliths seen often in the pelvis and seldom elsewhere, veins rarely contain calcium in their lumens and exceedingly rarely in their walls. We mention degenerative disease frequently but we should also relate its severity and extent in the spine and in the appendicular skeleton. Metaphor is valuable as reckoned as the names of a treasure trove of radiologic signs (we have uncovered nearly 700 of them in a review of the imaging literature from 1895 to today). But outside of those hallowed references, appreciated for their linkage of two disparate realms of knowledge, vague metaphoric substitutes for relevant anatomic delineations are not helpful. Thus, the term region can be replaced by the more specific non-metaphoric anatomic site it refers to. The word "aspect" should also be avoided There is always a better term. Bilateral and bilaterally (a pseudo-adverb that modifies nothing) are frequently found in radiology descriptions. Almost always it is better to discuss right and left separately as the findings on each side are usually different to some degree. Such a commonly important distinction can be hidden under the "mask" of bilateral. We often report the constancy of a persisting pathologic condition by the use of "unchanged". But that is not sufficient there needs to be a more precise and specific demarcation of consistency i.e., unchanged in extent, unchanged in location unchanged in size, etc. Even unchanged in appearance may not suffice, say for a nodule that remains rounded but on successive images has grown or shrunken and yet its border describe a circle as before. Your reports are also not served by the inclusion of meaningless words, which can be excised from a report without altering its import. The word "significant" is only consequential when deployed as a statistical statement rather than as merely an emphatic one. The consequence of a finding should rely on its objective description alone. We do not need to modify the analysis of the images we view with the disclaimer "evidence of" because it is generally acknowledged that what we view is not the substance or the pathology itself but rather a depiction of it, as such a mere semblance of the actual reality. You will not be at a disadvantage in a malpractice suit by not including those two words in your report. We are expected to interpret sequences of images-one done now and the most recent one done some time age-and comment on the differences between them if any. The time between them is known as an interval. That goes without saying so it should go without dictating and the quality of your report will in no way suffer by omitting the word interval.

Not only do we strive for precision, we should also seek to be as accurate as possible. Here too, we have drifted into the use of cliches and terms that belie the truth even as we have come to accept them as standard. A frequent error is to ascribe some finding (e.g., the mediastinal contours as being "within normal limits"). But there are no such limits to be within or beyond, so it would be better to avoid this term when there are no measurements to support it. A mediastinum may be widened or not, without needing recourse to a phrase about it's supposed "limits". Similarly the word minimal frequently occurs in radiologists dictations. But that is not accurate at all. Pointing that out is not merely semantic nitpicking. Minimal connotes that what is seen is the smallest that could be seen. But that end point is hardly ever known. An abnormality may be small or even tiny (in either event it should be measured) but minimal is almost always a bad guess not an incisive estimation.

A finding often appears the same now as it appears at some time in the past. Are we justified in calling it stable? Absolutely not. For in the interval between the two studies, it might not have changed but then again it could have gotten bigger and then smaller, or smaller and then bigger or oscillated in extent or configuration several times between now and then. So stability cannot be ascertained by sequential imaging studies alone unless all time between image and images are also continuously demonstrated.

And while on the subject of changes in time, we must recognize that except for angiographic and tine studies, we look at snapshots, not movies. Therefore it is not accurate to employ the present participle in our descriptions of findings in our "snapshots". We should not report that the nasogasteric tube we see with its distal tip overlying the gastric air bubble is "coursing" through the esophagus to the stomach, because we are not seeing it moving. Rather it extends below the diaphragm on the left side or something to that effect which recognizes its position but avoids reference to motion.

Similarly, patients who are not well centered for an ICU chest X-ray, are not rotated even though we are apt to assert that ascription. In fact they are not in the act of turning at all. Instead they have not been properly positioned when the image is taken. So it is more accurate to indicate that the patient's chest is situated oblique (either right or left) to the film. Other examples of inaccuracy that find frequent lodgement in X-ray reports include the observation that bowel wall is called "thickened" when actually it is only not distended. Or "surrounding" edema is noted when a full evaluation of the neighboring sides, front, back, top, and bottom of the suspected anatomic reference cannot be made. It is better to say adjacent edema instead of surrounding edema.

And then there are neologisms, new words or new uses of words that are well known for other definitions in which they are employed not the special ones known to a small segment of the medical caregiver population. MSK radiologists, orthopedic trauma surgeons and rheumatologists know specifically what it means to aver that a joint is "maintained", but are all primary caregivers aware of that piece of jargon? Even fewer of them know what a joint has been "located" signifies, when relocated is a more apt term with its meaning more widely and properly comprehended.

And there are neologisms that obfuscate through the impress of tradition even though when carefully analyzed they are logically ridiculous on their face. For the most part we do not deal with color in radiology, rather only in shades of white, gray, and black, with a range of contrasting shades on plain films and CT that extend through a spectrum from radiolucent to radiodense. On CT we can measure this variable by the denotation of Hounsfield units. To be otherwise accurate our qualitative terms are limited. Things can be of normal density, or be lucent or be dense, or be less or more dense than normal. But they cannot be hyperlucent -there is no definition of such a term nor can they be hyperdense-there is also no definition of that term, and to refer to a shadow as hypodense or hypolucent is even more murky. Those four words have no meaning at all to be both precise and accurate about them. Radiographic shades, then should be described in comparative terms with respect to normal or in absolute terms as dense or lucent, not in the contrivances of these four neologisms beginning with the prefixes hypo and hyper.

Another broad area in which there is a tendency to confuse rather than to illuminate and educate in radiology reports is the intrusions of subjectivity into the written records. Our observations should be devoid of intimation of our personality, our emotions or our moods, and they should also avoid the rhetorical devices of attributing capabilities to parts of the body and to pathologies within them that cannot possibly exist.

Hence, it is not appropriate to offer your feelings in a report when they are more objective ways of stating the same consultative impression. It is an intrusion of your affective response, in place of your considered opinion, to label a finding as suspicious when you could better convey your insights by the labels of suggestive or indicative or some other non-emotion laden descriptor that indicates a deviation from normal. Likewise the word concerning is even more connotative instead of being denotative. A figure of speech, useful perhaps in fictional narratives, but out of place in radiology reports is the pathetic fallacy, so-called when the account ascribes human qualities to non-human subjects or even to parts of the body. Although it is generally understood in casual conversations that a pneumonia improves or my cold got better such formulations are out of place in a radiology report where objectivity should be the hallmark. Hence, your right lower lobe infiltrate increases in extent, lessens or resolves as revealed by an X-ray. On the other hand, you report that one improved or got well in accord with the resolving course of the pneumonia. Do not mix up the problem in the patient with the patient as a whole. Similarly your organs do not have the power to display, they have other virtues and susceptibilities. Thus the kidneys reveal nothing on a renal scan, the scintigraphic images do.

The most important attribute to be maintained on your dictated report is your reputation as an expert. Anything you do inadvertently to reduce your esteem in the eyes of your referrers will likely lead eventually to your detriment, if it's habitual. The way you construct your consultations, the definitiveness you can demonstrate to the extent the findings allow, the grammar, syntax, and vocabulary you choose can all generate the regard in which you will be held by your clinical colleagues. Consequently, the manner in which you related a normal study or one with abnormalities with which your expertise resonates can be crucial to your believability and sometimes even to your continued employment. Because if you are deemed wishy-washy or reluctant to make commitments as permitted by the evidence on the images you review, you will be diminished by it. So if you designate a normal study by the word unremarkable instead of normal, most of your colleagues may accept it. But a few and there always be at least a few of your referrers, will be mildly annoyed by the choice of that word. And if there are findings that are not definite please avoid the word some, because some could be a scant number or amount or many or much. As a referrer, you have not helped me with that manifestation of your supposed expertise. Nor is possible something that should inhibit your referrers. What does that mean? If anything is possible, is possible anything? Almost should be another verboten word. It is or it is not there. One or the other even if you are not sure of its significance. Avoid as well likely because it too, is too indefinite to be prescriptive. Even worse is "questionable" because it means you do not know if it is there or not and you do not know even if you could know. The worst of all is the phrase "cannot be excluded". Anything no matter how unusual cannot be excluded. The value of the phrase is nil, the implication for your ethos as a valued specialist can be immense. Also, "may represent" is to be shunned. Often it appears as it "may represent A or B", which implies that it could also represent something that is not A or B. But you really mean it is only one of those two possibilities. So instead you say it is either A or B. By the way, if you see it say it, don't say because you suspect it may appear or is developing. If it is present that is enough.

Now if you are unsure, words like suggestive, indicative of, compatible with or the more strong diagnostic of, are better alternatives because they are not subjective, they convey authority even if not definitive and as such they enhance your expertise not erode it.

Finally, there is one word never, never, never to be used. It should be obvious. The word is in fact "obvious" because what would happen to regard for you if it turned out not to be there.

Competence is required of radiologists. Dealing with uncertainty is a measure of it, but hubris is always a no-no! Rather, that, too, should be obvious.

Reference

1. Naik SS et al. Radiology reports: examining radiologist and clinician preferences regarding style and content. AJR Am J Roentgenol. 2001;176(3):591–8.

The Radiology Report

27

In the preceding essay on the radiology report, or at least my particular take on what should be in it and what should not. I began with a recitation of conventions or habits that should be subject to scrutiny. For the sake of improvement I will now continue with this roster of bad habits before considering at a later session what is our obligation as communicators in the radiology report.

Although vagueness can infuse many reports, sometimes there is too much exactness. For example, consider the rating of the degree of pneumothorax. When we say that there is a 50 % pneumothorax we are almost always incorrect, because we are making a linear inference about a volumetric phenomenon. If we would assume that the hemithorax is a sphere then with a reduction of the expanse of the lung to one half of its width the decline in volume is really one half times one half times one half. Hence a supposed 50 % pneumothorax is really a 7/8th or 87 % pneumothorax. Since we cannot on plain films make a precise volumetric ascertainment, there is inappropriate exactness in describing a percentage to it. Rather, I use the five M's, miniscale, mild, moderate, marked and massive to provide a semi-quantitative measure of the extent of pneumothorax as evidenced by its depiction on one frontal chest image.

I recently read a paper where an attempt was made to quantify numerically a pneumothorax on CT. Here, I think is an example of too much information. Unless a need can be satisfied by such a calculation it really is the demonstration of a distinction without a difference.

Another tendency is to personify pathology. For example, many might say that an infiltrate is improving. Yet, infiltrates having no personality cannot improve. They can only lessen or worsen. A patient can improve but the infiltrate can only change physically not subjectively. Similarly, we can mix up object and subject when we personify anatomy. On a CT one might say, the kidneys reveal a stone. Yet the kidneys have no capability to reveal anything. What is going on the kidney is revealed by what is seen on the image. It is the examination with images that reveal the pathology. The kidneys and all other organs have no intrinsic broadcasting facility.

Now moving on to style, there is a tendency to use a passive voice in dictating reports to the point of annoying monotony. The classic example is the word "there". As defined in the dictionary, one meaning of there is that it is a functional word to introduce a sentence or clause in which the subject follows the verb. That is the way it is used in radiology reports. Now if we say there twice, as in there, there, we employ a condescending phrase urging calm. If we would use there thrice, it could be in the form of an explanation referring to a place or thing or phenomenon some distance from you or your listeners. As in there, there, there! But if we use there 4 times or more in one paragraph, we run into the boring stylistically inappropriate radiology report. As in there is followed by there are, followed by there

S.R. Baker, *Notes of a Radiology Watcher*,
DOI 10.1007/978-3-319-01677-1_27, © Springer International Publishing Switzerland 2014

is, followed by there are. Try to avoid the passive. Also try to avoid too many theres, only one or two belong in any paragraph.

Another habit evident especially among junior radiologists is to include trivial information in the report with no further qualifiers. For example, it is merely to fill-up a page to say that there is degenerative disease in the dorsal spine on a chest x-ray if that finding has no clinical significance and if the extent of it is not described or its relation to other things in the narrative are not linked. Similarly mild scoliosis without any further acknowledgement of its import or lack thereof is inappropriate. Similarly, the isolated finding of spina bifida occult a does not need to be mentioned on the seventh consecutive daily ICU chest.

Now for ER and ICU patients it is very important each day to indicate where the catheters are. One must comment on the course of the catheter, where its distal tip is located and whether there are angulations or kinks in it. For central venous lines we should look carefully for pneumothorax. However, a very small pneumothorax usually is innocuous. Much more worrisome, but thankfully much, much less common is a perforation of a vessel by a catheter leading to a hydrothorax, which will continue to increase, as long as the IV is open and the infusate goes into the pleural space. Hence, I am concerned much more about a small pleural effusion than I am about a small pneumothorax. The latter will resolve but if the former is due to perforation by a central venous pressure catheter then even a small pleural effusion would be a deep concern.

How about some conventions that are not helpful in a description of the lungs. A bit of jargon formerly unknown to me but introduced by my residents was the mention of the term "low lung volumes". When a patient has not taken a deep breath the ascription of low lung volumes by itself is misleading. It is most often due to the fact that the film is obtained in the expiratory phase of respiration but previous surgery or ascites can decrease the size of the lungs as well—by itself the term is not informative.

Another habit which I believe is wrong in concept but rife in practice relates to incompleteness of reference especially for ICU patients. In reviewing emergency and ICU patient's every day, I find that in some instances, the changes that occur are subtle and are first manifest after a review of films over several days rather than from one day to the next. Thus, I instruct my residents evaluating an ICU patient's chest x-ray for which multiple films have been obtained to not only look at yesterday's films for comparison but also to look at some films from some days or weeks before to see if a subtle change has occurred even though it is not apparent within 24 h. Hence the report that we render should say a comparison was made with previous films, the most recent obtained, for example, at 10 pm 8/23/2006. Then I would know that the resident has looked at other films to find those possible subtle changes.

In the heart and mediastinum what are important features? Certainly width and contour for the mediastinum and configuration and caliber for the heart. Thus we must look at each of those areas in the thorax and we should mention each of those features even if normal. In essence, it should be a separate sentence on each.

Now for organs and lesions when a mass is recognized, it is not enough to say what that mass is. Rather, it should be measured in two dimensions at least, its homogeneity should be mentioned if that is pertinent and almost always it is. The density of the mass should be considered too especially in relation to the presence of calcification or gas.

And calcifications can be further defined not only by their location and mobility but most importantly by their morphology. For calcifications there are essentially four classes. These are concretions, conduits, cystic lesions and solid lesions. Concretions have a completed perimeter of calcification. They tend to occupy expected locations, and their internal architecture may be a peripheral rim a laminated interior or they may be homogeneously dense throughout. The only conduits that, in the abdomen at least, can be partially opaque are certain arteries and the vas deferens. Conduits seen in profile appear as discontinuous tracks of density. If the vessel is very small like the uterine artery, it may only appear as a single line but the larger arteries and the vas are revealed as discontinuous tracks along the expected location and their course. When seen en face they appear as an incomplete circle of density conforming to the diameter of the particular vessel. Cystic calcifications on the other hand has discontinuous curvilinear margins, but their diameters are larger for the most part than conduits. Cystic calcifications refer to true cysts, pseudocysts and arterial aneurysms. Solid calcifications have usually a speckled, whorled or mottled appearance. Like cystic calcifications they can occur anywhere in the abdomen. One caveat to this schema is that some calcified leiomyomas of the uterus look cystic even though they are solid.

When calcifications are very small or faint, they cannot be further categorized morphologically. Ossification can usually be distinguished from calcification by the presence of trabeculae interiorly and/or a cortex marginally. Each of these densities should not be confused with artifacts. The problem here is that the term artifact is confusing because it has two separate meanings, and it is often not clear whether one is referring to one or the other. One meaning is an extraneous finding, an error in technique that does not exist in actuality but is present because of the way the film was processed. Yet, a second artifact refers to a substance or object that actually exists within the field of view, anywhere along the path of the beam whether outside, on, or in the patient.

In descriptions of the bones, qualification must be part of any narrative. It is not enough to say there is degenerative disease. Rather the number of joints should be mentioned, the extent of change in each joint described and the specifics of the deformation portrayed.

A few points about the components of the report. As I propounded in the first lecture, the report should be considered as literature. That is, it should be held to the same standards of clarity, succinctness and veracity as any written word. The report requires preliminary information, the main narrative, the impression and possibly the recommendation [1].

Preliminary information should include demographics. In this category, one should know the date of dictation, the time of dictation and the age and gender of the patient. In this regard, human beings should be described by the nouns—men, women, boys and girls, whereas animals are males or females. It is dehumanizing to label your patient as a male or a female when they are also either a boy or girl or a man or woman.

What about ethnic identification? Is it a routine component of such communications? Maybe 60 years ago we could make a distinction in the US only between Caucasians and African Americans but what about people of mixed race? Furthermore, what if that African American is really an African who has only come here recently? And most importantly, what about the term Hispanic and Latino? These are wastebasket appellations that were introduced in 1972 by the Department of Health Education and Welfare, a precursor of the Health and Human Services department. What do we do about people with Spanish surnames? Well, some of them may be darker than white and lighter than black and some of them may be very darkly complected and others appear as white as anyone from northern Europe. The problem is that Latino/Hispanic could include mestizos from Peru, Indians from Guatemala, and Italians who migrated to Argentina and then to the US. There is no relationship by last name alone, about what diseases in such a diverse group of individuals may be more prevalent. The relationship of Spanish surnames to ethnicity is vague at best. Without further qualification Hispanic/Latino is misleading. I suggest that these terms not be included in the report.

Reference

1. Ridley LJ. Guide to the radiology report. Australas Radiol. 2002;46(4):366–9.

More Jargon

28

To an extent greater than any other activity in this era of P.A.C.S. we as radiologists communicate predominately through the radiology report. Our written consultation lays bare our demonstration of competence. Thus, how we frame what we see and interpret defines, in large measure, our ethos in the estimation of referring physicians who are our customers, if you will, in the knowledge transactions we participate in numerous times each day.

The report, then, should be something we care deeply about not just for its content but for its form and context. Do we say what we mean in a clear way without demeaning our function as consultants? Do we provide our consultation in a succinctly and ambiguously way? Do we infiltrate our commentaries with jargon and verbosity? Are we responsive to our referrers needs for answers to vital questions which the patient's condition imposes? Do we communicate crucial information to our referrers directly in addition to the written report? Or do we use the report to promote unnecessary studies to build our practice which is a euphemism for overutilization? The subject of this presentation is an elaboration of these issues. Perhaps you will find my positions controversial and in some cases anathema to your routine and predilections. OK then. The overriding point is to engender discussion about this critical aspect of practice which for too long has been essentially unexamined.

The radiology report is the record of many elements brought together in a few paragraphs. It is a document displaying our expertise as image interpreters. It is also a manifestation of our involvement in patient care. At the same time, it is a reflection of our consultative ability and it is a display of our narrative skill in relating findings.

Like the images it addresses, the report is permanent. We are responsible for everything put in or left out. What are some of the virtues we would strive for in an excellent radiology report? Well, its style should be journalistic, which means its points should be made without excessive verbiage yet be pertinent and comprehensive. We must also direct our communication so that physicians understand what we say so that they can then relate directly with patients, transmitting clearly the observations we make. And we must address the underlying issue of the appropriate utilization of imaging. Hence, the characteristics of an excellent report should be that it is germane, succinct, accurate and specific in the description of findings. Also, it must be anatomically correct, incisive in its analysis, humanistic in its concerns and stylistically unobtrusive.

In every report, your reputation is on the line. Thus your report must be focused and authoritative. Words that reveal your inadequacies will change the regard others have for you. Yet if you are unsure you must portray that uncertainty in a way that maintains your reputation as an expert. By that I mean that you may not know exactly what is going on, but you should express it in such a manner that you as the image interpreter have a better handle on the complexities and confounding issues than anyone else looking at the report or the images.

S.R. Baker, *Notes of a Radiology Watcher*,
DOI 10.1007/978-3-319-01677-1_28, © Springer International Publishing Switzerland 2014

115

Consider the differences between the generalist, the specialist and the wise expert with regard to the assessment of findings whose meaning is not quite clear. The generalist will say "I don't know." The specialist providing an opinion in the face of uncertainly will say, "It is not known". The expert who possesses wisdom might say, "I don't know" if it is not known or if it is not knowable. The point here is that if you do not know something, you should use the appropriate language to express it. Yet at the same time, maintain the concept that you are approximating an understanding to the fullest extent possible. And even when you do not know, you are wise enough to say that you do not. It is sometimes challenging to always act as an expert in a radiology report. It is easier to be the generalist and provide no information.

Now, a very important rubric in any radiology report or any medical communication is, if you wish to be understood by a few, use jargon but if you strive to not be misunderstood by many, use English. It is very easy for jargon to seep in to what we say and write but you must put yourself in the place of the informed reader who may not know your special vocabulary. Thus, statements must be clear in English even when incorporating the lexicon of Radiology.

Here are some definitions of jargon, I'll give you three. (1) it is the technical terminology of a characteristic idiom of specialists or workers in a particular activity or area of knowledge often a pretentious or unnecessarily esoteric terminology. (2) Jargon is a special vocabulary fashionable in a particular group or clique. (3) Jargon is language vague in meaning and full of circumlocutions with long high sounding words. If any of the terms and phrases that you are now using fit into these three definitions, you should expunge them.

Let's start with poor word choices. How about words that you might use that lack specificity? Aspect—there is always a better word than aspect. Aspect is a garbage word. You should find something more suitable. Some. Well, some is a word that could mean anything from a 1 to 99.44 % extent. A more specific term should be used. Possibly. Possibly is the same problem as some. What do you mean? Our expertise should

rely on the assignment of the more apt word, probably which is, certainly more specific and focused. Might and may. Why use the subjunctive tense instead to answering the question is it likely or not?

What about some commonplace euphemisms? Unremarkable is a euphemism for normal. In fact, because we are remarking on something, unremarkable imparts a logical contradiction. If we remark on it how can we say that it is unremarkable? There is nothing to be gained by using that word vs. normal. Now what is normal? Normal can be a condition of perfection when we are talking about an organism. But when we are talking about a finding, normal means that there is no pathology. To say it is unremarkable is in essence the same thing except it damages our ethos to remark on something by saying there is nothing here to remark on. We should avoid redundancies. Typical of that is a phrase relating to the ribs. They are symmetric bilaterally. Obviously symmetric refers to two things on either side of the middle. Patients suffer traumatic injuries, yet all traumas can induce injuries and all injuries are traumatic.

Next, beware of temporal confusions. A small infiltrate does not mean it is early, it could be recurrent. Hence do not confuse time with space. It may be metaphorically seductive, but it is often not apt. It would be misleading to say that because something is small it is early if you do not have previous images. Also we might succumb to the opportunity to substitute vague qualitative terms for anatomic position. A typical example is to say that ET tube is in good position. What does good position mean? That is a vague value judgment. What we really need to establish is some anatomic relationships, preferably a numerical one. "The distal tip of the tube is 3 cm above the caring", is much better than "in good position". Furthermore if we present ourselves as being anatomists, the term vascular calcification is insufficient. Vessels can be lymphatic, they could be veins or they could be arteries. With rare exceptions when a calcification is in the wall of the vessel it is in an artery. When we observe arterial calcification, we should relate what vessel it is rather than merely say vascular calcification. We should also report on the extent of that calcification in that artery. So vascular calcification by itself would not suffice. One must state which artery and bear in mind that only some arteries calcify and arteries are usually in a position that we can determine their identity.

Here are three reports done by one of my residents. On the day 1 chest x-ray, the patient was rotated to the right. Day 3, chest x-ray, the patient continued to be rotated to the right. On day 7 chest x-ray, the same patient is persistently rotated. One gets the idea that the patient is really a kabob on a spit. In actual fact the patient was not rotated at all but merely positioned oblique to the central x-ray beam. It is better to say that the patient has assumed the right or left posterior oblique position than that he or she is rotated, which is not true.

are responsible for everything put in and left out. The report should be journalistic in its aptness and brevity. It should be pertinent, accurate, specific, anatomically correct, incisive in its observations, humanistic in its considerations and stylistically unobtrusive. At the same time it should be free as much as possible of obscurantism [1].

A good rule of thumb is if you want to be understood by a few, use jargon but if you don't want to be misunderstood by many, use English. Things to avoid in the report are nonspecific words like some and aspect, euphemisms, like unremarkable, neologisms like hyperdensity and non-informative phrases such as "the ET tube is in good position". A carefully crafted report requires as much care as the observation of findings. Both are essential components of our expertise.

Summary

The written report is the key document with which radiologists communicate with referring physicians. What we write is permanent and we

Reference

1. Hall FM. Language of the radiology report: primer for residents and wayward radiologists. AJR Am J Roentgenol. 2000;175(5):1239–42.

This is an unsettling time for Radiologists. We have become an issue for public attention not just for our capabilities but also for our connection to the matter of dose deposition-a subject generating many current newsworthy story lines. Most acute is the inadvertent excessive radiation received from perfusion CT studies but an issue with more "legs", so to speak, continues to be the perception and the reality of overutilization in imaging. No doubt, investigative journalists will continue to seize upon it and inevitably individual radiologists and the specialty itself will be deemed, by some self-appointed opinion makers, to be in need of reform.

We are also being impinged upon by other specialties not just in practices and programs of self-referral but also and more cogently in the legitimization of curricular reform. As traditional procedures in surgery and medical specialties have lost their luster to be replaced by newer techniques that combine incisive probing with imaging, the requirements for training more and more will include an understanding of and facility with the generation of pictures using the devices over which we have hitherto exercised dominion.

Hence in order to maintain and even augment the special expertise we possess we have to provide better interpretations, more coordinated service and a closer spatial, temporal and intellectual relationship with our referrers. At the same time as we undertake these initiatives we have to be aware of the centripetal forces that are tearing at the fabric of our essentiality as dominant interpreters of images. Teleradiology, sustained by the convenience it affords, nonetheless heightens the remoteness of radiologists as a common presentiment. We can do little about that because that innovation is too compelling to dismantle. Rather, efforts to enhance our availability and the pertinence of our opinions are in our control.

In the North Jersey region in the past 6 months I know of two radiology groups that have had their hospital contract severed and they have been replaced by an entirely new set of radiologists probably hired at a lower price. For one of them the bone of contention was the reports they provided were often indecisive, frequently and unnecessarily advocating additional studies. Also they were distant from their referrers so that no strong bond was created to enhance their reputation.

To avoid this unpleasant happenstance and in a sense to protect us from an indictment of irrelevancy, it is worthwhile to examine how we manage uncertainty. Do we render impressions that bespeak confidence in our estimations even in light of not being certain about what we see in an imaging examination or do we, unconsciously perhaps, use words or phrases that undermine our status?

The matter of either is not emphasized in our training as imaging interpreters. Nor are they usually included in continuing education curricula. So correctives to habitual use of expressions we should avoid are not part of our canon of good practice. As a result we are apt to diminish estimation of our expertise by relying on well-accepted terms that nonetheless reduce the difference between our knowledge and that of our

S.R. Baker, *Notes of a Radiology Watcher*,
DOI 10.1007/978-3-319-01677-1_29, © Springer International Publishing Switzerland 2014

referrer. Ethos is defined as the character of disposition of a person. In radiology reports our ethos is sustained by our maintenance of a sense of authority in how we choose to describe things we are not certain about.

Here are some terms we should avoid. To say that there is a "possible pneumonia" is really not saying much that is helpful. Inasmuch as anything is possible does saying possible mean anything? Surely one can provide a more definitive statement than it is possible. Using this word as a manifestation of expertise does not elevate ourselves. It implies you are as indefinite about it as is the referring physician. Similarly to include in the report the phrase "cannot be excluded" is another example of the diminution of your value as a consultant in the eyes of a clinician. Something that rarely occurs and is then termed "cannot be excluded" gives it similar potential validity to something else which is much more common and is also labeled "cannot be excluded". The referrer seeks more discernment by the radiologist in his rendered report. "Cannot be excluded" offers none of it.

Another locution to be avoided is the word questionable. Here uncertainty is married to vagueness. What is a referring physician to make of such a contribution to a supposed expert's report? What is in question? Is it the significance of the finding or the existence of the finding? Is it real or not and if so is it significant or not? Here too, we fail to inform and we fail to impress.

A presumption of the dictated expressions of the radiologist is that they represent the conclusion of an objective analysis. Subjectivity is not a helpful ingredient in the written discussion because it imposes further ambiguity as well as magnifying uncertainty. Hence, the word suspicious should be eliminated from the radiologist's lexicon. One who is suspicious suspects something; he or she is wary or disbelieving. But that is not the point of a rational estimation of the import of a series of images. The impression offered by the radiologist should be by temperament and, therefore, by testimony devoid of emotional content. Something seen may have unclear significance but it should not elicit suspicion.

So if all these words and terms are to be avoided what should go into a report when the finding to be commented upon cannot be assessed unequivocally. Semi-quantitative expressions are needed to the extent that one can draw inferences if not conclusions. It is therefore better to say that an abnormality is consistent with or compatible with or even is suggestive of. Each of these terms is not definitive but each allows a distinction to be made. Moreover, each expresses a degree of particular competence that does not detract from the ethos of the radiologist for with each a tacit notion of special knowledge can be inferred.

The difference between a generalist (a referring physician) and a specialist (in these instances a radiologist) can be summarized by this disjunction. The generalist says "I don't know" whereas the more expert specialist retorts "It is not known". Saying that something is possible and cannot be excluded or is questionable places the radiologist at the level of the generalist while the use of expressions that underscore the capability to make an educated guess preserves the radiologist's position as one more knowledgeable than the clinician in this regard. Inasmuch as our expertise is our currency we should not squander it with articulated intimations of inadequacy.

The Radiology Report: The Value of the Impression

30

Now we come to a final component of my ruminations about the Radiology Report. In the preceding essay, I talked about inappropriate words and phrases that create ambiguity or worse. Also I went through the various components of the report including preliminary information and the main narrative. I now wish to discuss the most important parts of the report, the impression and the resulting recommendations.

The impression should be considered like a headline, encapsulating the key information to be transmitted to the referring physician. Therefore, one should not repeat verbatim what was stated in the body of the report which will only disconcert the reader by redundancy. Another point of frustration told to me by referring physicians is the inclusion of the phrase "as above" in the impression. It is silly. There is no point in having an impression if you put that phrase in. By the way, you could put the impression on top which would make proper journalistic sense akin to what is displayed in newspapers. Could you then imagine having a headline in a newspaper that would state 'as below' referring to the accompanying story? If that sounds ridiculous, so does 'as above'.

How about what you put in the recommendations? I did an informal survey of about 50 of my clinical colleagues regarding the radiology report. It revealed three things that they loathed (I mean really LOATHED) about impressions rendered in radiology reports. The first thing they do not like is an impression that includes the phrase "clinical correlation requested or suggested". For some referring physicians, this may just be standard claptrap that they ignore. But others, with slightly heightened sensitivity about propriety will resent such a statement. After all, isn't their business clinical correlation? That is why they request imaging studies. That is why they do a history and physical. That is why they seek lab data. For you to gratuitously suggest that they do what they are supposed to do could be resented by some and appropriately so.

The second phrase that they do not like is suggestions for further non-radiology tests specified in the impression. For example, for a patient who exhibits findings of pancreatitis a "detested" recommendation by us would be to get an amylase. Referring physicians regard as anathema even more than merely the recommendation clinical correlation suggested because now you are specifically telling them what they should do when they know what they should do. This is gratuitousness "squared".

Third, they expressed opposition to suggestions for further imaging tests specified in the impression. Well what is the problem with that? Isn't that a manifestation of our expertise as consultants to suggest further imaging tests? If you take a narrow view of the relevance of imaging, I guess that is true. But if you care for the whole patient, which is our responsibility, it is assuredly not true because we as radiologists know how to interpret imaging tests to be sure but we generally do not know the patient very well. If there are no old studies available, for example, and there has been no previous discussion about the patient with referring physicians, which is often the case, you know very little because you have not done a history except for the one or two sentences that have been told to you in the radiology request, you have not done a physical exam, you have not examined old records, you do not know extenuating circumstances and you do not know how the patient regards his or her disease. So how could you then make a request for imaging studies which is regarded by referring physicians as tantamount to an order when you do not have that information?

The end result is that you will promote unnecessary utilization. Perhaps you may regard that increased utilization as valuable because you will gain more information about that patient. But not all information about a patient is necessary to the patient's betterment, even though it might be good for the generation of revenue to your department. As I mentioned, it has become commonplace for your suggestions to be regarded as tantamount to an order. However, this misapprehension as I have discussed on previous essays in this volume is based upon the conventional but incorrect wisdom about the frequency and likelihood of malpractice suits in particular clinical situations. In a study that we have reported previously, as assessed from data in the National Practitioners Databank which lists malpractice claims whether they were resolved favorably for the plaintiff or for the defendant, of 3,231 cases in which we could find a primary allegation against a radiologist, failure to diagnose was overwhelmingly the primary allegation. The radiologist had only a peripheral role in a few complications of therapy were the cause of even fewer actions, and failure to communicate occasioned less than 2 % with contrast reaction even fewer than that. Surprisingly, perhaps, failure to do additional testing, which is what we are talking about here was the primary allegation in only 21 of the 3,200 cases, less than 1 %. Now it is possible that failure to do additional tests may be bound into the issue of failure to diagnose, but if it was the main issue it would be listed as the primary allegation. So 20 out of more than 3,000 cases indicate that this was rarely the main reason

for malpractice suit, 20 times more of the claims were due to a failure of therapy or misdiagnosis. Hence, suggesting a test in the impression to forestall worry about malpractice is pursuing a conventional notion that is not true.

Yet, what is the importance of bringing this up? Let us look once again at the American College of Radiology guidelines for communication of diagnostic imaging findings. Although guidelines are the term we use, plaintiff lawyers and perhaps juries regard this as equivalent to standards. Whatever word you want to invoke, you know that this recommendation from the ACR is determinative of practice in many regards. The ACR also states in their general disclaimer about guidelines that an approach at variance from the guidelines does not necessarily imply that the approach is below the standard of care. Going on they state, "to the contrary a conscientious practitioner may responsibly adopt a course different from that set fourth in the guidelines if such course of actions is indicated by the condition of the patient". A practitioner who employs an approach substantially different is advised to document it in a patient record. I absolutely agree with these principles.

So let's apply it now to the ACR guidelines about the impression in a radiology report. There are four components to their remarks about the impression. The first three I agree with and the last one I do not. (1) Unless the body is brief, the impression is necessary. (2) There should be a precise diagnosis. (3) The differential diagnosis when appropriate should be listed. (4) "Follow-up or additional diagnostic studies to clarify or confirm the impression should be suggested when appropriate". On this last point, I respectfully differ. Why? Because of the general concern about overutilization that I discussed before, and (just as importantly) because of the particular matter that since we do not know the patient directly in most cases, we should not offer up a roster of additional tests because that suggestion is interpreted as a command. What we should do instead is that when we perceive a need to indicate that more studies might be helpful we call the referring physician and document that call in the body of that radiology report.

Many of you may bristle at this statement claiming that it is very difficult with all of the cases that we do to find and call the referring physician each time. And we cannot always find the referring physician or we get a recording, etc. All of these are logistic difficulties. I am sure. They may be very challenging in many circumstances. Nonetheless, lawsuits in radiology are initiated and won by the plaintiff often because direct communication was not established with the referring physician. So a scenario more likely than not which will happen sometime is your career is a test performed on the basis of an "order" from you but you did not know the extenuating circumstances about the patient. On that basis something bad happens i.e., a contrast reaction a complication, a misdiagnosis etc. Hence the challenge before us is not to conduct business as usual, but to find ways in which we are able to make sure a direct line of communication by phone or in person is established with the referring physician. In this era of text messaging and fax and paging I believe the argument that you cannot speak with a referring physician is somewhat self serving and perhaps just a little bit lazy.

The evaluation of the appropriate format and content of the radiology report in all of its dimensions—preliminary data, the body of the report, the impression and recommendations—is an objective that we have integrated as part of systems based practice and communication skills for our radiology residents. Each month, 10 reports are submitted to me by each of our 20 residents. They are evaluated under a 12 point scale in four categories. (1) Whether the report was verbose or succinct three points being the best score. (2) Whether grammar was used correctly and jargon avoided- three points (3) whether the report was clear instead of ambiguous—three points being best and (4) whether there were utilization issues related to recommendations for additional studies. On this 12 point scale on the average, the minimal score for a first year resident is 7, a second year resident 8, a third year resident 9 and a fourth year resident 10. As a result of this repetitive exercise there has been a remarkable improvement in the quality of the reports

of residents in each year of training and in each class through the year.

Finally I would like to cite another statement of policy, this one by European Association of Radiology, in their standards on communication. I agree with every one of these components and I quote, "Communication of the report of the exam is an important source of error". When an urgent clinical situation is present, whether it is a major unexpected finding that involves urgent patient management assistance, the radiologist opinion should be transmitted to the attending physician. It is the responsibility of the radiologist to ensure that the information is received precisely and unambiguously, that it is fully understood and that a clear record of the conversation is made in the report. Given this policy, it is much less likely you will be sued if you undertake a conversation with the referring physician. But the report must document the conversation about the finding specifying the receiving doctor's name and date and time of day. You may find as we have that more dialog equates to more congeniality and less distrust with your referrers and most probably better care for your patients.

Summary

The impression with or without accompanying clinical recommendations is the most important element in the radiology report. As such it should be presented in much the same way as a headline relates to a news story, no matter if it precedes or succeeds the body of the report [1].

Recommendations included in the report should avoid reference to clinical correlation per se and advice about non-imaging tests. It is far better also to discuss by phone or in person considerations for further diagnostic imaging examinations and relate that conversation in the report rather than merely listing other possibly helpful studies inasmuch as you do not know the patient. It should be remembered that suggestions in the report unassociated with a conversation with the referrer are often regarded by the latter as tantamount to an order.

Despite ACR guidelines allowing for recommendation for further studies, the above approach is congruent with good care and is not contrary to the ACR's position on the matter because communication is enhanced not avoided by the process.

Reference

1. Clark JA. Language of the radiology report. AJR Am J Roentgenol. 2001;177(2):468. doi:10.2214/ ajr.177.2.1770468.

Metaphors in Radiology

31

Radiology is the most visually oriented of all medical specialties. Because the patient is reduced to a set of images viewed remotely, cues provided by sound, touch and even smell are denied to the radiologist. Thus learning is gained not just from observations directly but also from radiologic signs, many of which are metaphoric. Is knowledge engendered or merely decorated by reference to figurative connections? This essay provides data and some answers to the enduring speculation on the power of metaphor and its pertinence to diagnostic imaging.

How do we learn things in Radiology? Our specialty is now recognized as probably the most dynamic in all of medicine. Characterized by the implementation of both new instruments and new observations, it has revolutionized diagnosis. But we must understand some limitations. We deal only in images. Images are not reality. Reality is the patient or organs in the patient, or the supporting structures attached to those organs, or the cells in both parenchyma and supporting tissue, or the flow of substances and impulses throughout the body. Aside from interventional radiology we gain knowledge only through visual depiction of those structures and phenomena. In essence, we are narrowly informed, having at our disposal only a fraction of the sense data that could be acquired, interpreted and assimilated in order to gain and retain knowledge.

Other specialists interact more fully with the actual human being they assess. They speak with them as they look at them. They see their gestures and predominately they learn from speech what the patient is complaining about. Aural cues also include the sounds they have been able to discern from auscultation of the chest, heart, and abdomen. All other physicians directly involved with diagnosis also touch patients. Physical examination with its tactile observations allows inferences to be drawn about the presence and particularities of disease. In some instances, olfactory clues also have relevance about mental and physical conditions that are specifically associated with distinctive smells.

But for radiologists, we just have pictures to go by. Incisive images for sure but they are merely simulacra, to use a fancy word, not the thing in itself. Unlike other physicians we cannot, at one encounter, look directly, or hear or touch. Having each type of sensual information can reinforce, question or refute our professional opinions. We are remote. We can only see and reflect, usually at a distance in space and often after an interval of time.

So how do we learn through the process of image-gauging? Is it merely pattern recognition, an entirely non-verbal imprinting on our brains of distributions of white, black and gray? Surely it is more than that. Every picture has an arrangement of constituent parts; every image is examined, not in abstraction but refracted by some context. At the least, we should have available to us, name, gender, ID, type of study, and body part. But for the sake of patient care, we want more—including history, physical exam, laboratory data, old films (if available) and the referring physicians' comments that instigated the study.

S.R. Baker, *Notes of a Radiology Watcher*,
DOI 10.1007/978-3-319-01677-1_31, © Springer International Publishing Switzerland 2014

All of these are pertinent to help us make the relevant findings and whittle down the differential diagnosis. In a sense, radiologists inspect scenes and words. The lexical element is crucial to the visual. We just don't remember patterns, we classify and organize and we assign labels. We must have a vocabulary to describe what we see and the words we use must be intelligible to our fellow radiologists and to referring physicians. Hence, despite being bereft of much of the information that a patient could present to our ears, fingers, and nose, we can to a degree overcome this deficiency of input by employing a sophisticated rhetorical system allowing for intricate and formal taxonomies. We are compelled to articulate what we observe in order to communicate to our fellow physicians the import of differences and particularities in appearance that inform an insightful, consultative report.

In radiology, one may gain mastery in part by compiling learning signs. It helps us come to know the name of things, each identified with a specific assemblage of features deemed to be diagnostic and often unique. Probably no other branch of medicine is so sign rich. How many signs are there? Well, a lot to be sure. But their multiplicity should not daunt us. A monograph by Eisenberg published in the early 80s was in essence a compendium of signs. It was fun to pore through yet it was essentially a descriptive work. Several students and I thought there may be some value to categorize well-established signs and also to recognize in the 20 years since Eisenberg published his work that there had been many more signs introduced. So we counted them up, divided them by organ systems and tried to further organize them by nominal identity. That is, they were grouped by whether the sign was directly related to the body part to which it referred, whether it bore the name of its coiner or discoverer or whether it had an appellation with which a novel relation could be made between a pathologic condition or anatomic derangement and some other object or notion. In other words, were the signs anatomic, eponymous, or metaphorical? [1]

All told our roster of signs numbered nearly 900 different entities. 183 were anatomic, 675 metaphoric, and only 19 bore a persons name. The signs encompassed the GI, GU tracts, the heart and lungs joined together, and the musculoskeletal system. In the GI tract, thorax and the bones and joints, anatomic and metaphorical terms were nearly equal but in the GU tract, metaphors nearly doubled anatomical references. In each of the four, eponymous terms were sparse. In fact, self perpetuation through naming is quite rare in radiology in comparison with many other specialties where eponymous designations are rife. And we stand out in marked contrast to surgery where the predominant practice is to associate the developer with the novel procedure he or she introduced. Dorland's Medical Dictionary lists 366 operations in which are known by is the surgeons' surname. So modest we may be, but immoderate are we in the employment of metaphor.

Before going further, one would ask what precisely is this figure of speech. According to the American Heritage Dictionary, it is described as a rhetorical device in which a word or phrase that ordinarily designates one thing is used to designate another, thus making an implicit comparison. Another definition is a trope or figure of speech for seeing something in terms of something else. In a metaphor a thing is at once what it was and what its new meaning is. In a simile a thing is like another thing and in analogy something is portrayed as if it were something other.

Throughout history there have been those who felt that a metaphor does not inculcate meaning, but merely decorates it. The great Roman orator Cicero considered metaphor as a literary ornament employed by skilled wordsmiths to replace a literal meaning with a figurative one employed for the sake of charm or because of lack of a proper word. However, now rhetoric and science have been claimed by most postmodern theorists to be at least complementary in the creation of knowledge. The cognitive power of a metaphor has come to be recognized. The science writer Ken Bakke has shown us with an auditory metaphor of his own that the magical value of a metaphor is inherent in its harmonic virtues—how like certain tones it has overtones,—additional reverberations that harmonize and frame the note played. Another investigator of this subject (which now has a vast literature) has maintained that metaphor can touch a deep level of understanding for it points to the process of learning and discovery by an analogic leap from the familiar to the unfamiliar which rallies imagination and emotion as well as intellect.

A recent functional MR study has shown increased brain wave activity with the hearing of a metaphor when compared with reception of a simile, a finding that underscores the harmonic concatenations of metaphoric pronouncements. The etymology of the word itself comes from transfer or transport. It is no wonder, harmonic references aside, that metaphors are predominately spatial and often geographic. For example, we may say his condition has gone south, or refer to a stream of consciousness or claim that she can move mountains. The spatial affinity explains the popularity of metaphor for a visually-related epistemology like radiology. Yet in fact, there is no geographic majority or even plurality in the subjects of metaphors used in diagnostic imaging. In any event the power of most metaphors is invested in the revelatory effect of the figurative element to be transported to its new meaning. A key is that the psychologically new relation to observable pathological alterations and/or anatomic arrangements rests in the fact that its original meaning is generally familiar to the audience of learners.

An effective metaphor in radiology counters Cicero's claim of mere decoration. Its meaning resonates with us. That is the source of its retentive effect. Yet a few caveats need to mentioned. It is a reference not an identity. I have noticed on several occasions misdiagnoses abetted by uncritical evaluation of some signs. Here is one example. The bowel abnormality closed loop obstruction is associated with the coffee bean sign. It was not diagnosed in one instance because the observer demanded verisimilitude not similarity. Because the abnormal gas shadow did not exactly look like a coffee bean, the possibility of obstruction was rejected. Therefore, the metaphor overwhelmed the condition instead of revealing it.

A further requirement for metaphor is that it is understood in its literal meaning by more than a few cognoscenti. An egregious non-apt metaphor is the Phrygian cap sign which refers to a flopping over of the fundus of the gall bladder. To its popularizer it simulates the hat worn in ancient Phrygia in Asia Minor. In actuality the history of Phrygian cap is fascinating. It was adopted by the Roman slaves and their emancipators. In the Revolutionary War it came to be the hat worn by the rebelling Americans and it is now commemorated in the state flags of New York, New Jersey and West Virginia. Yet, soon after it came to be adopted also as a sign of the French Revolution. Marianne, the stock character representative of republican France wears it as a distinctive identifier. Now all of this is wonderful but is of no aid to those trying to learn its radiological connection when they do not appreciate its historical references and cannot remember its shape.

On the other hand, the Northern Exposure sign is a more apt metaphor. It refers to the migration upward above the transverse colon of the sigmoid colon as a pathognomonic marker of sigmoid volvulus. The metaphor is geographic but the resonating references are abundant. The transverse colon can be considered through the mediation of a corresponding metaphor to be the equator of the abdomen. In the abdomen, a raft of geographical metaphors comes quickly to mind. Food is transported from above to below through a winding tract. Upper in conventional understanding is associated with North. This is in a sense a persisting spatial relationship known to everyone. It makes the transference of northern to above easy to remember. What is more, the Northern Exposure sign further emphasizes the relocation of the sigmoid colon rostral to the transverse colon as being abnormal, an invasion of territory if you will and a sure sign that the sigmoid has volved. So learning this sign helps one make the relevant observation for sigmoid volvulus because it truly illustrates the power, harmonic and otherwise, of metaphor. It underscores why this figure of speech, often colorful and vibrant, is also enriching and necessary for the dissemination of radiologic knowledge.

Reference

1. Baker SR, Partyka L. Relative importance of metaphor in radiology versus other medical specialties. Radiographics. 2012;32(1):235–40.

Metaphor: Redux

32

Metaphor in Radiology is a subject of continual fascination for me. As a hobby, if you will, I like to explore the role, value and extent of the use of metaphor as a learning tool in diagnostic imaging. I and my coworker, a recently graduated resident in our program have mined the indexes of the major encyclopedic texts in Radiology and six other specialties in order to develop specialty-based lists of referenced metaphors which are well established as being denoted as signs of imaging appearances. We found that Radiology far more than any other specialty depends on these metaphors to transmit meaning and understanding. In surgery, in contrast, metaphoric signs are few but eponymic markers are abundant as both diagnostic signposts and as identifiers of operations. Apparently, surgeons are eager to commemorate their specific contributions whereas radiologists are not so impelled to commemorate their insights with their names. And Radiology's predominance as a metaphor-information discipline is not emulated to anywhere near the same extent in the two other predominantly visual specialties of Dermatology and Pathology.

A metaphor creates a linkage between two distinct and otherwise separable realms of knowledge, not by imposing the relationship as an exact identity characteristic of a simile but by revealing a connection of hitherto disparate notions and/or objects. The result of a good metaphor, one that by its freshness and incisiveness creates a novel bridge between the familiar beyond radiology now linked to the revealed perception of an imaging manifestation. It attaches that radiologic fact to the general substrate of established memory so that the new insight, too, can be long retained.

We were stimulated by our initial work and now with a new cast of helpers i.e., several fourth year students at my institution and also a recent graduate from abroad, we sought to delve further in our specialty's long interaction or should I say dependence on metaphor to illuminate the often emotionally-laden and enduring content of an imaging pattern as a reflection of a disease or abnormality. So we decided to search the radiologic literature from 1895 to the present to record when each metaphoric sign was initially reported. That means that we examined the table of contents of every issue from the beginning of their respective runs of most radiology journals in English including the AJR, Radiology, Clinical Radiology, the European Journal of Radiology, European Radiology, the Journal of the Canadian Association of Radiologists, Clinical Radiology, Acta Radiologica Scandanavica, Radiographics, Abdominal Radiology, and JCAR as well as textbooks that included lists of signs. The purpose was to accumulate as comprehensive roster as possible so that we could analyze the particularities of metaphoric signs in greater depth. Twenty-five years ago there was published a monograph on this subject by Eisenberg which was essentially a list of them not further analyzed but replete with pictures. He recorded over 250 such signs. We are not quite done with our research. To date we have found more than 700 [1].

S.R. Baker, *Notes of a Radiology Watcher*,
DOI 10.1007/978-3-319-01677-1_32, © Springer International Publishing Switzerland 2014

From Roentgen's discovery until the early 1970s radiology consisted predominantly of plain films, GI contrast studies and intravenous dye distribution imaging procedures. Diagnostic imaging became the more encompassing term for what we do now starting 40 years ago because nuclear imaging, angiography, ultrasonography and CT came on stream to be followed by MR in the early 1980s. With these advanced techniques using new energy sources for the rendering of pictures, the way was clear for a panoply of observations as more of the body's spaces, contours and vessels were revealed. The newly recognized spatial configurations opened by these techniques raised the possibility of the observation of linkage of similar shapes, contours and internal arrangements from other knowledge domains, some esoteric and others mundane. Hence the metaphor repertoire widened.

In fact, the golden age of new signs reported in the radiology literature was the decade of the 1970s, Bone, GI, GU and Chest were the four subspecialties in which the compendium of metaphoric signs expanded markedly. In contrast neuroradiology had a relative paucity of new metaphoric citations. These trends persisted to a slightly reduced extent in the 1980s and have gradually lessened in intensity after 2000. No doubt the new anatomy that CT uncovered was largely responsible for the boom in the late 70s and early 80s. The revolution created by MR with respect to the pictorial differentiation of soft tissue structures led to the primacy of MSK as the subspecialty whose store of metaphoric signs increased to the greatest extent. In the first decade of the twenty first century, the chest has been the locus of most newly described metaphoric references, no doubt influenced by the gain in both static and dynamic imaging afforded by improvements in CT which were introduced between 1995 and 2004. Since 1980, the last year perhaps when plain film-related procedures predominated, CT and MR are now the modalities from which most new metaphors are described, albeit at a much lower rate than conventional radiology in its heyday. But overall, the descriptive era in Radiology may in fact be drawing to a close as all the modalities we use mature and as the roster of

diseases to be described by their spatial manifestations have been intensively explored and as the consequence of anatomic changes by surgery and drug therapy have been largely recognized. And like other science-related disciplines that have a century-plus legacy of discovery, descriptive elements eventually give way to more precise analytic estimations. We may now be passing through this anticipated transition.

The candidates for metaphoric references are as broad as the full range of knowledge discernable by humans and recorded any time from the remote past to the present, as long as it has been shared through common parlance or through written permanence. Even with just such a vast array of possibilities among the subject of radiology-related metaphors we have found they can be aggregated into general categories. By far the most frequent referent are man-made objects. Some examples are the rugger jersey sign of hyperparathyroidism and the lead pipe fracture which is a combination of a greenstick and a torus fracture. In second place are food metaphors such as the lollipop sign of the bile ducts in Crohn's disease and the apple core lesions emblematic of a colonic carcinoma. In third place on our list are signs related to general shapes such as the crescent sign in greater curvature ulcers and star-like stones in the gall bladder and urinary bladder. In decreasing order are metaphors that connect plant forms, like the coffee bean sign of sigmoid volvulus and weaponry, an example being the arrowhead sign in appendicitis. Also having representation are supernatural or mythical inspirations as demonstrated by the medusa sign of ascaris infestation and the Phrygian cap appearance of the fundus of the gall bladder. These signs in their totality bespeak a fascinating diversity that enriches radiologic description.

In our residency program, we try to make learning fun and stimulating with unorthodox assignments from time to time to enliven the acquisition and retention of facts and relationships. In that spirit we completed our first "creativity day" project using metaphor creation. Each resident was assigned a day free of clinical responsibilities. His or her obligation on that free day was to devise two metaphors from his or her experience as an imaging interpreter. One metaphor related a well-known object to a radiologic appearance, the second metaphor linked an imaging appearance to a more recondite object. After each trainee had his separate day off we met collectively to share each one's metaphoric formulation and then to pick the best ones. Everyone was able to come up with two examples, and the three best ones will be submitted for publication. One I particularly liked was the Cape Buffalo clavicle sign. The appearance of this bone when the patient is x-rayed in the apical lordotic projection resembles the curvilinear horizontal course of the horns of that fearsome animal.

Reference

1. Baker SR, Noorelahi YM, Ghosh S, Yang LC, Kasper DJ. History of metaphoric signs in radiology. Eur J Radiol. 2013. ISSN 0720-048X. http://dx.doi.org/10.1016/j.ejrad.2013.04.005. Accessed 16 May 2013.

Electronic Health Records and Expectations of the Transformation of the Work of Radiologists

33

A key component of the American Recovery and Reinvestment Act of 2009, popularly known as Obamacare, has been the provision within it entitled Health Information Technology for Economic and Clinical Health or (HITECH). The law expends federal money for the adoption by health care facilities of information technology, specifically for the utilization of electronic health records. The impetus for the initiative is the expectation that by having a patient's health care record immediately available, the decision making process will be influenced by the ready access to data. Consequently, unnecessary tests, especially perhaps those related to expensive imaging, will be reduced thereby ultimately decreasing health care costs [1].

On its face, this notion is compelling. We are far behind other well off countries in the comprehensive use of the electronic medical record. Finland and even neighboring Estonia have, for more than 5 years now, been completely wired and most of their health care indices surpass that of the United States despite the fact that aggregate cost of care as a percentage of gross domestic product there is less than two thirds of the 18 % of GDP we pay for here.

Two recent studies, contradictory in their conclusions, require us to consider this matter not as an article of faith in the redemptive power of instantaneous comprehensive access, but rather its adoption as a testable, measurable process involving incentivisation issues as well as electronic capability. The first study "Giving Office-Based Physicians Elective Access to Patients Prior Imaging and Lab Results did not Deter Ordering of Tests" by McCormack et al. appeared recently in Health Affairs. Examining the records of a sample provided by office-based physicians, they found that electronic access did not lower but actually increased the rate of ordering of imaging tests. The authors acknowledged that in academic institutions the presentation of recent results electronically could reduce redundant imaging test ordering but they suggested that for the totality of outpatient facilities the opposite was true. In contrast, a year earlier in the same journal in a study entitled "The Benefits of Health Information Technology: A Review of the Recent Literature shows Predominantly Positive Results", Bernstein and her co-authors claimed that in both large and in small practices and in other care-giving organizations, the electronic medical record does change test-ordering behavior and therefore can reduce costs. Yet the authors also acknowledged that the incorporation of the electronic medical record into standard practice will meet with resistance before adoption becomes commonplace.

What might make its virtues more manifest in the American system of care? I refer specifically to its putative effect on the proper rather than the excessive use of imaging. For one thing, perhaps the most important, accompanying operational innovations should require the central participation of the radiologist. Now let me be clear here. By such participation I emphatically do not mean remote decision support schema and programs which incidentally are regarded by the ACR and by some well-meaning prestigious academic institutions as the perfect accompaniment to the EHR. The notion that resort to recipes i.e., the reliance on appropriateness criteria as a panacea is fundamentally wrong.

It rests on the assumption that offering referrers data will provide answers to their queries and/or provide relief from their befuddlement about the exemplary sequencing of imaging tests and, as such, costs, dose and discomfort pertinent to specific patients will be minimized. Why is it wrong? Because like other recipes, it assumes a standardization of ingredients. But good care cannot be successful and will often be mischievous and even deleterious when a patient's condition becomes subsumed into just a chief complaint or a single symptom or an aberrant lab value.

A radiologists' expertise is bound to his or her interpretations of images and, equally important, to proffered assessments of relative risks and utility of imaging tests. If his or her encounter with a referrer is limited to just a few dollops of information instead of a comprehensive presentation of an illness its antecedents and its confounding peculiarities much that could be essential is bypassed. Patients have histories that bring with it a richness of detail calling for a nuanced assessment of diagnostic tactics and strategy. Many patients have comorbidities that bear upon their disease and the approach to a diagnosis. Moreover, some have anxieties and some others have allergies that must be taken into account. Also, they can be often immersed in social situations that should inform workups. The effective radiologist must be aware of these complexities before rendering an opinion. Often such cognizance will result in accommodations that consider the patient as a subject rather than an object who has an organ or two that maybe abnormal and therefore is apt to get a test or a series of tests to study it. Yet, without a detailed history you cannot "phone in" a carefully directed workup by a simple or rather simplistic resort to a predetermined diagnostic algorithm.

For the last 35 years, every day I do on the spot, face-to-face consultations with referring physicians. I have published my results in three separate articles that appeared in JAMA,

Radiology and AJR in 1984 and 1985 well before the idea of an electronic medical record was more than a gleam in some futurist's eye. I have not been compensated directly for this function which I have performed for both internal medicine and general surgery teams. But I know I can reduce unnecessary tests and can avoid avoidable care without harming patients because my dialog with referrers gives me more than a chief complaint upon which to make a recommendation.

And my capabilities have been enhanced by PACS, which provide not a complete medical record but one that gives me immediate access to not only all imaging tests performed in the last 10 years at my hospital but also vital historical material. Face to face discussions with the patient and referring physician should elaborate current history, including, when asked, relevant medical, social, family and travel information. Physical findings and recent lab data are also related to me at my daily meeting with the medical staff which takes place in our radiology conference room where the images are shown on a large screen. And it is both the older images and the historical data as well as the large screen that have made me realize that together my diagnostic acumen has increased.

Two recent cases illustrate the insights I have gained. They occurred on the same a day and both remain for me a vivid example of electronic display in the context of face to face consultations. Marshall McLuhan, the famous Canadian media theorist 50 years ago coined the phrase "the medium is the message". I believe him. By observing chest-X-rays daily on the big screen in conjunction with discussions with referrers I came to appreciate now what for all my career I neglected to consider before. I have noted that the width of the "flesh" lateral to the ribs reflects the degree of obesity. We all know this after a fashion. It is such a mundane fact but we have not appreciated its deeper importance. It is more starkly evident on a big screen than a small one. And by rapidly viewing a series of film we can tell qualitatively whether one is gaining weight or losing it or maintaining stability. We are, by the way, now doing a study to determine if we can make quantitative statements about the change in actual weight from the change in the width of soft tissue between the lateral lower ribs and the skin surface. But no matter, for significant weight change, this cognitive advantage by comparative viewing of past and present images can be significant for enhancing our awareness of a patient's condition over time.

The first case was a 78 year old man who was demented and came to the hospital short of breath. The chest X-ray showed pulmonary edema which resolved with dialysis. He had been cared for at home by his niece, his only caregiver, who visited once a day but she had to work two jobs to make ends meet. I noticed now in my new routine of observing at my consultation session with the medical team that he had been losing weight over the past 2 years gradually but probably inexorably by measurement of his "flesh width" on films taken roughly every 4 months. His renal failure was thus not his only problem besides his dementia. He also has been underfed or had not eaten well enough. His treatment? Social service was called. His niece realized she could not properly care for him and he was placed in a nursing home.

The second patient was a 48 years old man who was admitted from the E.R. to the medical services for his complaint of a 40 pound weight loss over 4 months. But a review of six chest X-rays we had of him over 2 years demonstrated no change in the width of his soft tissue lateral to the lower ribs. In fact his weight had to have been more or less stable. After that observation, the presumption of likely expansive weight loss workup was aborted. In this instance the radiologist's observation as a consultant obviated the need to commence a fishing expedition for which there were no fish. If we had accepted the chief complaint and resorted to a routinized "decision support" recipe the evaluation would likely have been prolonged, costly and non-productive. Without the physical presence of the consultant radiologist engaged in a dialog with his referrers, electronic records would not cut costs.

Incidentally, I then went to the E.R. to ask what the patient's weight was. To my surprise and chagrin, they admitted they do not have a scale. So everything about this admission was based on the patient's misrepresentation and you know that deceitfully or unwittingly people will lie about their weight. Now we will buy and place a scale near patients and so we will have objective evidence of weight loss.

Radiologists are physicians. Their relevance depends not only on electronic means at their disposal but also on an institutionalized colloquy with primary caregivers. That is where their value ultimately lies and that is where the electronic medical record can be utilized to the utmost to realize the opportunities it affords for optimal care, not unnecessary inappropriate care which sometimes is the inevitable effect of transmuting a complex history into a chief complaint.

Summary

Recent studies have led to contradictory conclusions about the value of the Electronic Medical Record as a controller of the costs of care. Nonetheless, the availability of such records can afford the opportunity for radiologists to advise referring physicians remotely through a program of "decision support". Yet most decision support protocols reduce a patient's clinical history to a chief complaint which then directs suggestions for further workup. This approach is wrong and may not lead to savings of money or radiation exposure because the considerations that inform a diagnostic evaluation often multifactorial and irreducible. This requires the radiologist to be physically present and to communicate face-to-face with referring physicians as part of a mutually educational colloquy. Also, visualizing various studies on a big screen helps illuminate seemingly inconsequential but really profound findings such as chest wall thickness when presumptive weight loss is a putative component of the presentation of illness.

Reference

1. Jha AK. The promise of electronic records: around the corner or down the road? JAMA. 2011;306(8):880–1. doi:10.1001/jama.2011.1219.

Telling Patients Results

34

A well-remembered article which appeared in Radiology, October 2006 entitled, "The State of Radiology in 2006, Very High Spatial Resolution but no Visibility" by Ruiz and Glazer, raises once more an important issue in Radiology—one that has appeared often in old clothes but now has shown itself in a new guise. I am speaking specifically about our role in the delivery of information. The subject is the radiologists' involvement or lack thereof in relating to patients the results of recently completed imaging tests.

One of the problems for a radiologist in his or her capacity as a deliverer of care is where to position ourselves. The capture of most diagnostic workups in the past decade and a half by cross sectional imaging studies, particularly CT, but also to a lesser extent MR has placed the imaging interpreter at the fulcrum between the uncovering of abnormalities and the initiation of therapy. Today, by and large, the radiologist renders his or her diagnosis at a remove from the patient, increasingly so in space, yet, also decreasingly so in time. Advances in communication and the electronic rendering of images can mean that the radiologist can be placed anywhere in the hospital, as well as even anywhere on earth. And the twin advances of PACS and voice recognition mean that a report, soon after it is dictated and approved, can move instantaneously to the primary physician. Given the diagnostic incisiveness of imaging why shouldn't a radiologist make known his diagnosis even faster—by telling patients right there before they leave the imaging suite about what are the findings and what they signify. Proponents of this idea, like the authors of the previously cited paper, maintain that it is not enough to be the doctor's doctor as we portray ourselves, dispensing our expertise exclusively to the referring physician. Rather, we should take the opportunity to confer with the patient at hand. The justification for direct face-to-face communication with the patient stems from the notion that we as radiologists know more about the test we perform, specifically, and more about imaging in general. Thus, so as the logic proceeds, we know best what to tell the patient.

This view is informed by what I would call a mechanistic and ultimately dehumanizing view of medicine, even though it is portrayed incorrectly as an advancement in humanism. Could we really be criticized for an urge for direct interaction with the patient? I say yes, not for our good intentions, of course, but because of the inevitable untoward consequences for some patients. What are we really doing with when we review a CT study? In actuality, we have reduced the patient to an object when we do a computed tomography examination. Personhood has been replaced by a series of slices through the body, providing intricate anatomic detail, to which, if we were to pursue the author's notion we will now attach an ear to the assemblage of slices by having the patient receive the news about what the pictures reveal. Yet, how do we gauge the receptiveness of patients for what we have rendered in cross-sectional images and from those images made observations and conclusions, which we will now express to them through verbal interchanges? However, for the most part, we as radiologists really do not know much about that subject, i.e., the patient, who is often a worried and frequently medically uninformed individual.

Despite the virtuosity of sophisticated imaging, before the test is performed, we usually do not see the patient. We have not taken a history, so we do not know the patient's story, except for a few words on the request form. We do not hear the patient relate that story. Often we do not know if there are old images from other facilities which if made available would allow our assessment of the implication of present images to be more apt and our advice more pertinent and less misleading. We do not examine the patient so we have not touched them or listened to their heart or belly. We have not smelled them. We do not know their apprehensions, their preconceptions, and their fears. We are in the dark about their personhood even though we may be enlightened about the configuration of their pancreas.

So how can we give them bad news? I am boarded in both diagnostic radiology and radiation therapy. So I am very aware that providing a dire diagnosis is not something to be done matter-of-factly. You have to size up the patient, as well as his or her family, pick the right occasion, and sometimes perhaps, you should make the announcement obliquely, letting the patient ease into it slowly so that what is said by the physicians is acknowledged and more readily accepted. Disclosing bad news to someone for whom you have had no prior relationship can be a brutal experience for the sufferer, one that need not be made necessary or inevitable just because a radiologist invokes the doctrine of a compelling need to tell.

That having been said, I do recognize three instances for which the radiologist could inform the patient about a diagnosis immediately. We are required to do such when we perform mammography and the patient has no physician of record. In this scenario, the patient enters our care by her initiative alone and we must be both film interpreter and the information disclosure. To delay a communication of the diagnosis when breast cancer is found or suspected is unconscionable. Therefore, we are compelled to tell the patient what we have found. When we do obstetrical ultrasonography the patient, of course, is right there as interested as we are looking at the same pictures that we create. It is likely that we have for the most part, formed some personal relationship in this encounter mediated by conversation and the laying on hands along with the transducer. The patient is often anxious. Hence, allowing a delay when the diagnosis is clear, is unnecessarily unsettling. A third instance is when we perform angiography. Usually the patient is awake looking at the images, the operator's hands are on him or her, and an occasion for a dialog has been established. Moreover, even before the study a visual and aural connection should have been made in the preliminary interview in which the procedure is explained to the patient. Thus an ongoing professional colloquy having been instituted, the radiologist is able to continue it in the context of diagnosis disclosure.

However, how could we become so closely involved when we do a routine CT? Often computed tomography studies are done elsewhere in the department and a group of them are batched for our review. Typically, the patient has usually left the premises of the imaging site when we examine our slices. Should each patient wait around for us to come out and chat with them? We cannot do that routinely because we are too busy viewing other images. Moreover, the usual CT case involves a patient we do not know, we have not touched, we have not talked with. How can we find the time and more importantly the quiet, unhurried setting, to give them news, hopefully good, but sometimes, awful? How then could this be a practical arrangement? Even if realizable it is no improvement over directly calling the primary care physician and telling the results to him or her as soon as possible so that the primary care doctor can tell the patient expeditiously?

It is stated in that article that rendering bad news will not be so frequent given the fact that there are about 30,000 radiologists and about 1.25 million diagnosis of cancer per year. Well this is an example of fuzzy math, because the initial diagnosis is not the only time that radiology is involved in the assessment of patients with cancer. Many of these sufferers come back for repeat studies to determine if the therapy has worked or if the disease has advanced or retreated. Every PET/CT deserves a prompt diagnosis and a call to the primary care physician. After all, what are the stakes of a PET/CT examination? In essence the patient agrees to the examination in the fearful expectation that when the results are in they will know if they are likely to die soon or not. If you have never seen the patient, why should you, instead of the primary care physician, give that information and give it on the spot. Advocates of the policy of radiologists providing information directly to the patient should also make provisions in their daily schedule for follow-up calls for clarification or emotional succor—just like if they were oncologists. Furthermore, what about abnormal results of imaging studies reporting infectious, traumatic or metabolic diseases for which the radiologist might be the first to discover? The authors are silent on the communication of the results of imaging examinations referable to these illnesses.

I am a firm believer that communication and consultation are both key in radiologic diagnosis. However, the means by which that information is transmitted is crucial. The recent review of the American College of Radiology guideline on communication is a document I fully agree with. Malpractice suits are sometimes sequences of incomplete information or, in fact, the information is lost on the way to the referring physician, because there is no direct communication of (1) immediately important results, or (2) correction of a prior misdiagnosis, or (3) a finding which not causing immediate harm, if left unattended to and untreated, will lead to dire consequences. The interaction between a radiologist and the referring physician must be frequent, collegial and readily achieved. Such a dialog should also be included in the radiology report documenting a direct verbal communication either in person or by phone.

Nothing in the ACR guidelines mandates that there should be direct communication with the patient except in the unusual instance when the primary care giver is unavailable and a backup is unassigned or unreliable. The crucial elements for communication in radiology are the speed in which the radiology report is transmitted and the certainty that it will be received by and understood by a responsible caregiver. Except for the circumstances that I have mentioned, institution of the idea that the radiologist must engage in primary discussion with the patient without knowing much or anything about that individual, I believe will not become an advancement of care but rather it can often be an instrument of misunderstanding and, in many instances, can induce unintended, unforeseen dismay [1].

Reference

1. Berlin L. Communicating results of all outpatient radiologic examinations directly to patients: the time has come. AJR Am J Roentgenol. 2009;192(3):571–3.

Part VI

Radiologist Responsibilities

The essays in this part are connected by the way radiologists present themselves, how they reason and how they interact with other physicians. In the first two chapters common fallacies are presented. In the third and fourth, the nature of our relationship with our colleagues is explored in greater detail.

Fallacies in Reasoning: Part 1

35

In this report, I would like to delve into the treacherous and unforgiving fallas sea (pun intended), a region of analysis where all hypotheses are subject to the Draconian test of logical estimation. In the search for the presence of falseness biases are exposed and hitherto comforting propositions which seemingly cover a supposed truth are eroded away leaving gaping holes and even unbridgeable gaps in the assumption of veracity. In other words a search for fallacies can be a refreshing exercise for critics and a withering one for authors who have failed to think through their positions. In everyday activities fallacies are rife in all measures of reasoning and in fact are crucial for existing in the world without becoming suffocated by anxiety. After all, many rationalizations are really fallacies and yet belief in them can get one through the day. For example we want to believe that we were lucky when our car was totaled but we weren't hurt even though the persons luckier than we weren't even in the auto accident. What a relief to escape injury but your equanimity has been disrupted while others not involved nary give it a thought. We want to believe that every cloud has a silver lining, that wishing and hoping will make something good happen even though that sensibility alone will not influence external events. In that context, fallacies give us buoyancy even though they are often full of baloney.

In medical science as well, we wish that our suppositions will be borne out by facts congenial to our predictions, that our methodology is not flawed and our data is derived and analyzed through disinterested objectivity. Sometimes that can happen but more often than not, and especially in Radiology, where the impetus for verification is based on the force of use, fallacies intrude. And eventually the errors in our fallacious formulations will be exposed when looked at afresh by those who perhaps have not a vested interest in the conclusions we had reached. Along the way and nearly at every step a fallacious obstacle is likely to get in our way. One source lists 107 separate forms of fallacies and misconceptions from incorrect reasoning or argumentation. Many of them can relate directly to radiology [1].

Consider the following examples:

An event occurs singly or repetitively and an explanation for it is then given after the fact. The cause of the occurrence is then provided with the expectation that it is predictive, i.e., when similar circumstances occur, similar outcomes will also occur. That may be true for a simple procedure like coin flipping where after a while the numbers of heads and tails will converge. But with more complicated eventualities, the same result will not necessarily occur each time because the impress of externalities is too diverse in space and time. In other words it is a situation with multifactorial impingements and influences. Thus what happened once need not happen next time although you might want to believe that an imputed cause and observed effect are invariably linked. This is known as the hindsight bias or the fallacy of retrospective determinism. For instance, ultrasound is diagnostic of pancreatitis because in the first case report of this condition

S.R. Baker, *Notes of a Radiology Watcher*,
DOI 10.1007/978-3-319-01677-1_35, © Springer International Publishing Switzerland 2014

the patient had no gas in the stomach or colon to impede the visualization of the inflamed gland. But with the next 15 patients with a similar diagnosis but also with each having a collection of intestinal gas near the pancreas, ultrasonography becomes non-diagnostic. The virtue of the test in this circumstance is elusive by virtue of its inconsistency.

A corollary is the fallacy of small numbers in which enthusiastic presumptions are made because of encouraging results as derived from the outcome of a few tests but, later, with more cases, the numbers and percentage of positive and equivocal results increases, ultimately dashing hopes that a promising diagnostic implement or maneuver or sign is reliable. This fallacy could be restated as the fallacy of the case report in which an observation of one or two cases becomes considered an established truthful relationship when it is merely a preliminary observation. It might, with time and repetition, become accepted and even hallowed as lore, which in many instances, is really phony knowledge dignified by age and repetition. For example take the matter of the calcified gallbladder, silent clinically but recognizable by imaging. One small report from Argentina years ago related that some patients with a porcelain gallbladder harbored cancer in the organ. A well remembered association was then created, derived from a small number of people in a remote country which revealed a finding corroborated by cross-sectional imaging. There was no longitudinal analysis of these patients to assess the temporal consequences of a calcified gall gladder wall and no follow-up study in another population. Nonetheless this one and only study has led surgeons everywhere to become further enriched by removing the offending rock hard organ yet without gaining confirmation that what they were doing was any good. This fallacy is so common in American medical practice that it constitutes a "normative" response to information which provides no more than an inkling, not confirmation of an hypothesis. Actually the natural history of gallbladder wall calcification is unknown. What is known is that cholecystectomy causes a risk small in the young and healthy, increasing with age and that the operation always incurs a cost even if it confers no benefit.

To now move from anecdote to a more rigorous ascertainment of understanding of pathologic susceptibility, we can set up a controlled experiment. For therapy we engage in data accumulation through clinical trials. Surely this is an advancement over the reporting of a series of cases which for the most part remain the customary means of information presentation for the expansion of the corpus of knowledge in Radiology. Yet clinical trials by themselves are subject to the fallacy of illusory verisimilitude. That is an infrequently recognized problem intrinsic to prospectively designed, seemingly unbiased population studies from which generalizations are made. Yet subjects in clinical trials are often specially selected, like unbruised apples at a fruit stand. They are each ideal specimens for the issue in question because they lack confounding intercurrent conditions. Such subjects are usually confined to one age group, often from one socioeconomic status and one geographic area. Hence clinical trials, even large ones, are not conducted on two generalizable random populations distinguished by one possessing and the other lacking the attribute in question. So is the consequence of a diagnostic investigation or therapeutic intrusion performed in a clinical trial predictive of its outcome on the next patient (who is probably somewhat different from the stereotypical ideal subject)? Do the trial groups vary from him or her in some profound but yet undeciphered way? In other words, relying on the results of a trial presupposes that similarity between the study group on the patients has been taken for granted. Often this is a fallacious notion.

In Radiology we do not do many clinical trials but some leaders in and out of the ACR are proposing the implementation of appropriateness criteria. Moreover proponents of health care change are floating this concept as the latest administrative nostrum to reduce the intensity of care and at the same time reduce costs and supposedly increase quality. Nonetheless inextricably in accord with the compulsion to apply such overarching criteria, is the danger of succumbing to the same fallacious notions implied in clinical trials although the opportunity for dysfunction is worse.

It must be recognized that every disease has elements of space and time in both the metaphysical and actual sense. The space of a disease relates to in part to its depiction by imaging tests in full view, or in cross, sagittal, coronal or oblique sections at a specific moment in time. For some, the expanse of tissue is too large as the patient is too heavy, so the "appropriate" CT scan cannot be done even though it is foreordained by an algorithmic designation directed to the so-called average patient. Furthermore, such criteria as listed in appropriateness criteria are ahistorical, never in the cascade of tests is a call made for a review of old films which if available still constitute the most informative next study to look at. Such longitudinal aspects do not enter into appropriateness formulation, nor do careful reviews of medical records, lab results and the attitudes and cultural constraints of the patient. Hence it is a fallacy to give primacy to appropriateness criteria which by themselves are not a sacrosanct directive but only an adjunct to diagnostic planning which is sometimes instructive in the fuller context of seeking optimal care and sometimes not applicable and even occasionally mischievous.

I now want to turn to another area of inquiry pursued by radiologists, one that is rife with fallacy. This is the quest for knowledge through information gathering by survey. I am concerned here not just with data gathering per se but also with the topic of the exercise itself. One must consider the anatomy and physiology of surveys. I have some knowledge being an active reviewer for radiologic and emergency medicine journals as well as an investigator utilizing surveys and also as a critic of radiology investigative maneuvers in general. Surveys have been modified by technological innovation which some claim have made the laborious process of data mining easier through the wonderful capabilities of the internet.

Before getting into the fallacies liable to snare a surveyor, here is one verity. All technological advances trumpeted initially as an improvement over past practice will be subject to the more mournful, regretful tones of risk, i.e., complications and uncertainty in the medium term. The wonders of the repeating rifle on the prairies in the 1870s led to the near extinction of the buffalo by 1890. Similarly, the CRT tube manifest in its capabilities is now a cause of ergonomic difficulties by those whose job it is to sit in front of it every day. In like fashion, survey monkeys and other programs of similar ilk allow for a wide ingathering of information accomplished with limited output of time and expense. And yet here are some fallacies about the virtues of electronic questionnaires.

Since an e-survey can be repeated with regularity without recurrent physical mailings and stamp licking though the mediation of the postal service response rates should be higher than with conventional probings by letter. But one must acknowledge the fallacy of insistence especially when the subject is controversial. We recently completed a study of the attitudes of female urology residents towards their training, including questions about sexual harassment by patients and colleagues. Repetitive surveys easily done on-line would have been misleading here. In this context they would account for very few additional responses as we discerned that they would engender resentment by those who did not want to answer such questions in the first mailing of the survey because of the intrusive nature of the subject.

Yet surely web-based surveys are more efficient than conventional surveys by mail. Is this not the real value of electronic dissemination? This is another fallacy. For sensitive questions, many of my respondents have told me that they do not regard an email survey conducted by one who is a stranger to them to be free of hazard. They actually preferred the anonymity of a mailed survey to possible detection by savvy electronic snoopers. This is the fallacy of questionable confidentiality.

A third fallacy is that a paperless survey allows the collection of much more data as it preserves trees. Yet this very possibility in fact tends to corrupt the data received. One cannot expect that a multipage survey will be answered with equal alacrity on page six as it is on page one. It is to be expected that respondents have a limited attention span and may not answer at all the later questions or will reply with impertinence or anger after a few minutes of dealing with a subject for which they do not have high interest. Thus one should question the extensive internet survey for its inherent validity. For later questions no matter if responses can be transmitted by email or sneaker mail, fatigue may vitiate reliability. Hence for me, the old way is less fallacy-suspect, less subject to suspicion of quality of the data. The shorter the survey, the more reliable the results even if less expansive the scope of the investigation.

Yet I have only drilled down a little so far in my exploration of fallacies. In the next essay I will discuss among other points the fundamental insights of Tversky and Kahnemann, for which the latter won the Nobel Prize in Economics even though he is a psychologist. Their explorations in the presumption of hypothesis generation and the impress of fallacy bear noting for all intellectual disciplines, Radiology included.

Reference

1. Kahneman D. Thinking, fast and slow. New York: Farrar, Straus and Giroux; 2011.

A plea for the relevance of the topic of fallacies is that for me, and I hope for you, a discussion of errors and argumentation is in fact helpful for successful management of any radiological enterprise be it direction of a department or simply interaction between one radiologist and a colleague who may be a fellow radiologist, a referring physician or an administrator. The opportunity to engage in dialog is inevitable and commonplace even if some radiologists prefer the security of physical isolation. Making your position known is important for your business and I daresay your self-respect. So join with me in a recitation of a few mistaken notions your associates might make but you should not.

The watchword is fallacies, which can be defined as false reasoning often from true factual premises so that false conclusions are generated. Since the articulator of a fallacy is often convinced of the veracity of his claims, a fallacy is a self-deception. But it refers not just to one point made at one time on one issue but rather to a predilection to argue falsely repetitively in other circumstances. So a fallacy is not merely an error but a means of falling into error.

I have been guided in these thoughts by two sources. The first is David Hackett Fischer's book, Historical Fallacies published 40 years ago but enduringly relevant not just for matters of historical content but also for daily discourse. The second is the collective work of Tversky and Kahnemann whose insights into subjective assessment of probability, biases and judgments under uncertainty have exposed the fallacious reasoning within seemingly logical thought paradigms.

The roster of fallacies is long and I offer here a sampler that can be relevant to radiology. My first example is the fallacy of the exalted human. You are uncertain about the necessity or advisability of an imaging test. But your reluctance is challenged by the statement of the advocating physician. "If it was your mother, wouldn't you want the test?" Often this is a powerful pronouncement. You might in an instant picture your mother, ill, vulnerable and possibly to be helped by the examination in question even though you know it is likely superfluous and may incur some risk as well increased cost. Often you cave in to the emotional compulsion engendered by dragging your mother into the scenario.

Yet what is that argument based on? It is a consequence of the fallacy that there are two types of humans. Class (2) everybody else; Class (1) your mother. She is more worthy, more important, more exalted. But should she be? Shouldn't we care about everybody the same, at least with a valuation of efficacy or a minimization of discomfort? Of course we should. Your mother's value to you is not germane to your patient's needs and concerns. You can only overcome the appeal of this fallacy by noting it. When you do, most often the proponent of the exalted human fallacy will beat a hasty retreat.

A second compelling fallacy relates to a lexicographical error. Unfortunate does not mean unfair. They are by no means equivalent although they are often considered to be synonymous, sometimes

S.R. Baker, *Notes of a Radiology Watcher*,
DOI 10.1007/978-3-319-01677-1_36, © Springer International Publishing Switzerland 2014

with bad tidings for radiologists. It is crucial to recognize this fallacy but you must be attuned to it. For many it has been an effective conjunction learned by children and carried to adulthood in both private and professional life. A child loses a game and claims her defeat is unfair; a young adult loses a job possibility because others who interviewed had better qualifications yet he calls the proceedings unfair; and a 42 year old woman has breast cancer initially undetected by mammography. You missed it, she calls it unfair and seeks to sue you. But a bad outcome only sometimes is due to stacking the deck to not favor you, to willful action by a hostile decision-maker. Probably more often than not it is bad luck that befalls you. If you do not realize the distinction you are likely to accede to the conclusion if not the demands of the complainant even though you are not at fault.

The mammography example is front page news at this writing. Breast cancer in a woman in the fifth decade of life is often a rapidly progressive disease. The popular belief in the omnipotence of medical technology is that bad things should not happen and if it does it should be detected so it can be cured. Many women believe it is their right to live to the average life expectancy of female Americans, about 80 years. They say it is unfair that I am now likely to suffer much and die young.

Hence, it is your fault that I got this disease. Even though my breasts are dense, you erred. Well, this is a classic case of the substitution of unfair for unfortunate, a distinction society at large tends not to see. As radiologists it is incumbent on us to make that differentiation, to expose the fallacy which if left to "fester" will harm not just the unfortunate patient but the physician who ministers to her.

A recent article regarding the regulations of the Radiology Resident Review Committee, of which incidentally I have been a member, criticized the six competency requirement in particular and the surveillance project of the ACGME in general. Instead the author argued for the removal of regulatory strictures, replacing them with a plea for freedom in curricular opportunities to create a model of education based on trust. Here is the either/or position. Abandon what is now for what I propose. This is the fallacy of the false dichotomy question, an invidious device which if accepted leads to conclusions that are sometimes dangerous if followed as they are based on a logically incorrect premise. There are very few mutually exclusive, collectively exhaustive dichotomies save for mathematical constructs and the distinctions of life from death. In all other instances there is an overlap of the two presumed polarities or there is a middle ground between the two having elements of both or neither. A dichotomy proposal is not correct when what is demanded is a demarcation that is not exclusive or exhaustive in its separateness. In fact the competencies if embraced as a means of introducing innovation and experimentation can foster creativity in curricular design and stimulate investigative activity. And even if such possibilities were not so obvious, there would still be in nearly every instance no way to perfectly bisect actuality into two neat halves. Compelling in its strident advocacy, a plea to opt for the unrealized choice in a dichotomy is false on its face [1].

These three examples are but a few examples of the kaleidoscopic facets of fallacy. They relate to how a question is framed. Often such fallacies have seductive appeal at the outset. Once detected, their illogic can be revealed. But fallacies can also result from error in fact specification and from mistakes in generalization from motivation and from the presumption of the pertinence of analogy which is a referential tool at best and not a simulation of reality. The point here is that fallacies occur in many rhetorical formats and can be discerned only by inserting skepticism before acknowledging acceptance.

Reference

1. Kahneman D. Thinking, fast and slow. New York: Farrar, Straus and Giroux; 2011.

We Are Radiologists: What Business Are We in?

The title of this essay on its face seems contradictory. Of course we know what business we are in. Don't we? Well how should we answer that? You and I are experts in the interpretation of images of the human body generated by a variety of energy sources. We are also experts in the implications of the abnormalities we recognize and in the appearances of the spectrum of normality. And increasingly in both of these manifestations of illness and lack of illness, we gain perception of both its static and dynamic configurations.

Well, that is the substance of our intellectual labor but our main business is consultation and communication. Such a distinction is important for how we comport ourselves, how we make ourselves and our expertise available, how we relate to referrers and patients, all of which are dimensions of our job as important as and separable from our capabilities as diagnosticians. Fundamentally, the distinction between our craft and our business is akin to that of animated movie makers who possess special knowledge to create alluring images but whose salable product is wonder and diversion.

So how do we perform in a very specific environment; a large hospital. Do we tend to our business as I have defined it?

Radiologists tend to decry the incursions of other medical practitioners into the territories we consider our own. We all hear the litany from many of our leaders about how much (some say even more than half of imaging) is done by physicians in other specialties who purchase and use their own machines for their enrichment. True enough but radiologists presentiments and the exigencies of our partially regulated market place do not necessarily have to coincide. We also rightfully complain about intra-hospital competition by others such as E.R. physicians who after a few days of attending at a course claim competence in ultrasonography and by vascular surgeons who want a piece of the angiography pie.

Yet, by and large, in major hospitals and in their associated outpatient clinics and imaging centers, radiology remains a monopoly. No one else is allowed to do breast imaging. The CT and MR machines are ours by ownership or usufruct. PET/CT is almost always a province of radiology and so forth. Yet, too often as a monopoly we adopt and maintain the business ideology of one who has no competition, especially when it involves our core functions of communication and consultation.

I have spent considerable time traveling abroad, occasionally to less developed countries whose governments are controlled by dictators or cabals. These leaders make sure they control public means of communication, a reality best understood, perhaps, by watching daytime TV there. The fare on the tube is humdrum, consisting of programs the leaders want you to see which glorifies their accomplishments. Everything else is so boring you want to turn off the set. And you know what passes for real news is censored. That is because information is not free on the media, it is not customer oriented, it is subject to the practice of the monopolist in charge. Remember when there were just three networks in American television and AT&T was the telephone monopoly. Now the airwaves are wide open, the means of image transmission have expanded and customer enticement and satisfaction is a key feature of any entertainment and news enterprise. In fact the two are often connected. Hence, when the providers of information are not directly accountable to their audience, the products they provide might not be suitable to their listeners and viewers needs and wants.

So let me return now to your radiology department if it is a large hospital where your group is in charge of pictures and their interpretation. How do you get the news out? Who do you send critical findings to and how quickly? How do you locate referrers? What standards do you use to determine if a finding is critical? How do you document that you have made the communication and initiated a consultation when the situation requires it.

At an annual Radiology Intersociety Conference several years ago, which incidentally used to be called the Radiation Summit, the subject was communication. There it was expressed, by several speakers, and acknowledged by the attendees, a nearly unanimous view that the transmission of results of imaging tests had gotten exceedingly complex. The conventional wisdom was that telephone numbers of referrers were changing all the time and one could often not be sure who the ordering physician was and even, if that was known, it was too frequently not clear who the results of a test with emergent findings should be sent to expeditiously. And even if that could be determined in any one instance there was no consensus on how the relevant information should be relayed, in person, on the phone, by fax, email or by an expanding roster of new systems that automatically register when a prompt communication was received even without a conversation between the radiologists and the pertinent caregiver.

I have come across several research papers which attempt to quantify this vexing problem. Together, there is among them a consistency of frustration. The majority of respondents, resident and attendings, assert that it is difficult to reach referrers, that they did not receive guidance as to what results constitute the need for immediate communication, that they were unsure who was the appropriate individual to receive an important result before the receipt of the dictated report. For some a medical student was an acceptable link and for others a call to the ward or clinic without specifying a designated individual would suffice as an indication that the radiologists had fully discharged his or her responsibility. In one study I had the occasion to look at, the maximum number of crucial findings per morning or afternoon readout was not many, at most five with the average just two. Some even stated that they often did not call in critical findings because they were too busy with their work. One should wonder what work at any one time would be more important than the prompt dissemination of a crucial finding.

What this catalog of inadequacy says to me is that in the context of hospital practice we as radiologists are content with this sorry state of affairs. We explain away our inadequacy by pleading overwhelming complexity. It is not that at all. Rather it is blatant management failure because by the way we do our work and the lack of competition for it, one can be dismissive about our core mission.

Do you think a patient would be satisfied with a system in which he or she could not reach his caregiver emergently? Such physicians would not be in business very long or maintain their reputations if they were deemed to be unreachable or did not have coverage. Because we are those physician's consultants it is incumbent on us to know how to reach them at all times or get in touch with their covering caregivers or support team at all times.

This is not difficult. It only appears that way because many of us choose not to make an effort. With email, Facebook and other social networking systems readily available, there should be no excuse not to relay important findings immediately. Moreover, the manager of the radiology department should know much more about the communication particularities of every referrer in the same way and with the same diligence that a successful company knows much about its customers, their predilections, habits and idiosyncrasies. It is easy to do if you have the will. The excuses that hospital monopolist radiologists provide should be regarded as nothing more than laziness.

Now what findings should be transmitted immediately? Here I take issue with the latest ACR recommendations. I agree with their insistence that life threatening findings must be communicated verbally and immediately. But then they make a distinction for important but non-emergent finding like the discovery of a lung nodule for which it is deemed acceptable that the direct conversation with the referrers take place after a while. Some even say that a 72 h delay is OK.

For those who regard this up to 3 day delay as constituting a standard of care, I refer you to examine judgments made against radiologists as revealed in summaries listed in the National Practitioners Data Bank. A frequent scenario is the patient who has died or is near death from lung cancer which first came to attention as a lung nodule years before. But the radiologist's report never reached the referring physician or the primary provider never acknowledged receiving it and claimed to never received a call about it. The typical circumstance was the presentation to the E.R. on the weekend at which time both the emergency physician and the radiologist on duty were part-timers. The report never got to the physician who could follow the patient and the 3 day delay enabled the dictated report to lie fallow. As a result, the cancer grew undetected despite its initial recognition in time for a cure.

There should be no difference in the rapid personal responding of a crucial result with respect to the present conditions of the patient, whether he or she is now at death's door or will by neglect get there later but prematurely [1].

OK maybe you agree or maybe you are not in accord with these specifics. Nonetheless you should concede that collectively we have to do a better job of communicating urgent findings. We must set up procedures prospectively and monitor

them as key Q.A. indicators so there will never be a lapse for any reason including the woeful excuses I stated before. How can we do it? We have largely instituted a range of procedures in our facility to overcome the inertia.

We know the number of all our referrers both in hospital and beyond the hospital. Mostly this is accomplished by lists generated by our radiology subspecialists interacting with their roster of referrers. Our policy is to call in all critical results regardless of the supposed latency of their clinical expression. Our hospital policy is to only direct our verbal declarations to doctors (attendings and residents) and designated nurses and P.A.'s, never to medical students or other personnel. The record of the communication is included in the dictated report. An appropriate documentation in the report includes the conveying of the diagnosis, the name of the physician or appropriate physician's designee, the location of the receiving care giver and the date and time of the day- A.M. or P.M. or military time. We also are specific about time of day. If the conversation took place at 1:14A.M. we don't write at night, at 1 o'clock or at 1:15A.M. but the actual time, 1:14A.M.

How do we monitor compliance? As Chair of the department, I regard surveillance of communication of reports as one of my main administrative responsibilities-one I do not delegate. Thus I review 10 reports of each resident every 6 weeks for style, accuracy and for adherence to our communication standards. It is a major error for a resident to report the presence of an important finding in the dictated report but to not include also in that report a record of the verbal communication with the relevant caregiver. And I do the same review every quarter with each of my attendings even if they have a close relationship with their cadre of referrers.

It is amazing how clinical colleagues can become adversaries when a significant finding is supposedly reported but not acted upon because there was no record of verbal communication between the radiologist and clinician. As consultants there is nothing we do that is more crucial. And today even though we may remain the only image interpreters on the scene, we should not assume as acceptable an effort of direct interaction that is longer than the minimal response any consumer servicing organization would provide to its customers.

Reference

1. Baker SR. The transmission of non-emergent critical findings, communication vs. consultation. Radiology. 2010;257:609–11.

Communication vs. Consultation: Two Duties We Must Pursue

38

I would like in this essay to delve into the subject of the radiologist's interaction with referrers. In the preceding discussion I hinted at this obligation. What is most important about our tasks for the sake of our patients was not just the interpretation of findings but also the character and quality of the physician-to-physician transactions that followed from your observations as manifested in your reports. Moreover, our responsibility is not limited to the recognition of abnormalities. It is concerned, too, with the integration of our expertise with other elements of care. For that we needed to consult with referrers and, more to the point, to make those exchanges central to our daily work.

But in our assessment of the essentials of practice, I have noted a subtle deviation from that aim toward another function that some might consider similar or, at least, analogous to our consultative responsibilities. Yet it is one which when substituted for consultation often lessens our value to a degree and therefore diminishes the excellence (or at least the pertinence) of the care we can provide. That distinctive outreach activity is verbal communication. It is such a common exercise why should anyone criticize it. Let me try.

Much is made of our relationships with other physicians through directed communication. It is the focus of policy statements by our leaders articulated through regulations and recommendations. Nonetheless, by itself a communication can certainly disseminate information but it also, in its conventional format, imposes uncertainty

and risk, two untoward consequences consultation largely obviates. I will attempt to explain this issue by undertaking a detailed analysis of the ambiguities inherent in the ACR's guidelines for the Communication of Diagnostic Findings, specifically the latest iteration of them promulgated in 2005.

In the first paragraph of the preamble to these guidelines a disclaimer is provided. "They are not inflexible rules or requirements of practice and are not intended, nor should they be designated to establish a legal standard of care". Unfortunately, that is wishful thinking because these guidelines are often invoked by plaintiff lawyers as the written embodiment of the standard of care, useful in providing a touchstone to which a defendant radiologist may fail to adhere. So with the specter of legal proceedings in mind we must regard them for their prescriptive implications and not merely as advisory messages.

Here we have the crux of the matter. It is the replacement of our potentially consultative role supplanted by an often more flexible means of offering information, through pronouncement instead of colloquy. In that regard, my attention with this set of guidelines is focused on section C. 2 entitled Non-routine Communication. It is described as occurring in "emergent or other non-routine clinical situations" for which "the diagnosing images should expedite the delivery of a diagnostic imaging report (preliminary or final) in a manner that reasonably insures timely receipt of the findings". There are three distinct situations in which there would be a need for non-routine

S.R. Baker, *Notes of a Radiology Watcher*,
DOI 10.1007/978-3-319-01677-1_38, © Springer International Publishing Switzerland 2014

communication. The first two are obvious i.e., first a finding in which is demonstrated a need for immediate or urgent intervention and, second, an observation that is different from a preceding interpretation. The third situation is the one that stimulates the most malpractice suits. It relates to "Findings that the interpreting physician reasonably believes may be seriously adverse to the patient's health and are unexpected by the treating or referring physician".

The next paragraph with respect to the third situation is the most problematic one. The words are pregnant with ambiguity and as such are the basis of contentions if and when such findings are either not reported or if reported are not received by the referring physician or if received are not perceived, understood or acted upon by the recipient caregiver.

The key statement in this section of the guideline is "These cases may not require immediate attention but, if not acted upon, may worsen over time and possibly result in an adverse patient outcome".

Allow me to ponder with you that last sentence. First, what does "may not require" mean. The dictionary definition of require is clear and unequivocal. It is to have need of; to place under an obligation or necessity. In other words, to require is to demand. There is no wiggle room with require. Thus, the phrase "may require" creates a potentially confusing antithesis which annuls the import and impact of require. There is no volition in require. To make it contingent renders it non-operative. So according to the guideline one must definitely or just as plausibly need not at all report such a finding. In other words here is a guideline that provides no guidance.

What is it one may or may not require? It should be an immediate response in order to make the referrers aware of the presence of a finding promptly. Yet the recommendation allows the deferral of the communication of information from radiologist to referring physician to some later time. Now many have interpreted the acceptable delay to be 48 h. But the record of lawsuits related to the missed reporting of a newly recognized pulmonary nodule is replete with delayed and then uncompleted connections. The longer the interval between detection and attempted communication the more likely the referring physician or his designee or his replacement will not be informed.

Moreover, if one is uncertain about the obligation to report, one is still left with the problem that the abnormality "may possibly" result in an adverse patient outcome. However, what does "possibly" mean across the spectrum of eventualities? Perhaps nothing terrible in the next case. But given many such cases, "possibly" assuredly means inevitably. So for many of us working every day the ambiguity inherent in the phrase "may not require" will at some time by immediate choice or delayed consideration turn into the tragedy of a recognized and treatable abnormality becoming an untreated fatal condition.

The fault here is both the overly permissive but actually inconclusive guideline (an oxymoron in effect) and the flawed process for the transmission of information. These guidelines have been conceived with communication as a goal and are thus aptly named. The presumption is that by such communication we are pursuing a normative practice as we participate as caregivers. But by doing so do we do our best'? Is supposedly normative optimal and if not is optimal achievable?

Whatever their or your political views, many people regarded Ronald Reagan as the Great Communicator. He spoke to us and made his positions clear even if we did not agree with him. But did you have the opportunity to talk to him? No, because communication need not and rarely is a reciprocal engagement. Communication, according to the dictionary, is to divulge, announce, disclose or reveal. The process imparts knowledge from articulator to hearer or reader. In a communication something is sent and presumably received. It is unidirectional. Comprehension, analysis and feedback are not integral to it. The emphasis is on transmission. Thus, an excellent communicator is adept at the timely and cogent transfer of data and opinion to a responsive referrer who is expected to take it from there.

But is that enough or does expert care on our part demand more? As a communicator of radiologic information a standard scenario is as follows: You find a nodule on the one chest film and recommend a CT for further evaluation. Your advice is received and the CT is ordered. Have you really fulfilled your obligations to the patient here? Sometimes maybe but surely not always, because you have communicated but not consulted.

Consultation is defined as an encounter involving a conversation. Its setting is a meeting in which occur deliberation, discussion and often decision. It is bidirectional. Intrinsic to it is a dialog permitting an interchange. Perhaps if you had consulted with the referring physician about that nodule you would have found out that the patient had a chest x-ray somewhere else two years ago and the density is the same size and shape now as it was then. So no CT scan is needed nor would a biopsy be necessary. The scenario of tests and procedures often diverges when consultation replaces communication.

In consultation, one finds a multidimensional interaction between the radiologist, who in the present knows about imaging findings and the referring physician with access to old studies, current lab data and a record of part illness. Together the knowledge possessed by each of these two physicians complement each other and enriches the diagnostic enterprise, as they jointly bring vital data and expertise to the process of clinical decision-making.

Part of the allure and power of Radiology over the past 40 years in which its scope and reach has expanded so greatly has been the adoption of new technologies for the generations of images and the movement of information. But every innovation welcomed initially for its utility is inevitably accompanied by untoward consequences in the middle term. The phenomenal growth of CT has now engendered concern about deposition of radiation dose. The growth of imaging in general has brought with it increasing costs which if they continue to burgeon may make healthcare as we know it unsustainable. And the electronic movement of words and pictures has been fostered by the widespread deployment of P.A.C.S. The C in this acronym stands for communication not consultation.

In fact, communication is now so easy it can be done at anytime from anywhere. It does not have to place the transmitter of information in verbal contact with the intended receiver of his or her message. But the ease of instituting consultation even by electronic means has not matched the versatile application of communication programs. Dialog demands the coexistence of the radiologist and referrer whereas simultaneity of attention is not a requirement of communication. Consequently, the impetus for the substitution of communication by consultation must overcome an energy and intention gradient. The change can be relatively inconvenient even if vital. To establish the primacy of consultation in the Radiologist's armamentarium demands leadership, operating under the realization that mutually informing discussion between referrer and radiologist is better than unanswered directives issued from cyberspace.

It is informative to evaluate how the communication-consultant dichotomy has expressed itself in policy generation. In the recent history of Radiology this can be discerned by reference to authoritative statements by radiology organizations about it and by the extent of contributions about each of them as presented in the major journals in our specialty.

Much work has gone into the elaboration of principles and practice of communication by radiologists. In this report I have evaluated my assessment of the flaws in the ACR's guidelines on the subject. Yet there are no such detailed guidelines for consultation. We have searched the titles of Radiology and AJR over the past 50 years and evaluated the meager assemblage of articles that deal with either consultation or communication. For the latter we have excluded titles that refer to mechanical issues about communication functions such as articles on PACS implementation. Rather, we have compared only the frequency of reports that deal with the concept of communication and consultation. Over the last 50 years there were 74 articles which have been concerned with consultation. Only a very few provided data, the remainder were in the main speculative and even wistful rumination about consultation as a desideratum. The number of such contributions to these two journals has varied little with each decade [1].

On the other hand, communication-focused articles were rare until 1990, with only 12 titles in 30 years. And for the past 20 years, they were the subject of on average just one article per year.

Yet during the past score of years, policies and practices regarding communication have been presented and revised in response most often to the opportunities and challenges offered by PACS and related innovations. For consultation, the thrust of published reports has been more atmospheric than substantial. In effect, overall the literature offers lip service to the notion of consultation and little else.

Yet even if consultation is what we should do, communication is what it seems we want to do.

The result is that major manifestation of our special skills and, in great measure, our legitimacy as experts has not been fully realized. Too often by relying on well-meaning communication alone we foster overutilization and subject patients to risky studies. And equally important, in the face of the broadening incorporation of imaging into the contemporary practice of all specialties, we place in jeopardy as well the vitality and vibrancy of our specialty.

Reference

1. Baker SR. The transmission of non-emergent critical findings, communication vs. consultation. Radiology. 2010;257:609–11.

Part VII

Quality Considerations

Quality must be a hallmark of what we do. In this section specifics are provided and innovative initiatives, both in general and in particular, are described.

The issue of quality is a radiology imperative. Some of you may not know that there are almost 75 various organizations in Radiology, which I call "balkanization" in the extreme. Nonetheless each year about 45 societies meet to discuss a particular topic, At a recent meeting quality was the subject. There the participants were placed in three large committees for the purpose of providing recommendations on metrics for quality. 78 proposals were proffered by the committees which were further distilled into 48 separate notions that could each frame a metric. Bear in mind that results of this meeting of minds should not be regarded as a document which stands on its own as authoritative. Really what it represents is a set of preliminary statements to engender focus on matters of quality. Whether these proposals will be implemented by the American College of Radiology or any other group depends upon a consensus about their pertinence and validity which frankly requires widespread rank and file Radiologist impact about their merits or lack thereof.

The 48 different recommendations were placed into four groups (1) Access and Appropriateness, (2) Patient Safety, (3) Radiology Report, and (4) Satisfaction Surveys. In this discussion, I will not go through all of them. Instead I will discuss a few, providing some comment reflecting my opinion with either approbation or criticism. As I pointed out in the previous essay, appropriateness is an admirable concept but without committed participation by referring physicians it will be difficult to implement any such measures related to algorithms for the choice and sequencing of imaging examination- no matter how noble and farsighted they may appear to be in concept.

Nonetheless, even though the task is daunting there should be some movement in this area beyond the mere promulgation of a recommendation. In essence, a sanctioned, structured dialog with our clinical colleagues for "buy in" is essential.

On the other hand, access issues have been made more clear cut and well defined. I believe some of the measures here should be implemented promptly by every department. The first three relate to quality measures for the initiation of a radiology transaction. They are, respectively, the percent of phone calls answered within X minutes, the percent of patients scheduled within X minutes of initiating a phone call, and the percent of time for which the third available time for an imaging exam appointment is available within X days. The third available time for an imaging exam is standard for other practices and other specialties. It reflects the outer limit within which schedulers most operate to serve patients. Remember this is not the first or second available time, but the third time which must be accommodated to merit adherence to quality.

It has been very rewarding at our institution to carefully monitor the percent of phone calls answered within a certain period of time. We restrict it to six rings before labeling the call an outlier. The tardy response must be investigated. As you know from being a patient or consumer, waiting for someone to answer a phone call can

S.R. Baker, *Notes of a Radiology Watcher*,
DOI 10.1007/978-3-319-01677-1_39, © Springer International Publishing Switzerland 2014

be exasperating. Moreover, it is rude and will likely initiate a negative comment on a satisfaction survey. The second metric, the percent of patients scheduled in x minutes from a received phone call reflects the quality of the reception staff and the scheduling staff. In terms of the esteem of your operation, these individuals are probably just as important as the radiologists themselves in relation to patient satisfaction. Such are a few of the matters to be considered and measured in terms of the initiation of a visit to radiology. How about when a patient comes to your facility, how is he or she taken care of? In this context a valid metric would be the percent of patients who begin an examination within x minutes of registration at the examination facility. Some of you as patients may have experienced this scenario. You went to a very successful physician and had to wait for a long period of time before being served. There the insensitive nurse or physician might have said—well we were very busy that day in order to explain away the delay you suffered. But that is an admission of failure not of success. Our job is to take care of patients expeditiously. Of course, it is certainly true that unanticipated delays can interrupt a carefully planned schedule. But that should be deemed an aberration not an acceptable, commonplace standard.

Metrics related to the internal operation of the department with respect to access were also proposed. Included in this category were (1) the frequency with which equipment is down, stratified by modality and (2) the frequency with which information technology infrastructure is inoperative.

We are highly, dependent upon very sophisticated devices for the production of images and the transmission of information. These metrics are important as a way of valuing how effective is the equipment and how effective is your staff in servicing that equipment, especially in relation to IT. Furthermore, how much down time you experience relates to how you are dealing with vendors inasmuch as service is just as important as purchase.

Several of the 48 metrics are germane to patient safety. A few I do not mention here because I believe they lack measurability. But others are absolutely critical. The ones I cite are couched in terms of frequency, yet it is probably best to state that even one deviation from the metric should be regarded as grounds for generating an incident report. Moreover, for each, such a deviation could be the cause of a malpractice case with you as a defendant. Here is a sample: the frequency with which patients are screened for pregnancy before using ionizing radiation in women of child bearing age. You must have an ironclad assessment procedure so that in the absence of truly special circumstances, women who may be pregnant are not irradiated to their chest, abdomen, or pelvis. And the next one, the frequency in which patients are screened before intravenous contrast administration is equally crucial, given the fact that for in-patients at least, contrast induced nephropathy is the most common cause of renal failure. A recent review in JAMA stresses this issue in detail. In our facility we get a BUN and creatinine for every patient who has not had each of these lab measures in the past month. We enforce this rule strenuously despite the occasional protestations of referring physicians. It is our responsibility not to induce contrast nephropathy and if that means the study is not done until the laboratory data is in then so be it. A third patient safety initiative in this regard is the frequency with which patients are screened before undergoing a MR exam. Obviously here, screening is critical. One untoward event could be dangerous to the patient and if it occurred, it could shut you down forever. The likelihood is low, but the consequence of an MR event could be dire.

Another class of safety measures should not record, God forbid, even one violation. They are the frequency in which the exam is performed on the wrong patient, the frequency in which the wrong side of the correct patient is examined, the frequency in which the wrong examination was performed on the correct patient and the frequency in which less than two forms of patient identification were inspected before the examination occurred. For these any deviation from proper procedure should stimulate a careful analysis so that such mistakes can never be repeated.

Consider if you will an anecdote from our own institution; we had two instances of the wrong examination being performed on two separate patients over the course of 3 weeks. Well we can play the shame and blame game and fault the receptionist who caused the error. However, the mistakes were inevitable because placed on duty alone she had to answer the phone and perform several other tasks nearly simultaneously on her watch during the lunch hour when we are the most busy. We learned the hard way from this event to stagger the lunch hour so we have at least two people in this capacity at any one time. Neither is therefore so hurried that such errors are likely and each checks the other. Yet by careful planning you need not have to learn as we did.

Quality: Measures in Radiology

In other essays in this monograph, I touched on some of the difficulties radiologists face in trying to determine if what they do is best for patients. The focus of my criticism was not the concept but rather the measurement of appropriateness criteria, the product of a noble effort undertaken through the auspices of the American College of Radiology to offer what some may view as the most proper sequence of tests to reach a diagnosis for many clinical applications. I viewed the methodology as flawed, especially because the criteria are based on radiologists, if you will, "speaking to" but not "conversing with" referring physicians. As a program, appropriateness criteria are deployed in a manner both insular and distant, consistent with our customary practice patterns. We are a special type of medical consultant. Typically we do not see the patient or even know much about him or her before making a judgment about a diagnostic plan. In its present iteration appropriateness criteria will be ineffective until we also establish a formalized reciprocal dialog with referrers. Our remoteness is by itself self-defeating with respect to affecting change for the sake of better rather than more utilization of imaging resources.

Yet, the impetus behind the creation of appropriateness criteria is compelling. American medicine is pluralistic (perhaps a virtue and vice at the same time), inordinately expensive so that it continues to take a large and enlarging piece of the national economic pie and not necessarily of the highest quality despite the repeatedly articulated self-congratulating messages that "it is the best in the world".

Well, consumers may believe that we are doing very well but payers and government, payers too, in their own right are increasingly skeptical. By now, nearly everyone knows about the IOM indictment through the publication of "To Err is Human" in 1999, focusing on preventable errors and patient safety. In 2001 the IOM report "Crossing the Quality Chasm" offered means for initiating value-directed purchasing which lead to further publications related to financial incentives to achieve a higher level of performance.

Even before 1999 innovations for the sake of quality were being tested. Most of them concentrated on patient management, not the diagnostic interval. Before proceeding we should recognize that quality can be understood in relation to a tripartite dynamic involving (1) structure, an arrangement of facilities and interactions among them separate from patient encounters, in a sense the anatomy of quality (2) process—the actions taken in the delivery of medical attention which could be considered the physiology of care and (3) outcome—the result of structural and process change with respect to the efficiency and efficacy of both diagnosis evaluations and the treatment of the ill and injured.

Outcome research, especially focused in diagnostic imaging, is now and has been very limited. Force of use and economic incentives are the engines driving most of us to do more. Both not only enable us to maintain income in the face of declining reimbursement per procedure, but also to do more expensive tests to alter the mix of reimbursement in our favor and especially to promote and adopt new radiology technology so as not to lose out in the battle for sophisticated toys and market share as we contend with other specialties. In outcome studies quality improvement initiatives have not been predominant considerations in our specialty. For example, the evolving concern for dose has arisen slowly and tentatively amidst the rapid deployment of new CT equipment, each notable for their enhanced imaging power occasioned by the production of more closely packed slices, each providing an additional measure of radiation.

Three mechanisms have been presented to achieve quality improvement. The center of excellence model seeks to identify facilities showing the best results for a particular treatment or procedure so as to direct patients there. This could be accomplished by payers contracting only with these sites or by urging patients to seek care at those facilities to the exclusion of other clinics and hospitals. For example, the Leapfrog Group, a coalition of employers including many large corporations providing generous health benefits to their workers, directs cases to hospitals successfully pursuing evidence-based medicine for five surgical procedures. For each of which a minimum component of quality is the realization of a volume benchmark. Yet, such initiatives often do not take into account variations in patient population with respect to risk as a component of decision making and resource allocation.

More popular than centers of excellence is the concept of pay for performance abbreviated as P4P. This mechanism has as its goal the rewarding of good performance with financial incentives. CMS has taken the lead here. For example, appropriate use of antibiotics with respect to treatment of particular clinical presentations could result in more money for a hospital. Obviously, behavior will tend to follow the money. Yet many P4P proposals may include structure and process change, but we don't really know if outcome is altered. And the process can be gamed to the detriment of patients. Like any other innovation unforeseen and unintended consequences can ensue, especially for P4P in which a reductionist approach is necessary to isolate a particular treatment regimen so results can be measured and providers rewarded or punished. For example CMS has mandated that when a patient comes to the ER with signs and symptoms of pneumonia, a chest X-ray must be done expeditiously and after a positive image, antibiotics are to be administered within 4 h. So now at our ER nearly every asthmatic gets a chest X-ray because after all they may have pneumonia. Yet data from studies in the 1980s have shown that in otherwise healthy asthmatics presenting with a fever below 101 °F and no elevation in WBC, the likelihood of pneumonia is *very* low. Our extremely low positive chest X-ray rate in such patients confirms this clinical fact.

Moreover, patients with CHF also can be short of breath and have infiltrates on a chest radiograph. Nonetheless, to practice according to this quality directive, many patients are receiving antibiotics but do not need them. A simple quality measure can be helpful with respect to a simple problem. Yet patients often suffer from several diseases together for which close attention to the use of antibiotics could be a distraction and may be deleterious if ultimately not indicated.

A third mechanism of quality improvement is known as pay for participation. This strategy for provider-led quality enhancement is to encourage groups of physicians and hospitals to collaborate with each other to undertake large prospective studies relating to the institution of scientifically established best practices. Providers are paid for their participation not for their performance. The prospect is to develop meaningful outcomes data that can be broadly applied, including some measures of risk stratification and risk adjustment. Registries would be developed. Pay for participation requires cooperation not competition. Outcome experience will become available in the medium term, not immediately. Public reporting, not often a palatable notion for many facilities is central to the process. As such pay for participation schemes may not find favor.

The ACR knows that among the three strategic ploys P4P is the most immediately attractive and available for implementation. Accordingly it was the subject of their annual intersociety meeting. At that session performance indices were agreed upon for further development and possibly wide-scale use. In the next essay I will present those measures and discuss their relationship to structure, process, and outcome. Some I strongly favor. But for others I will describe what may be unanticipated and perhaps controversial consequences related to their adoption as a quality standard.

Quality: Initiatives You Should Know About But May Not Have Heard About

41

Unless you are spending your working time under the protection of and within the shelter of the proverbial rock you should be aware of the advancing impress of the concept, methods and policy demands of quality as it impinges on the practice of Medicine in the U.S. in general and the practice of radiology in your facility in particular. The facts and the folklore relating to quality are no longer recondite matters. Whatever your views on the Affordable Care Act, you know that measurements of quality are going to be matters for which you must become knowledgeable. For example, in a recent issue of JACR there is an article entitled "Medicare's Physician Quality Reporting System: Early National Radiologists Experience and Near-Future Performance Projections", which is a report on the utilization of Medicare's Pay for Performance program known under the acronym PQRS. The program enables bonuses to be paid by those who comply with reporting and documentation obligations which are detailed and specific. The earliest bonuses to those who comply, that is those issued from 2007 to the present, will then reduce in amount through 2014. Then the "stick" of penalties will replace the "carrot" of financial awards by 2015. In the following year it will amount to 2 % of Medicare payments to individual physicians. It is clear that this program has "teeth" and that all of us, current participants and non-participants alike, should be aware of them for their financial implications for one thing and for the maintenance of our professional qualifications including MOC satisfaction for another.

But while this particular initiative will garner our attention, more and more, I wish to alert you to another one, a program I suspect most of you have not heard about unless you actively (1) practice in an academic environment and (2) are intimately involved in resident education and their accreditation obligations.

I am referring here to the newly announced C.L.E.R. program, which was developed by the ACGME. To explain the alphabet soup of acronyms before proceeding onward, the ACGME stands for the Accreditation Committee for Graduate Medical Education, a government sanctioned but independent organization charged with monitoring compliance with accreditation rules for all allopathic residency programs and by 2015 for all osteopathic training programs as well.

The ACGME has on its board public members, a government representative and delegates from a range of organizations including the AMA, the American Hospital Association, the Council of State Medical Societies and the American Board of Medical Specialties. Under the ACGME's board are separate RRCs or Residency Review Committees for each specialty. The Radiology RRC for example is responsible for the oversight for all primary diagnostic programs in our specialty, all fellowships in neuroradiology, pediatric radiology and interventional radiology and some programs in abdominal radiology and musculoskeletal radiology. Each RRC has one resident member. On the Radiology RRC there are nine other members- three members each chosen, by the AMA, the ACR and the ABR respectively and approved by current RRC members as replacements. ACGME-directed initiatives like the imposition of duty hour rules nearly 10 years ago are a result usually of policy initiatives spawned from the Institute of Medicine-which then influences Congress which in turn pressures the ACGME to institute change in the regulation of resident education. Now the emphasis is on quality and CLER, the acronym I mentioned, is one result of this political process. CLER stands for Clinical Learning Environment Review. Oversight of its activities will function much like a JACHO inspection process. With little advanced notification, outside reviewers from the ACGME will visit each teaching hospital and at random will engage residents, among others, in conversation with respect to how house officers and the administration of the hospital are in meaningful ways engaged in establishing and effectuating means of improving quality definitely, but not remotely nor in delayed fashion as measured by quantitative outcomes. The CLER scorecard has six categories. For the purpose of this discussion, two are paramount.

(1) What programs have been undertaken and what are its results with respect to enhancing safety and (2) (and it is not necessarily separate from the first) what programs have been undertaken and what are its results with respect to improving quality. Now, let me be emphatic. It is the residents themselves that are the actors here, in their responses to the site visitors and in their active participation in meaningful projects both within the confines of their specialty and across disciplinary lines.

CLER was recently announced. Widespread involvement is imminent. One might ask how I got to know about this seemingly arcane intrusion, if you will, which might once again disturb established routines to pursue a novel mandate for which there is no or very little experience to provide a guide to meet compliance.

Well, I happen to have three jobs in addition to editing reviews and providing commentaries each month. I have been and remain, a program director for 33 years, a Chair for 27 years and the D.I.O. or Designated Institutional Official for all

48 training programs here at New Jersey Medical School for the past 12 years. It is my obligation to create meaningful opportunities to pursue the program to satisfy the CLER requirements in both letter and spirit.

So if you are still listening what does that have to do with my practice? For many of you who are in private practice and maybe both physically and philosophically detached from the problems and prospects of academia what does this mean for you?

Well, the only way we can meet the rigors of CLER is to have every resident every year participate in a hypothesis-initiated, data driven quality and safety project. It is really the essential mandate of CLER. We have been doing so in our program for several years and our residents have learned to both speak and act with quality and safety in mind. So have residents in other departments. CLER forces us to have each program share their data, their innovations and to implement programmatic change, with other programs in allied specialties. In effect this will be its lasting effort a key part of training of all residents. It will engender an awareness of the need and the formulation of the means to enhance quality.

Here is now the key point. Soon these quality-sensitized trainees will be entering the job market. You will hire them if there is a clinical need, of course. But you will also need them because of their sensitization to the essential protective mechanism of continuous quality initiatives not just for PQRS demands but for the preservation of your practice. Why such a Draconian projection? Because there are many ways of reckoning money. Wherever there is an opportunity or an obligation the response to either is never uniform. Differentiation will be made between those who can deliver the product or service and those who cannot or choose not to. In essence quality will be codified, commoditized and commercialized. And there will be competition to provide it. Because it will be a public issue, you cannot hide within an existing practice agreement with your hospital or hospitals to preserve the status quo unless quality is addressed in a continuing and active way. At first, if you do not get on board bits of your enterprise may be outsourced. Perhaps, before you know your whole operation may be re-sourced that is replaced by those-likely more junior to you who have the means, energy, attitude, and aptitude to play the quality card from the top of the deck.

Hence, there are impresses from the establishment that bear watching. Also there will be newly graduated young radiologists who will join our workforce as well. Their training will be different from yours. They bear watching too for what they can bring to your practice and the practice of your competitors.

Quality: Some Simple Things You Might Change

42

The prolonged national debate about health care has led to specific passage of functional changes mandated by Obamacare. Given the vagaries of its many new segments, the most salient has been the modification of insurance coverage. Of the triumvirate of access, cost and quality, the emphasis of the legislation has been on the first, the critics have focused on the second and to some degree quality has taken a backseat. Yet it is still on the bus!

It may be a sidebar issue, but the Obama administration has acknowledged that the quality of medical care can improve. And when coupled with cost considerations, the target is utilization and the bull's-eye is imaging. For radiology, the increased attention on too much of what was once thought to be a pristine good thing translates into an impending assessment of inappropriate CT and MR studies. In fact, that surveillance which may be a stalking horse for all radiographic tests in general. Such heightened scrutiny will open opportunities for research studies on apt imaging protocols and at the same time mandate that we examine traditional paradigms for even mundane uses of radiological tests to determine if what is customary is really necessary.

Therefore, I endeavor here to consider some common practices most of us do and offer suggestions derived from published studies and my experience as a radiologist that reflect on quality and at the same time may be accomplished with the same or less reliance on imaging. I confine myself to examples of the seemingly humdrum daily work that many of us who do general radiology do often.

The first example encompasses an exploration of an imaging question in a patient with recurrent congestive failure who will most likely be admitted and who presents with shortness of breath. He may have just CHF or CHF and concurrent pneumonia. If these are the possibilities why do we get a chest X-ray routinely on presentation to the E.R.? The elaboration of abnormalities in the lung fields can vary in extent but is markedly limited in its patterns of expression. There can be interstitial infiltration with its accentuations of linear densities. There can be pleural thickening and/or effusions and in frank edema there can be replacement of air in the alveoli by extruded fluid. Yet, the alveoli in other conditions can be infiltrated by blood, pus or tumor. Thus the radiographic appearance of each of these other circumstances evaluated over a section of the pulmonary parenchyma will look the same as edema fluid.

So if the diagnosis of pulmonary edema is suspected or if it is masqueraded by a widespread pneumonia or if both edema and pneumonia infiltrate are present together, if you will, a chest X-ray obtained at entry in the E.R. will look the same for each.

The key point here is to wait and examine the lungs by chest X-ray after diuretics have been administered to expunge the fluid. If the initial chest X-ray is delayed by several hours during which time a presumptive diagnosis of recurrent CHF is suggested and treatment administered, then clear or clearer lungs observed on chest X-ray will confirm the diagnosis of CHF, now resolved at least for this episode. And if the delayed initial chest X-ray after diuresis reveals a pneumonia then the diagnosis of lung infiltration in the face of congestive failure will be established.

Why is the several hours delayed chest X-ray not routinely obtained and the immediate X-ray a matter of course? The reason, I believe in most cases relates to administrative decisions between the emergency physician and the hospital-based service to which the patient may be admitted to for completion of surveillance and care. The inordinately prompt chest-X-ray is less revealing than a delayed one in this scenario and it is ordered routinely. However, if more attention was paid to quality than to jurisdictional decisions between services, the patient would benefit.

For example two let us stay in the emergency department. We all know that with advances in multi-detector CT technologies we can now diagnose pulmonary embolus with much more certainty than with the previous protocol of chest-X-ray and lung scan. We also know that as the capabilities of CT have become widely known the utilization of computed tomography for this purpose has grown and ultimately the percentage of positive cases has decreased as strict criteria for CT study have been abandoned. Hence in many E.R.s the real operative instigation is not carefully vetted evidence-based considerations but merely because the referring physician wants it. Forget about D-dimers and other clinically relevant criteria. Pulmonary embolus can be lethal but it also can be treated-together these constitute an explanation but not a justification for its overuse.

But given that the patient will get a CT, why do we often also get a chest X-ray first and then move the patient to the CT table where the examination entails among other things a digital scout view along with the generation of "CT slices" of the thorax. In this context since the usual CT protocol provides full frontal and lateral chest views, the preliminary standard radiographic series is unnecessary, requires more time and superfluous transportation of the patient. In truth in such patients the initial chest X-ray is not needed.

Why not stop doing it? I am sure quality will not suffer. Turnaround time will improve and nothing essential will be lost by eliminating such a pro forma maneuver.

A third customary but unnecessary imaging study is the daily chest X-ray for the ICU patient. Certainly frequent surveillance of the lungs and mediastinum of a very sick patient is valuable, but by what standard must it be every 24 h. Of course, after the placement of tubes, catheters and drains, a chest X-ray is mandatory. And the initial placement of an ET tube or a tracheostomy tube should be assessed by a frontal chest X-ray to locate its course and its distal tip. Moreover for any untoward change in the patient's condition, a chest X-ray may be part of the workup. But for maintenance purposes alone, a recurrent chest X-ray done daily has no clinical justification in and of itself.

Furthermore, the interpretation of daily films with reference only to yesterday's image as part of a lengthening skein of chest X-rays obtained roughly 24 h apart for days, weeks and even months on end often engenders a laconic conclusion i.e., "No change from yesterday". Thus ending the analysis.

In my department, such an abbreviated quotidian and rote dictation is not allowed. The radiologists must put in the report "Examination of this image in comparison with a series of prior images, the most recent obtained on (blank)". "Both the date of yesterday's film and the dates of representative older studies are listed in the report." That is our standard language.

This requires the interpreting radiologist to look not just at the last images but several of them done before that to detect subtle changes that may not be apparent from day to day but can be perceived when compared with images performed over a wider interval. One may get a myopic restricted view of meaningful change when looking at only today's and yesterday's films. In fact the latter or the former may each not be necessary and quality need not suffer.

Hence for the ICU, there should be a clinical indication for the chest X-ray. And for the interpretation of that image, temporal context is important. That context may only be established if a retrospective protocol becomes standard, requiring the radiologists to compare the present with a series of older images and then report on the discrepancies between the former (there may be more than one of these) and the latter, today's image for example. By referring to a specific time and not just the day before or thereabouts, we have enhanced quality through standardization of recording of time of image generation.

These three modifications are examples of bread and butter studies we all do but can do better to engage us more meaningfully in the pursuit of quality. Small steps to be sure, but ones taken, I believe, in the right direction.

Part VIII

Malpractice Apology and Appropriateness

The threat of malpractice looms large in the general consciousness of radiologists but the subject is liable for misunderstanding. Here are discussed data-supported evidence of the causes and demography of malpractice. Also analyzed are the value and risk of apology and a critique of the appropriateness of appropriateness criteria.

Medical malpractice has become such an insistent and important issue that it should now be considered a national debate topic. Everyone with an interest in the provision of medical care has a stake in it. It is a cause of concern, of course, to physicians and lawyers and it is also a topic of conversation engaged in by the public in general and presidential candidates in particular. The fact that we deal with images generated by machines gives us no protection or immunity from assertions of negligent care. In fact, it has been stated that unlike other specialties radiologists produce their own mistakes and store them for eternity or, at least for several years.

Radiologists rank sixth among all specialists in frequency of malpractice suits. It is not just the prospect of a judgment of malpractice that is disconcerting, it is the specter of a putative action i.e., the recording of you and it in the National Practitioner Databank that is unsettling. Moreover, now that such information has become public in some states, including my own in New Jersey, the mere registering of a possible suit is enough to besmirch a reputation because inclusion on such a list can be perceived as a stain on an otherwise spotless record of service and accomplishment. Due process has been forsaken because for many people the allegation itself can be considered as a prima facie assignation of guilt even when no wrongdoing is eventually demonstrated or if the suit is dropped or even if the radiologist is separated from it. Yet what do we know about the likelihood of actions being taken against us? Are there geographical differences between regions or among the states? Are some of the various imaging modalities subject to more malpractice allegations than others? Are there gender differences with respect to the frequency of suits? What about the failure to communicate as a cause of a malpractice action? How about the rules attendant to our obligations or our predilection to suggest additional tests on our reports? Is that a good thing or a bad thing?

In this context, we decided to examine a large cohort of radiologists, some of whom had a record of no suits and others for whom malpractice suits were listed in the databank. I am fortunate to be associated with One Call Medical, a radiology broker for workman's compensation cases, for which I provide the credentialing. This gives me the opportunity to look at credentialing and re-credentialing files for a vast number of individuals as this company has gained a large number of recruits. In the listing of credentials, allegations of malpractice are reported. The majority of such cases included a short summary of pertinent clinical information contributing to our ability to make these analyses. The variables extracted from the available data included gender of the radiologist, state where he or she practices, the year in which the lawsuit occurred, the reason for the malpractice action, the radiologic intervention involved in the suit, and the specific diagnosis occasioned. The database was then analyzed to identify correlations between the aforementioned variables.

Thirty-five percent of the radiologists in this sample were involved in 2,676 lawsuits ranging

S.R. Baker, *Notes of a Radiology Watcher*,
DOI 10.1007/978-3-319-01677-1_43, © Springer International Publishing Switzerland 2014

from 1 to 16 suits per individual. Seven percent of the sample of physicians were female and the proportion of women with lawsuits to all women (23 %) was significantly better than the proportion of men with lawsuits to all men without lawsuits (37 %). We found this to be an unexpected and remarkable result. Is there is a bond between women patients and women radiologists that restricts the pursuit of supposed wrongdoing through civil action? Interestingly, 25 suits concerned fetal abnormalities, claimed to be misdiagnosed. For all of these, a male radiologist was the defendant. Of the types of suits filed 47 % percent were related to a failure to diagnose, 9 % were filed against radiologists for peripheral involvement in the case (that is, a roster of physicians were initially named including the radiologist and then eventually dropped from the case), 6 % involved complications of therapeutic intervention with imaging, 3 % were related to the problems pertaining to communication of findings. In only 1 % was the matter a patient reaction to contrast material, less than 1 % together encompassed instances of administrative error including failure to follow up, failure to order additional tests, failure to perform a procedure and failure to treat.

Despite a general perception that radiologists have an obligation in their reports to suggest additional tests because it is presumed failure to do so may put the radiologist at risk, in only 14 instances of these several thousand cases was this a matter for a lawsuit. This is a non-intuitive result and one that raises questions about the efficacy and appropriateness of defensive medicine and the risk and costs of unnecessary tests. Twenty-nine percent of lawsuit causes could not be determined by the available data.

Among failure to diagnose, the four leading causes were breast cancer, lung cancer, followed by other cancers and fractures. Of the failure to diagnose cases, all other causes account for 27 % of the total but in this group each individual cause accounted for no more than 3 % of the 1,270 failures to diagnose cases. One Call Medical has contracted with radiologists in 40 states. In some states there are only a few individuals that have gone through the credentialing process but in all the more populous states, California, Texas, New York, Florida, New Jersey, Illinois, Ohio, Michigan, Pennsylvania, Maryland, the numbers of radiologists in this network were significantly large. The states with the greatest number of cases included Florida, New Jersey, New York and California. However, the percentage of radiologists being sued was not found to be highest in these states. The leaders were Pennsylvania (51 %), Mississippi (51 %), Louisiana (50 %), Indiana (50 %), and Missouri (46 %). When stratified by gender, male radiologists had a 50 % greater chance of being sued in Indiana, Oregon and Pennsylvania. In those states where there are a large number of radiologists associated with One Call Medical the female percentage of suits was higher than the national average as discovered by our data.

As our analysis proceeded we discovered other interesting findings that will need further investigation. The number of women radiologists subjected to mammographic malpractice suits was slightly higher than the number of male radiologists so affected. This is probably related to the relative increased number of mammography examinations performed by women compared with those done by men. We are now looking into the issue of whether female physicians are less likely to be sued for supposed mammographic errors than male radiologists per mammographic study. Assessing the data by modality, chest x-ray was the most frequently performed imaging study followed by mammography, CT, and MR. Ultrasound was slightly behind MR and all other procedures were much fewer. However, relating the frequency of suits to the overall national number of examinations for each modality, mammography will most likely turn out to be the riskiest exam among the major studies but barium enema with a much smaller number performed, may turn out to be just as significant a threat to a malpractice action as breast imaging studies, as measured by the rates of suits to studies.

Our data has provided us with a rich source of information for further analysis in greater detail. Our larger investigation on causes and on demography were published in the February 2013 edition of Radiology. Focused studies on spinal and nonspinal-related malpractice suits with radiologists as defendants will be published soon as will studies of breast disease, chest, GI suits and suits in which the patient was elderly [1].

Reference

1. Baker SR, Lauro C, Sintim-Damoa C. Malpractice allegations and apology laws, benefits and risks for radiologists. JACR. 2008;5:1186–90.

Malpractice Suits Against Radiologists

44

I wish to bring to your attention information we have accumulated and analyzed from the malpractice data I have been fortunate to have gained access to in my capacity as director of credentialing for One Call Medical, Inc., a broker for workman's compensation cases which, at present, has over 9,000 active American radiologists on its panel of image interpreters. That is more than one quarter of all the radiologists in the country and I would imagine includes many of you.

I must state to dispel any anxiety about specific information about any of you, that when we evaluated the data collectively the information was thoroughly deidentified. Hence, I do not have at hand nor did my researchers during these investigations have particular data about any one of you. Of course, in my capacity as a credentialer, I looked at specific information about each new prospective enrollee on One Call's panel and I looked again at longer term enrollees too because there was a mandatory 3 year recertification requirement. Yet individual case histories with respect to malpractice were removed from the data assessment process.

The information we had available was I.D. number, location, gender and an abbreviated listing of all claims made against a radiologist from the beginning of his or her career. The narrative of each case consisted of one or two sentences outlining the primary allegation of the claim as well as the outcome i.e., if the claim was aborted initially or abandoned before judgment, or judged to be in favor of the plaintiff either before the trial at settlement or by verdict by jury. Also listed was the settlement or verdict amount if the decision was against the radiologist. This emphasis on the abbreviated information made available is important for an understanding of the meaning of the relative frequency of the various causes of each case. There may have been subsidiary issues informing the claims but our conclusions were based on what we had, the primary allegations which for the most part, constituted the motive for which the patient or the patient's family sought redress by instituting a lawsuit.

Case histories in which a payment was made by a third party-and this was most of the cases unfavorable to the radiologists-were garnered from the National Practitioners Data Bank which also provided the amount of the award. Cases in which there were no negative judgments were provided by the radiologists at initial credentialing or re-credentialing. If the radiologist dissembled and did not divulge his or her malpractice history and then those additional undisclosed cases were made known to the credentialing staff at One Call, then this radiologist was subject to losing his or her status as an enrollee and thus as a film interpreter eligible to be reimbursed. So the impetus was compelling for the radiologist to reveal all claims, including those for which there was not a transference of funds to the plaintiff after a judgment or other resolution was made.

With these terms now presented to you it will be easier to understand our data on the causes of malpractice suits against this large cadre of radiologists. Before analyzing them, I too believed in the conventional wisdom that includes the

S.R. Baker, *Notes of a Radiology Watcher*,
DOI 10.1007/978-3-319-01677-1_44, © Springer International Publishing Switzerland 2014

following supposed verities. Two of the most persistent notions are (1) if I do not do the test I will be sued and (2) most cases involve communication deficiencies between either or both the radiologist and the referring physician or between the radiologist and the patient and/or his family. There is a certain comfort or convenience in this assumption, one because it confers an ancillary benefit that is congenial to contemporary medical practice in a fee for service environment. Hence, the narrative may be "I will recommend another test to dispel the prospect of malpractice"—a fear often shared by the referring physician as well. Thus by these stimuli the unnecessary test is likely to be ordered. So to deny the implicit secondary gain from this notion is to be naive.

The second assumption-failure to communicate-is as different as sloth is to fear. The radiologist's job at the very least is to communicate important results. Communication is a unidirectional process from radiologist to referrer and failure to conclusively make that connection places the onus on us. That is why careful reading of the ACR communication standard, as vague as it may be, is crucial to avoid the patient being deprived, at his or her peril, from your expertise. But actual communication while necessary is not sufficient in some instances. There are those that call for true consultation in which is demanded a mutual interaction, a bilateral exchange requiring the verbal interplay between imaging physician and treating physician.

The literature on the cases of malpractice emphasizes such a breakdown in communication as being a major instigator of bad practice and subsequently claims of malpractice. A comprehensive study published last year in the Annals of Internal Medicine looked at most major specialties, including Radiology, and noted how prevalent communication errors and insufficiencies were in the instigation of lawsuits. Included in this large group were the records of 808 radiologists. Moreover, among physicians in Boston in the Harvard-affiliated hospitals it is presumed that communication errors are the predominant precipitant causes of malpractice claims.

Well, with that prolonged preamble what have we found? By far the most common generic

causes of malpractice cases against radiologists was failure to diagnose. It was about 10 times more common than the next most frequent general allegation which was procedural errors. Of the category of errors in diagnosis, accusation of malpractice referral to imaging of the breast was most common, encompassing about 23 % of all suits in which a diagnostic error was claimed. Non-spinal bone diagnoses were about 18 % followed by spinal misdiagnoses and pulmonary diseases at about 10 %.

In second place among categorical causes of malpractice were procedural errors. The rate of malpractice for all radiologists for failure to diagnose per 1,000 person years of practice was 14.83 but for technical mistakes or allegation of such mistakes it was 1.76. Third was negligence of some sort at 1.26, followed by the radiologist having only a peripheral role (and likely dismissed from the case) at 0.92. Failure to communicate with another provider was fifth at 0.71, about one twentieth as common as error in diagnosis. Failure to communicate with family was seventh at 0.40 per 1,000 practice years about one fiftieth as common as failure to diagnose. So while it is necessary to relate findings seen on imaging to referrers and their patients, it is nonetheless not a major cause of malpractice action against radiologists. Inasmuch as radiologists do not directly interact with patients as a matter of course except for interventional and breast radiology, it is then logical to expect that communication issues would not be a predominant initiator of malpractice as claims they might be for primary caregivers. Now, to reiterate, our data related to the primary allegation. Communication failure may have made an error in diagnosis or a procedural mistake seem even worse but that possibility while very real for some cases could not be captured by our data.

Only in sixth place was the claim that there was a failure to recommend additional testing. There were only 41 such allegations among nearly 5,000 suits in our data set. It is likely that there were a greater number of procedural based results engendered by the assertion to perform additional testing than there were suits consequent to tests not suggested. It could be claimed that since radiologists always suggest additional tests, then that is why this cause is so infrequent. But there is an underlying cynicism animating that view, i.e., that radiologists exercise no discretion, that all are "drum majors" if you will for more tests. Some may be but in my experience many are not so inclined. Hence, the worry about being sued because you have not suggested to do more because you can is, from our data at least, an unsubstantiated notion no matter how widely it may be trumpeted and accepted [1].

Reference

1. Whang J, Baker SR, Luk L, Patel R, Castro A. The causes of malpractice suits against radiologists in the United States. Radiology. 2013;266:548–54.

Radiology Malpractice: The Demography of Medical Malpractice Regarding Radiology

45

The specter of malpractice action remains a matter of concern for the specialty of radiology in general and for individual practitioners in particular. Allegations of breast disease misdiagnosis remain the most common cause of claims against all physicians in any specialty, with the radiologist often the only defendant. Other common initiators of malpractice suits include a variety of errors of diagnosis, defects in communication of findings, and procedural complications. The details on the frequency of suits and their distribution by state, gender, and age of radiologist have not been subject to extensive analysis involving a large cohort. Moreover, responses by radiologists often involve retrospective comments which have tended to emphasize the opinions of those who have at least once been sued or have been the subject of a claim that never becomes a formal tort action.

For example, a 2004 American College of Radiology Malpractice Survey attempted to describe radiologists' experiences and concerns with respect to the medicolegal climate. This study found that 58 % of respondents had been defendants in a medical malpractice lawsuit. Many of the observations concerned the subjective experiences and attitudes of the radiologists they surveyed. However, of the 17,000 radiologists sent a link to the survey, only 9 % responded. The authors noted that those who responded were likely to have a history of a lawsuit and to feel more strongly about malpractice issues than radiologists in general.

Thus, the tendency of such studies is to highlight concerns about malpractice and perhaps exaggerate its frequency. To get a balanced view, one would need a large sample of radiologists to include the demographic characteristics of those who have and have not been sued. It would be helpful to determine the frequency of suits, their distinction by state, gender, and age of radiologist, and also to chart the percentage of claims that result in a settlement or judgment against the defendant radiologists as well as their distribution according to the same parameters. Such a study would require the recording of pertinent statistics independent of the radiologists' opinions about the circumstances of such impositions.

A dataset unbiased by radiologist's perception has become available from the credentialing files of One-Call Medical, Inc., a specialty preferred provider organization offering diagnostic imaging services for the workers compensation, group health, and auto insurance industries. All radiologist network members of One Call are subject to initial credentialing and re-credentialing on a strict 3-year cycle. For each participating radiologist, data is recorded with respect to radiologists' gender and age, primary state of practice, patient gender and age, legal outcome (judgment, settlement, dismissal, pending, etc.), payment amounts, and reason for lawsuit. At present One-Call Medical has contracted with 8,401 radiologists in 47 states, which represents approximately 32 % of all active radiologists in the United States.

S.R. Baker, *Notes of a Radiology Watcher*,
DOI 10.1007/978-3-319-01677-1_45, © Springer International Publishing Switzerland 2014

An analysis of data from this source constitutes an examination of the demographic constituents of claims, not settlements or verdicts, and therefore will include all actions directed against radiologists as derived from two sources. For each enrollee in OneCall Medical, the malpractice history as recorded in the files of the National Practitioners Data Bank is continually made available to the credentialing committee. This national repository records all settlements and verdicts greater than $10,000 against the defendant radiologist in all American jurisdictions subject to review from even before 1980. Also, initially and for recredentialing, each radiologist was obligated to list all other claims initiated against them to include settlements and judgments in their favor and all other claims whether announced only or processed to some degree and then aborted. Together, these two sources provide a malpractice history for each physician. From this information one could compute the percentage of radiologists in the network who were subject to at least one claim, the difference in the number and percentage of radiologists sued in the various states, the frequency of claims in each state disaggregated by age and gender, the course of the claim and whether the defendant radiologist was judged to be responsible for recompense to the plaintiff, and the size of the award. Here I will discuss the major demographic variables among the large assemblage of practitioners which undoubtedly include many of you.

By 2010 One Call Medical served patients in 47 of the 50 states and was also a presence in the District of Columbia. Hence its potential reach extends to over 98 % of the population of the United States. For data analysis we confined our investigation to states having 50 or more radiologists enrollees. Hence, we remove from consideration Iowa, Rhode Island, Washington, Idaho, Delaware, New Hampshire, Montana, West Virginia, Alaska, Wyoming and DC because their numbers of participants in One-Call are too meager. Seven of the 11 states each have less than 1.3 million inhabitants. Hence, by removing them we did not significantly affect the broad reach of the study with regard to the total U.S. population. For the other states, the ones with a sizeable

cadre of enrollees, the distribution of radiologists broadly reflects the percentage of radiologists in each state and the state's population as a whole with a few exceptions. Texas is the second most populous state but ranked fourth with 379 radiologists in One Call's panel. Participation by radiologists in Maryland is disproportionately high whereas the ratio in Massachusetts is lower than expected by both number of radiologists and number of people. California with 1,025 radiologists credentialed has only 200 more on One-Call's file than New York although it has twice the population. Yet, overall the number of radiologists there is not twice the radiology contingent active in New York.

The mean age of enrollees is remarkably similar with the oldest group of radiologists from New Mexico averaging 54 years of age and the youngest in Arkansas at 48. The mean age nationally is 51. Although there is a homogeneity in age of these radiologists there is great variability in the percentage of enrollees with at least one claim nationwide. The overall percentage nationally is 32 %. The most litigious state in relation to malpractice actions against them is Utah where 55 % reported at least one claim. In contrast, the state with radiologists least likely to have been sued at least once is Wisconsin where only 14 % have been so affected. States that have been generally considered particularly susceptible to plaintiff initiation of malpractice actions like Pennsylvania and Florida have claim percentages of 37 % and 36 % respectively. They are exceeded by Kansas at 49 %, New York at 48 %, New Jersey at 42 %, Missouri at 40 % and Indiana at 39 %. At the low end of the scale, i.e., under 20 %, is Arkansas at 15 %, North Carolina at 16 %, Mississippi at 19 %, Nebraska at 20 % and Virginia at 20 %. Mississippi and Louisiana have gained notoriety as the "jackpot justice" states because of the very high awards granted to plaintiffs. But at this juncture I am only considering the subset who have been recipients of claims at least once, not the percentage of those who had actual judgments as related to claims with regard to the dollar amount of such settlements or verdicts.

Overall women comprise 15 % of all radiologists. And in our cohort which collectively approximates one third of all radiologists, the percentage of women is 15.1 %. But there is great variability among states in the percentages of female enrollees, ranging from 4.8 % in Nevada to 26 % in Maryland. Nonetheless, 25 of the 36 states with sufficient numbers of enrollees for comparison have a female percentage between 10 and 20. So while the spectrum is broad, most states percentages bunch up near the mean. In a future review I will delve into gender differences with respect especially to the dissimilarities between male and female radiologists with respect to the most common error in diagnosis subject to malpractice actions, that is diseases of the female breast.

The explanation for differences by state in the percentage of claim initiations must include many variables. Legislative initiatives, jury predilections, the behavior of insurance companies, plaintiff attorney competence and award amount all play a role. But one statistical artifact in addition must be mentioned. In small states specifically the ones that have sufficient enrollees to make the list of 50 or more One Call radiologists, the make-up of this cohort is not necessarily a broad representation of the distribution of radiologists in the state as a whole. One Call contracts first with an imaging center and then seeks to register all interested radiologists that serve that facility. Over the past 20 years the tendency throughout the country is for radiology groups to enlarge. Yet this phenomenon is occurring unevenly. When a smallish state is dominated by several large groups and it is the practice of plaintiffs lawyers to first attempt to sue everybody in the group before refining their case to only those directly involved in the alleged malpractice or to abandon the case altogether for want of evidence or declining interest by the plaintiffs or plaintiff's family, then no money may change hands and no adverse judgment rendered against many yet the percentage sued as registered by the criteria used here and the annoyances caused will be high.

Among the states with the most successful lawsuits, the reputation realized over time about Louisiana and Mississippi is justified. The ratio of payment to no payment in Louisiana is 7.2. That is, in Louisiana of 33 suits initiated for which further information is available including resolution of the tort action, 29 resulted in payment to the plaintiffs. In Mississippi the ratio is 6.6, Yet in Maryland it is only 1.01 and in Kansas and Indiana two states with relatively high claim frequency the ratio of payment to no payment is merely 0.54 and 0.37 respectively [1].

Reference

1. Baker SR, Lauro C, Sintim-Damoa C. Malpractice allegations and apology laws, benefits and risk for radiologists. JACR. 2008;5:1186–90.

Apology: It's Elements and Legal Intrusions

46

Over the past couple of months many of you may have heard about a new initiative in malpractice legislation. This innovation is responsive to the notion that patients would be less likely to sue if we said to them, "Yes, an error was made, we regret it but please accept our apology". The intent then is that the patient would get some measure of satisfaction from an admission that doctors are human, too. They would acknowledge by accepting the apology that an untoward result was occasioned by unfortunate error not malicious or incompetent action. The hope would be that the impetus to sue would be reduced. Recent articles in the Wall Street Journal and Time Magazine have played up this initiative. In this discussion I will lay out some arguments that lead to the conclusion that an apology is a great risk for radiologists particularly [1].

The stimulus for using apology as a technique to minimize malpractice stems, in large measure, from the famous report in the Institute of Medicine with which I am sure most of you are familiar. It concluded that up to 100,000 deaths per year in hospitals are due to errors made by doctors and other healthcare workers. In 2001 JCAHO demanded safety standards requiring the disclosure of unanticipated outcomes. They further clarified that statement in 2004 with the regulation that patients, and when appropriate their families, be informed about untoward, unanticipated events. Furthermore, when questions arise about the breadth of treatment, a JCAHO-accredited organization must tell patients when harm comes to them in respect to their diagnosis and their therapy. Now, if JCAHO demands that we should tell patients when our actions induce injury, illness, discomfort or worse, one might conclude that we are further exacerbating the possibility of malpractice suits since we acknowledge that a deviation from expected results has occurred. Nonetheless, disclosure of harmful outcomes is both a regulatory requirement and, one might argue, an ethical obligation. Yet, only three states have passed laws mandating written disclosure of adverse or bad outcomes to patients and families, Pennsylvania, Nevada and Florida.

So, given the necessity of disclosure, what is the value of an apology? Well, in some institutions this has become so important that it is being taught in medical school. In fact, at Vanderbilt, students and residents are required to take courses concerned with communication of error and apology. But, is apology an ethical obligation, a strategic ploy, a legal desideratum, or some combination thereof. Before proceeding we should really understand what is and what is not an apology in its truest moral sense. According to Tavuchi in his book, Mea Culpa, the elements of apology are (1) acknowledge, through speech, the legitimacy of the violated rule, (2) admit fault for its violation, (3) express genuine sorrow or remorse, i.e., repentance, and (4) there should be an explicit offer of restitution or promise to reform [2]. The tactical value of apology rests with the assumption that juries will be more apt to decide for the plaintiff when they have reason to be angry at the doctor. And, if the doctor apologizes, the incendiary issue of physician stonewalling will have

S.R. Baker, *Notes of a Radiology Watcher*,
DOI 10.1007/978-3-319-01677-1_46, © Springer International Publishing Switzerland 2014

been removed. After an apology everybody will be in a more conciliatory mood, supposedly. An authentic apology includes all of those four elements I have just mentioned and it is meant to stimulate a moral syllogism in which there is a relational process engendering a heartfelt discussion between the doctor and patient. It requires real repentance and remorse. Once an authentic apology is tendered the initiative shifts to the injured party to grant a measure of forgiveness to complete the moral exchange. According to the proponents of its efficacy, an apology eliminates the issue of liability and tends to minimize the damage award. But herein is the rub. Since it is no longer an issue of liability, but one of damages, that means there will be an exchange of money, usually in a settlement agreement. The outcome will go on the physician's record with no culpability assigned but with an acknowledgement for anybody reading the record that a payment was made. Now, as most lawyers and physicians see it, the four elements of apology will not be realized. Rather, there will usually be an incomplete or inauthentic apology which might include an empathic response alone with no admission of fault, no true repentance, no offer of restitution and therefore, no moral exchange. One may make the distinction between an apology and an apologia. Webster's Third International Dictionary states that an apology is a frank, regretful admission that one has been wrong whereas an apologia is an explanation of a course or belief without the suggestion of guilt or error. What most physicians seek to provide is an apologia only. Yet, an empathic disclosure alone without an admission of fault is a defensive maneuver, not a true apology. Will it ultimately render the effect sought? In an empathic disclosure or incomplete apology you *say* "I am sorry it happened to you", or something to that effect. Yet, there is really no accountability and no real confession. An apologia is a false declaration, a moral abandonment of what is presumed to be an apology. This inadequate gesture may lead to vengeance at a later date by the aggrieved patient or the patient's family.

Yet, bear in mind there is now no ethical or regulatory requirement that an authentic apology be included in the disclosure of harm.

JCAHO standards require only that the patient is told that harm has been done and is given sufficient information about it. So, one might conclude that an authentic apology involving all the four elements including repentance and restitution is really only for the morally courageous and may be a tactical mistake. But now state legislatures have gotten into the act. A growing statutory fad, that is right, a fad, is the apology laws that have been passed in 18 states [1]. The first one was approved in Massachusetts in 1986 and all of the others have come on board since 1999. That first law in 1986 stated that a benevolent gesture relating to the pain, suffering and death of a person involved in an accident shall be inadmissible as evidence of admission of liability in a civil action. The Massachusetts law encompasses all civil actions. Most of the newer laws apply just to medical procedures. The intent and consequence of each of these laws is that if you state that you are sorry (and that sorrow could be only in the form of an apologia), such a disclosure is not admissible in a trial. The next state to pass an apology law was Texas. It stated that empathic gestures are protected but admission of wrong-doing is not. The Texas law has been the model for most other statutes. Yet, in 2004, Colorado extended the protection even further. I provide you the first couple of sentences of the Colorado law. "In any civil action brought by an alleged victim of an unanticipated outcome of medical care or in any arbitration proceeding related to such civil action any and all statements, affirmations, gestures or conduct expressing apology, fault (and the key word here is fault), as well as sympathy, commiseration, condolence, compassion or general benevolence, which are made by a healthcare provider etc., will be deemed inadmissible". This Colorado law and the laws of the other two states, Arizona and Georgia, that have followed them now claim that not only do you admit sorrow without fear of penalty but also to admit fault is no longer admissible. So, what is a patient to do given the fact that you as a healthcare provider are covered by a broad blanket of immunity for the expression of apology to one class of people-patients and their families?

Given the appearance of apology laws, is the radiologist protected? I say, he or she is not. Let me explain why I regard apology laws as a gaping trap. What happens when an apology is made and there is a suit with multiple defendants, radiology being one of them, but a primary caregiver being one of the others? What do you think will happen? The primary caregiver can apologize and say do not blame me, blame the guy behind the tree, which happens to be the radiologist. Radiologists are by situation often remote from patient interaction. We often do not see the individuals whose images we interpret, we may have not even been in the hospital at the time the study was done, and we may have reviewed the images from far away. Yet, our interpretations often are the cause of the malpractice action. So what will it mean when someone who does not know the patient or the family makes an apology and that apology does not express any real repentance and no offer of anything else including restitution? Will we really be protected by such a gesture? Mostly we will never even have the opportunity to even express empathy, that being the opportunity alone of the referring physician. Furthermore, there are instances when an untoward result occurs and yet no apology is really required. What about those extremely rare circumstances when the patient has a serious and unanticipated reaction to contrast material? Can a true apology be made? Can anything, even an apologia, really be morally defensible when there really was no error and no fault? So, given these circumstances you will be confronted with apology laws that malpractice lawyers on the defense side think are a panacea. Primary care physicians may agree but radiologists could be even more vulnerable than before because of these laws. Beware.

References

1. Baker S, Lauro C, Sintim-Damoa A. Malpractice allegations and apology laws: benefits and risks for radiologists. J Am Coll Radiol. 2008;5(12):1186–90. doi:http://dx.doi.org/10.1016/j.jacr.2008.08.003.
2. Tavuchis N. Mea culpa: a sociology of apology and reconciliation. Stanford, CA: Stanford University Press; 1993.

Is It Appropriate to Have Appropriateness Criteria for Radiology Testing?

47

The proliferation of imaging tests in number and variety has stimulated an effort to present guidelines directing the best way to work up a particular clinical presentation. This notion has been codified in the elaboration of published appropriateness criteria which seek to offer algorithms purported to reveal the best sequence of tests to reach a diagnosis. Is this approach valid or are these reasons to doubt its credibility or effectiveness?

According to Webster's New Universal Unabridged Dictionary—Appropriate is defined as suitable or fitting for a particular purpose, person, or occasion. On the surface this is an entirely plausible and simple definition. Yet what constitutes the opposite, i.e., if you do not do what is deemed appropriate, should it be considered to be anti-appropriate or a-appropriate. Are alternatives acceptable or is everything outside the paradigm inappropriate? The American College of Radiology Appropriateness Criteria do not really touch on this question which, in my view, is really crucial to their validity. Can personal preference be accommodated in such a schema without labeling that less than competent or even inimical to patient care? Are extenuating circumstances permissible informants to the formulation of a diagnostic plan? Is no imaging an option depending on the particularities of care? Should such variety be acceptable or will it be so at variance with consensus to thereby put an individual radiologist at risk for a prospective malpractice suit for his/her "deviation" in relation to what is the supposed "right" way. The problem is that appropriateness criteria depend not only on an available roster of tests and the order in which they are performed, but also on many other determinants which makes the uncritical application of the concept often not germane, sometimes mischievous and even ultimately dangerous to one's reputation [1].

In this part of the discussion, I would like to cite some data which perhaps will render the mist thicker because uncertainty necessarily beclouds even the most sharply defined imaging plan. We must ponder the question; do radiologists really know what is appropriate for the next patient they see, even though there are guidelines that seem to snugly accommodate every patient? Let us consider patients with abdominal pain, an area which I happen to know something about. What has been written to be deemed appropriate or optimal often differs often from what I claim to be a better imaging sequence placing my routine in opposition to a standard paradigm sanctioned by the title of appropriateness.

We recently conducted a study which posed two clinical presentations to two groups of physicians—ER physicians and college health officers. The first question was what would you do for a patient between 18 and 21 years of age, either male or female, who came to you with right lower quadrant pain, fever, and an elevated white count? The responses from 500 college physicians indicated that 75 % of them would get a CT. Asking the same question of emergency physicians, with again about 500 respondents 75 % affirmed that CT was a crucial test. However, when the clinical issue was changed in

S.R. Baker, *Notes of a Radiology Watcher*,
DOI 10.1007/978-3-319-01677-1_47, © Springer International Publishing Switzerland 2014

18–21 year olds to one day of non-specific abdominal pain, no fever, no white count, and no localizing signs, 40 % of the emergency room physicians indicated they would order a CT but only 10 % of the college physicians would request that test. Now, which was appropriate for the second group of patients? Were the ER physicians right but the college physicians misguided or was it vice-versa? My predilection is to say that patients with one day of abdominal pain and no fever, no white count, no localized signs need to be watched but not necessarily imaged. Yet, emergency physicians might well mention when that individual comes to them, we therefore have to rule out even an unlikely but potentially devastating disease. For after all, what if the patient went away and his/her condition worsened. So 40 % of them would advocate getting a CT "to see what is going on". What is appropriate here? Really it depends upon your point of view. Perspective may be as important for proper imaging according to a prearranged formula depending upon the clinical setting, the patient's access to care, and even his or her economic situation [2]. All of these are variables which may require a modification of appropriateness criteria to be more realistic.

Another indication for the construction of sets of appropriate sequence of tests is the fear that if you do not do any one of them or do not get them is correct order, eventually you will be sued for malpractice. So therefore, it becomes a canon of accepted practice to pursue a stepwise imaging assessment favoring completeness over restraint. Yet, information that we have culled from the records of nearly 25 % of all the radiologists in the country through malpractice claims data indicates that not getting an additional test is rarely the cause of a lawsuit against the radiologist. Yet performing an examination that may not be indicated from which complications ensue is a more common stimulus for a tort action. These facts are contrary to the conventional wisdom about what is appropriate in light of malpractice considerations.

Let us examine another issue that can be related to appropriateness or the lack thereof. It is commonplace among radiologists to request in their impression, an additional study. In fact, in an assessment of the behavior of our own radiologists with respect by their suggestions in the radiologic report, we found two distinct cadres among our body imagers i.e.,—one group who hardly ever suggested another test and another group that more than 30 % of the time indicated the value of additional tests in their written impression. It was proposed to the latter group that perhaps it would be better to call the referring physician before mentioning further workup in the report because a suggestion of an additional test is regarded by many clinicians as tantamount to an order. When the value of personal communication was emphasized the percentage of reports with suggestions for additional studies in the impression decreased slightly. And when it was then further pointed out to those with very high rates of test promotion that they were behaving as outliers with respect to their peers, a "suggestion" by me to get in line served to decrease the percentage of written solicitations for further studies. In fact, suggesting a test in a radiology report may not in itself really ever be appropriate because one does not always know the clinical context of a patient who may submit to an imaging test. To say on the basis of a radiologic finding alone that an additional test is necessary negates other important factors such as overall health, records of previous visits, etc. which will determine whether the test is truly appropriate or merely another image whose pictures might be interesting to look at. So appropriate depends not only on the perspective of the referring physician, but on the situation of the patient.

Do we know that what is established in the medical literature is really helpful in terms of appropriateness? I quote here a study performed by Dr. Claude Serlin from the University of California in San Diego entitled "CT of Appendicitis—What do we not know?" Dr. Serlin examined 123 original articles from a list of about 200 published in the last 10 years on the subject of CT for appendicitis. He included references in the ER, health service, pediatrics, radiology and surgery literature. All told, 45 journals from 17 countries were consulted. The settings of the patients were academic, academic plus community or community alone. The populations consisted in these various studies of adults, children and adults and children alone. The purposes of the article included an analysis of findings outcome, diagnostic performance, what to do about an equivocal CT, expert or not expert interpreters, clinical indications, technical comparison, and visibility of the appendix. The study designs include meta-analysis, retrospective studies, prospective studies, and surveys.

What do we <u>not</u> know on the basis of these studies? Well we yet do not know how accurate is CT because the radiologic literature and the surgical literature differ considerably in this regard. We do not know if a reader's expertise is crucial. We do not know what is the optimal CT technique, nor the value of reformation of images. We have no good criteria of as to who should get CT and who should not. We do not know precisely what to do with an equivocal CT nor do we know if CT improves outcome. And in fact, with respect to outcome there is no consensus whether CT decreases or increases the negative appendicitis rate. There are studies that revealed that CT decreased the perforation rate and others showing that perforation rate increased after a CT exam is done. With regard to CT and cost, there are references that conclude that reduced costs override expenditures but at the same time there are opposing references revealing how costs are augmented by it. Similarly you can find data whose conclusions favor the opinions that CT expedites surgery and others that claim it delays surgery. Does CT predict histological severity? Some say yes, and others say no. Take your pick. So how will we construct appropriateness criteria given the uncertainty as expressed in the literature about a technique that at least among radiologists is well established?

Putting all of these things together the situation gets murkier and murkier. What is appropriateness? Having studied the literature, and contributing to it, I find I do not know if the concept really has validity. Therefore, on that pessimistic note, I must go off to ponder the matter even more or perhaps such ruminations will only engender further doubt.

References

1. Baker SR. ACR appropriateness Criteria® on small-bowel obstruction: a critique of the term and its terms. JACR. 2007;4(7):443–5.
2. Jha S. From imaging gatekeeper to service provider— a transatlantic journey. N Engl J Med. 2013;369(1): 5–7. doi:10.1056/NEJMp1305679.

Authorization or Appropriateness or the Lady or the Tiger Redux

48

At the time of this writing and probably, too, at the time you are reading this, health care reform will remain a hot political issue. President Obama, having placed it at the top of his domestic agenda, will still have to contend with strident criticisms about it throughout his second term. The problem is both chronic and acute. Although health care costs are not rising as steeply today as they were several years ago they are still going up. The organizational problem inherent in the way we allocate payment for the ill and injured and how we seek to prevent disease in the United States will most likely not be ameliorated by any legislation because the philosophical polarities are too great and political infighting too intense to achieve anything more than piecemeal changes, obamamania notwithstanding. But one of those bigger pieces could involve radiology.

In fact a conventional metaphor that has now become a cliché is that imaging is in the "crosshairs". It has increased too much in volume and is now too expensive and, in contrast to drug therapies, it is too unregulated. By and large the remedies are two in number. First, policy wonks want to decrease imaging expenditures through the mechanism of prior authorization, allowing only certain tests in certain situations to be paid for by Medicare and Medicaid, with the expectation that private insurers would follow suit. Such an initiative for cost saving at first will work from an accounting perspective. It certainly will reduce test volume. And given the fact that many of these procedures are over-utilized and often, per case, lack medical justification, an across the board refusal to pay will stifle demand. But at the same time, prior authorization lacks sophistication as applied to medical management decision-making.

A one size fits all solution takes the referring physician and the radiologist out of the care-rendering scenario. It will undoubtedly lead to the harm of some individuals who may really need the "blackballed" test or procedure. Furthermore, authorization is so hostile to the status quo it is bound to have vociferous critics who will "hype" the negative consequences its implementation will induce.

Now for the second remedy. In response to the looming specter of arbitrariness, insensitivity and the denial of the reliance on physician judgment and expertise, implicit in the prior authorization bargain, the American College of Radiology, with the broad support of its members, offers an alternative approach. A panel of experts familiar with the capabilities, limitations, risks and uncertainties of the various imaging examinations formulates, for a wide range of clinical presentations, appropriateness criteria outlining a step-wise approach to diagnostic workups emphasizing the consensus about the best sequence of tests. Appropriateness criteria are proclaimed as advisory to both radiologists and referring physicians. Unlike authorization it is not coercive directly but by being exhortative it could be persuasive and thus indirectly coercive. The prospect is that it will save time and avoid absolutely unnecessary invasive tests and the ill effects they may engender. The appropriateness ambition optimistically

S.R. Baker, *Notes of a Radiology Watcher*,
DOI 10.1007/978-3-319-01677-1_48, © Springer International Publishing Switzerland 2014

portends more gentle examinations done more quickly saving discomfort and cost while leading to more incisive and correct diagnoses. It will, its proponents claim, reduce health care charges and improve quality.

Is such an optimistic claim justifiable? I believe a healthy skepticism is in order. In my view, the two competing philosophies for change I have outlined are reminiscent of the choices to be made by the protagonist in Ambrose Bierce's famous story "The Lady or the Tiger". Bierce tantalizes the reader with two possibilities to be chosen as the story ends either promising disquieting uncertainty or, more likely, dire eventualities.

The untoward consequences of authorization are clear for radiologists and perhaps for patients, too, at least in some situations. But the adverse effects or at least ineffectualities of appropriateness criteria must be acknowledged as well. Let us look into this in detail.

Should we consider appropriateness criteria to be authoritative? For guidance on this question I refer to an article and an accompanying editorial that appeared in the February 25, 2009 edition of JAMA. The article was entitled "Scientific Evidence Underlying the American College of Cardiology/American Heart Association Clinical Practice Guidelines". Cardiologists have been at the game for more than 20 years, far longer than have radiologists. They have devised a rating scheme based on varying levels of evidence to form the basis for their recommendations for diagnostic paradigm.

- Level of Evidence A—recommendation based on evidence from multiple randomized trials or meta-analyses.
- Level of Evidence B—recommendations based on evidence from a single randomized trial or non-randomized studies.
- Level of Evidence C—recommendation based on expert opinion, case studies or standards of care.

The record in cardiology has been that over the years there has been an increasing reliance on the so-called lower levels of evidence levels B and C. Moreover, recommendations have been made with increasing frequency for which the evidence is not conclusive. Cardiologists do not

use the term appropriateness, choosing instead to contain their official advisory statements as guidelines. Yet the science behind them has become more problematic even as the resources expounded on the realization of their recommendation has become more widespread.

So many of the guidelines seek to include change in the dispensing of expert opinion without scientifically valid data to support them. And in Radiology perhaps even more than cardiology the legitimizing of such advice-giving must be challenged on several grounds i.e., with respect to lexicography, credentialing, applicability, subjectivity and effectiveness. Together these are not an exhaustive list of concerns but merely, to this observer, the most salient ones.

Why was the term appropriateness chosen instead of guidelines or recommendations or some other more neutral term? As such appropriateness is a combative word. It implies that everything that does not fit this rubric is not appropriate. Should we call other pathways or diagnostic maneuvers if not appropriate then inappropriate, non-appropriate, or a-appropriate? Any way you slice it, to practice at variance with it connotes deficiency, a less than optimal approach, a deviation from the norm and most ominously when things do not go just right a pretext for a malpractice suit even though the alternative non-appropriate choices may be better for a particular patient. This could be the door that opens to the mauling tiger. Its subliminal message is my way has been determined to be the highway. Appropriateness is the route to follow, or else.

And who constitutes the committee to render appropriateness criteria? Bearing in mind that level (1) evidence is very rarely acquired in Radiology. ACRIN aside, for any issue we have few sets of multiple randomized trials to rely on in Radiology. And we have only a limited number of single randomized trials. So for the most part it is case studies, non-randomized reviews, and expert opinions that congeal around a supposed standard of care. Appropriateness committees are supposed to be constituted by presumed experts. But they must be representative, too, of various constituents-regional, gender-related and practiced-situated (small vs. big, academic vs. private). Hence are members really experts or delegates from inherent groups? Are their opinions state of the art? Is state of the art the state of humaneness?

Moreover, are appropriate criteria applicable? Not all facilities have the same clinical, instrumental and physician resources. Moreover, the appropriateness criteria are a-temporal. That is they are meant to be used at a point in time resulting from a cross-sectional analysis of a clinical presentation. The electronic medical record when widely used will restore the essentiality of history as a crucial component of the diagnostic endeavor. With the electronic medical record we will know about what the patient record was at another healthcare facility. We will know more about his multiple encounters at the home facility. For instance we may not need another CT now if we have access to the previous workup done elsewhere recently for a recurring condition [1, 2].

Shaneyfelt and Centor in their editorial response to the aforementioned critique of the ACC/AHA guideline paper, point out "guidelines (and therefore appropriateness criteria) are not patient-specific enough to be useful and rarely allow for the individualization of care or concern." They are often out of date, as well. Or they rapidly become so. The approval process takes time, the dissemination process takes additional time. By then the criteria may change because of new evidence or changing fashions or modification of reimbursement policies. Moreover, bias is bound to intrude. In Radiology we must deal with a range of inherent biases. Those who reach eminence in our specialty as investigators have often hitched their wagon to a particular machine, a CT or MR for example. And thus their recommendation for inclusion in appropriateness criteria deliberations may be governed by what they favor without proof or biased by what they are familiar with or slanted by a subliminal conflict of interest related to industry supported imaging research.

Finally if appropriateness criteria are to be considered an alternative to authorization initiative, heed must be paid to the effect of their adoption on the cost of imaging care. After all, the nation has acknowledged that health is too costly. Imaging expenditures are the fastest rising component of that cost. Any alternative system to rationing (for that is what pre-authorization is) must also save money. If it does not, it will be discredited on the basis of ineffectiveness alone.

So the choices are stark, no pun intended. There are things we can do though, to avoid to some degree our anticipated demonization as we become identified as recipients of the largess of a wasteful use of the taxpayers dollars, frittered away on the uncertain deployment of unneeded imaging. We must reintegrate ourselves back into the action of clinical workups not by computer or internet contact alone but by our physical presence in addition to messages from our PACS outlets. Without pursuing frequent colloquies with our clinical colleagues we may be culled from the herd to face the cost-cutters "music" alone. We must find a better alternative to appropriateness criteria to blunt the sharp effects of pre-authorization. That can only be done by radiologists becoming on site caregivers instead of just remote physicians.

References

1. Ravindran V, Sennik D, Hughes RA. Appropriateness of out-of-hours CT head scans. Emerg Radiol. 2007;13(4):181–5. doi:10.1007/s10140-006-0532-6.
2. Baker SR. ACR appropriateness Criteria® on small-bowel obstruction: a critique of the term and its terms. JACR. 2007;4(7):443–5.

Part IX

Opportunities for Radiologists

This grouping of essays explores novel opportunities for radiology. New initiatives in teleradiology are discussed. Medical tourism also can provide further practice possibilities. The emerging sub-subspecialty of geriatric radiology may enable us to develop new insights to apply heightened sensitivity and sophistication in the evaluation of the elderly.

Teleradiology: From the Confines of Place to the Freedom of Space

49

For most of the twentieth century teleimaging was a Buck Rogers notion. The idea that care could be directed by the inspection of pictures at a physical remove from a sick individual was regarded as science fiction even only a few years ago. Yet, developments in communication in the past decade have made it possible to manipulate pictures as easily as it has become to manipulate words. Now, as we know it, teleimaging is a reality so commonplace that it is no longer a strategic decision for most radiology practices and not even a tactical consideration for those acquainted with its virtues. Rather, it has become an operational necessity for many practices. I say this even as the use of teleimaging is only barely beginning for our colleagues in medicine, pathology and psychiatry. All of these specialties lend themselves very well to the transmission of pictorial information, be it an EKG, a pathological slide or a patient interviewed through teleconferencing. Yet, we in radiology stand apart as leaders of the application of this technology [1].

The digitization of information in the form of words and images has become the standard for all radiology practices. If you do not have PACS, you will probably get it soon. With it you will no longer have to worry about lost films or providing the space for capacious file rooms. You will link PACS into your RIS and HIS so that the free flow of information will not be encumbered at barriers between the providers of expertise at one end and at the other end the providers of payment for that expertise. Moreover, most likely you will integrate voice recognition into your PACS so that referring physicians will benefit from your interpretations without the delay attendant upon manual dictations, bound as they are by the transportation of words from you to the typist and then back to you, accompanied by a chain of events, each capable of engendering a delay.

At present, all of this can be accomplished onsite with the radiologist situated in proximity to the patient, but not necessarily so close as before. Because with PACS, the image, which heretofore as film was at the same time a diagnostic, archival and reimbursement document, can now in a digital form be ubiquitous and redundantly reproducible, so that each of those tripartite functions are eminently separable. Hence, with PACS you can interpret images remote from the patient.

You can situate yourself in your office and read from there, of course. Yet, you need not be positioned only at your office if away from the hospital. After hours, images can be available at home for you to look at. No wonder that today, more than 80 % of radiology practices have some form of teleradiology.

Mostly, remote interpretations are made in the context of intrapractice, extramural viewing. In effect, with teleimaging, you or your colleagues are theoretically available around the clock. Yet, you have to have a life outside of work and you have to sleep, too. Thus, the opportunity is there for a nighthawk organization to assist you (actually I prefer the term night owl, which is smarter and not so predatory). You hire someone to read for you or at least read first for you-providing

S.R. Baker, *Notes of a Radiology Watcher*,
DOI 10.1007/978-3-319-01677-1_49, © Springer International Publishing Switzerland 2014

preliminary interpretation from their place which is anywhere else. Mostly that distant place is in the continental United States. However, not everyone wants to spend a lifetime working at night, in temporal exile from the rest of the world. Hence, nighthawk firms have a high turnover. The product may be good but perforce the players are apt to change frequently.

Another option is to hire an offshore teleradiology outfit. Generally, this consists of an extracontinental group of radiologists whose time zone is so different from yours that their day is your night and your day is their night. Yet, in this arrangement, in addition to the issue of hospital appointments and state licenses, you need to be concerned that the images are not being farmed out to some sub-contractor. Keeping these very real concerns aside, the geographic fact is the same; the reading radiologist is fixed by the nature of his equipment to a certain place.

Or that is the way it had to be until now. Improvements in computers and telephonic transmission can now free the teleradiologist from the shackles of place. The viewing equipment is now so portable that he or she can be in Adelaide one week and Zurich the next, and then off to Hawaii for R & R, yet at the same time stay constantly on the job. Instead of somewhere else, the teleradiologist could be everywhere else.

Two centuries ago a well-to-do young English gentleman, as a rite of passage, would take the grand tour, spending up to 2 years on the continent learning to be worldly and sophisticated, an important complement to go along with the haughtiness that was a birthright of his class. Today, a young radiologist can sign up with a teleradiology company for a world tour of a year or more, serving a community hospital in the Midwest, perhaps, as he or she gallivants around the globe, computer in hand, enjoying life and fully employed too, serving anywhere he or she is needed but being in no place in particular. Faced with that possibility, enticed by the freedom to be in space free of the physical and psychological constraints of confinement in a rooted place, it could be difficult to get those with wanderlust to consider a traditional fellowship as the best of all possible options immediately post-residency.

As we have seen in our specialty over the past generation, many new technologies have been quickly incorporated into our practice, even if takes a few years to come to terms with the unexpected and often profound changes that that incorporation engenders. What was inconceivable in the past is now possible in the present and will become routine in the future. It is not to sound like a Pollyanna to say one should expect that unforeseen opportunities for our specialties will be numerous.

Yet there are also a plethora of scary risks out there too. That is a matter for the next essay, in which the technology that serves us today will be the technology that may render us obsolete tomorrow.

Reference

1. Baker SR. Teleradiology—from the confines of place to the freedom of space. Emerg Radiol. 2005;11: 125–6.

Medical Tourism, Opportunities for American Radiologists?

50

Prognostication in the configuration of the structure and economics of medicine is a risky business. Unlike scientific experiments, we do not and cannot know all the variables pertinent to the delivery of healthcare, because the likelihood that any innovation will enter practice is subject to many uncertainties. First to consider or confound is the trajectory of its further development, of course. Yet also one must pay attention to the impress of competing technology as well as legal, political, financial, sociocultural and now transnational influences, each of which may become compelling and even determinative almost overnight. For example, take note of how quickly the current fiscal crisis has transformed values, settled elections and stimulated legislation that might have revolutionary consequences about how, why and by what means care is rendered.

Nonetheless, the record of the past 40 years in Radiology could serve as precedent for what unexpected initiatives we should, paradoxically, come to expect, deal with and potentially considerably benefit from. In the 1970s and 1980s Radiology was transformed by the introduction of imaging techniques which fundamentally improved on conventional radiography, through CT predominantly, as well as the harnessing of other energy sources to create incisive pictures like ultrasonography with sound waves, various gamma ray generating imaging protocols in nuclear medicine, and the perturbation by radio waves of magnetic fields to form the basis of MRI. In the 90s there were further developments in nuclear medicine, MRI, and ultrasound.

Moreover, CT, particularly, advanced with implications for patient care and its costs. And interventional procedures with imaging added another dimension to the ascendancy of Radiology. It was also the time of the beginning of the information technology revolution, allowing images to be as easily handled as words, and all information to be free of the fetters of space and place.

The result of these multi-phasic quantum leaps of improvements afforded by the digitization of images and the deployment of web-based communication enabled the birth and then the explosive growth of teleradiology, which has gone from tentative beginnings less than a decade ago to near widespread deployment, becoming along the way a multibillion dollar enterprise.

And now the same thing is occurring with medical tourism. As conventionally understood, the term betokens the relocation for diagnosis and treatment of patients away from a reliance on local or regional care to opportunities for seeking such care in any and in many places in the world. What is the significance of this particular revolution for Radiology, or more specifically for radiologists in North America?

First of all, how big has medical tourism become? Two leading consulting companies, McKinsey and Deloitte and Touche have published recent analyses on the subject. McKinsey's report asserted that while medical tourism has a bright future its immediate impact has been "hyped". According to them less than 100,000 American patients sought care abroad in the past year. While McKinsey expects growth to be inevitable, it considers it at best a marginal player for the near term. Deloitte and Touche focused on all types of treatment rather than just surgery. Their consulting team put the roster of patients in the United States seeking care abroad at 750,000 this year. In this figure they included cosmetic operations, which made up the majority of patient encounters overseas or south of the border. They predict furthermore that in 4 years 10,000,000 Americans will seek care outside the United States, benefiting foreign countries by more than 20 billion dollars per annum.

The driver of this growth is the opening up of the market [1]. Some foreign facilities are like Bumrungrad, a hospital in Bangkok, which cared for 22,000 foreigners last year. It is state-of-the-art in every way, from excellent surgeons to cutting edge IT systems. Clearly, the product they offer is a distinct attraction. A push factor is the high cost and in some way the inhibitory cost of care in the United States, even for those who are insured. It is occasioned by high deductibles and co-pays, as well as by frequent denials of payment. In contrast, to offer for those with little or no insurance the prospect of reasonable charges, including even travel and excellent accommodations at the foreign site, is a lure that more and more are choosing.

Yet, the real engine of growth of medical tourism will not be the predilections of the individual patient, but rather the opportunities for cost containment by third-party payors and employers. Blue Cross and Blue Shield of South Carolina is considering reimbursing for care given at Bumrungrad. By one projection, up to a fifth of their business may one day-and that day may be soon-be relegated to care provided at offshore facilities. Aetna is partner with hospital facilities in Singapore for high-cost procedures. Hannaford, a grocery chain in New England, offers employees the option of foreign-based care. And as I mentioned in the previous essay, a medical tourism initiative was begun for West Virginia state employees.

Medical care in the United States is costly and inefficient, and now will be subject to competition. This is good for patients, and perhaps initially bad for American physicians and American hospitals. Nonetheless, ultimately it will be salutary because efficiency and quality are stimulated by competition.

The contraction of the American and the international banking systems, and the attitudinal changes regarding consumption engendered by the realities of the recent deep recession and its catalog of lay-offs and reductions in services, have quickly caused a sea change in our values about expenditures, credit and investment. Mostly likely, our once prevalent notions about spending and saving have been buffeted and probably fundamentally altered.

Yet, every challenge brings with it an opportunity. If medical tourism can jump-start foreign economies by providing a new industry, can we too in the United States also seek advantages? And particularly does American Radiology have possibilities for advancement or should it expect medical tourism to activate its decline? Well, I believe the former is the case. First, we need to embrace the inevitable and work with it. By that I mean that just as knowledge knows no boundaries, so too does medical care. National borders are no longer impenetrable, and really they should be breached to offer greater choices, and at the same time secure and maintain health at lower cost. Thus, we should anticipate universal licensure in medicine and universal board certification, as long as the criteria to achieve each are fair and sufficiently strict. Potentially, it can be effectuated with our prospective computer-based board exam which has now replaced the subjectively influenced, site-specific oral exam. Technically, we now have the capability to evaluate all radiologists from around the world. If sanctioned and implemented it will enable doctors from elsewhere to practice here. But it will make it possible for patients from elsewhere to become available to American radiologists, hitherto restricted access by national regulations and statutes. Moreover, with methodologies for teleradiology now ubiquitous, superbly trained American radiologists will be able to compete globally without leaving their offices. Medical tourism, which is now distance related, will remain so, but with liberalization and globalization of credentialing, the next innovation supplementing conventional medical tourism will be virtual tourism for imaging diagnosis. Can this be a new wave for American radiologists, allowing us to "surf" it for our pleasure and profit and at the same time provide enhanced patient care throughout the world? My view is that we should be prepared for this possibility and get ready to "ride" it as it approaches.

Summary

The growth of medical tourism offers both a challenge and an opportunity for American radiologists. The challenges are stark although not immediate. The frequency of hospital encounters for elective surgery by Americans traveling purposively to foreign hospitals is now a trickle but will likely soon be a flood for those with comprehensive insurance. The combination of high quality, amenity provision and low cost will be hard to beat stateside. A result could be the lowering of the price of hospitalization as well as physician charges, including those for radiologic interpretation.

A less obvious consequence of the free flow of patients to comparable facilities overseas or across the border will be an increasingly compelling urge to make licensure universal and thus to also make board certification universal, given that foreign training programs for both medical and graduate medical education meet tests of similarity with American programs. Then imaging services would become like other luxury goods open to global competition. And given the excellence of our training in the U.S. and the high quality of our radiologists, opportunities could abound for American radiologists to gain significant (even abundant) business from those seeking our expertise elsewhere.

Reference

1. Weiss EM, Spataro PF, Kodner IJ, Keune JD. Banding in Bangkok, CABG in Calcutta: the United States physician and the growing field of medical tourism. Surgery. 2010 Sep;148(3):597–601.

Geriatric Radiology
A Proto-Manifesto

51

Since 1995, a salient development in Radiology has been the emergence and growth of subspecialization as a defining organizational principle for the distribution of work and expertise. At that time, 18 years ago, more than 80 % of recent graduating residents opted to continue their radiologic education in a fellowship program. Today in the last survey we undertook of the 300 senior residents taking our annual board review course, 94 % of them will spend a year (for some even two) gaining knowledge and skill in one of the well-defined distinctive concentration areas of diagnostic imaging. About one half of them will be enrolled in an ACGME-sponsored program-all of those in IR, Neuro and Pediatrics—and a few in Abdominal radiology and MSK-while the rest will be in an unregulated non-ACGME fellowship including most abdominal and MSK programs and all MR and Breast subspecialty trainings, too.

The reorganization of the ABR board examination was a response to the imperative of subspecialty experience and competence which by 2000 had become essential for Radiology to distinguish itself, by dint of standards of education and superior knowledge, vis-à-vis other specialties who were vying for a piece of the imaging pie. Some of those impetuses had already been successful by them, and other such victories have been achieved by non-radiologists since then. But we have won even many more turf wars than we have lost because we have established to some degree that each subspecialty encompasses a fairly well defined corpus of knowledge that oth- ers could not possess and only we could attain by completing a fellowship.

And so to further legitimate subspecialty training, the reorientation of the board exam encourages the achievement of special compe- tence in a formal way through the passage of its certifying exam, which is designed to be flexible in content and subspecialty based orientation.

Well, it seems perhaps that all subspecialties are addressed by this compartmentalization of formal post-residency training. We have body organ fellowships-Neuro, MSK, breast, modality fellowships-MR-and special population fellowships-Pediatrics.

And yet, through both the absence of fellow- ship, and more important by an absence of an underlying agreed-to sense of and articulation of curriculum, one major and enlarging focus of attention has been neglected. We have given no consideration to, and perhaps even evinced no intellectual interest in, the fastest growing seg- ment of society both here and abroad in Europe and Asia. I refer, of course, to the elderly.

The baby boomers in the U.S. are aging, the first of them was 65 in 2011. It is reckoned that those over that age will comprise a quarter of the American population by 2050. In Japan, it has already achieved that percentage now. And the over-85's will grow relatively more numerous when compared with the more vigorous "young old", that is those under 75. There are about 50,000 centenarians in the U.S. today. In 40 years there will be four million!

S.R. Baker, *Notes of a Radiology Watcher*,
DOI 10.1007/978-3-319-01677-1_51, © Springer International Publishing Switzerland 2014

Are the elderly just adults who are like younger adults except that they have gotten on in years? Or do they have definable, discernible distinctions that merit specific investigations, focused concern and adaptations of attitude and practice. I believe the deficiencies of the maintenance of corporeal efficiency and safety are sufficient in each regard to set the elderly apart.

But let me be more specific. There are in fact two complementary ways to consider the particular needs of senior citizens, with respect to their encounters with radiology practices and with the analytic capabilities of radiologists. In fact they can be assigned to distinct fields of study- Geriatrics and Gerontology [1]. The former refers to illness especially prevalent in the aged. The latter refers to the normal or the expected decline in capability common to the process of aging. Geriatrics focuses on pathology. Its description for specific illnesses including its radiological manifestations as well as its treatments and responses to treatment, both of which can also produce distinct findings revealed by imaging tests.

Gerontology considers the changes brought about by living for so many years with anatomic markers appearing according to an expected chronology. But gerontology also refers in the context of accommodation by radiology facilities to the policies and procedures that acknowledge and serve this distinct population. In this category would be placed "falls protection", wheelchair access, elevation policies, and aid for the less mobile and those with diminished sight and hearing. In short, how do we manage the limited patient, in his or her way akin to how we adjust our protocols and design our department to appropriately serve infants and children?

To many of you, particular parts of the substance of a geriatric radiology curriculum are probably well known, with nuggets of information displayed in disparate sources. Probably you will be able to cull from your memory those bits and pieces relevant to the elderly. For example, you may recall that pseudogout arthritis is much more common in old people than in those in middle age and that its most common manifestation is bilateral glenohumeral joint narrowing,

although that feature is less distinctive than the meniscal calcification this disease engenders in the knee. Or you might remember that the combination of hypotension, intestinal obstruction, (appearing as a plain film pattern of gaseous small bowel distension) and unremitting abdominal pain is the triad characteristic of mesenteric ischemia, a condition which requires rapid assessment of the superior mesenteric artery by CT and the prompt administration of therapy to restore blood flow throughout.

Gerontologic radiology with respect to imaging should consider physiologic alterations in the brain and elsewhere. Yet sometimes the distinction with regard to radiographic display is not clear cut. Diverticulosis, one might say, in a society consuming a Western diet is in the province of gerontology, whereas diverticulitis falls under the domain of a disease of late middle age and the elderly. In other words, a geriatric abnormality par excellence.

In fact, the concerns of gerontologic radiology are often operational. Every department must be vigilant to prevent a patient from falling, perhaps a rare event but almost always a preventable one. One should follow restrictive criteria before allowing a patient to undergo such a common test as an upright frontal and lateral chest film. In a hospital or clinic how do you restrict it in patients at risk for a fall? Is the policy part of departmental QA? How do you work with your emergency department to avoid having a demented, a confused, a hypotensive or an otherwise unsteady elderly patient from standing up unaided in your facility when a fall is a possibility, we should have rules, which mostly are strictly followed to avoid this unpleasant and possibly tragic happenstance. Think creatively here. For example, we do not do upright chest films as a routine for elderly patients presenting with a wrist fracture. Why? Because they likely sustained the fracture when they fell somewhere "in the field" because their balance then and now is deficient.

Gerontologic radiology prospectively involves interior design and architectural input to secure safety for elderly patients. How to make the department accommodate expected frailties, especially of the very old, should be not just an abstraction but an agenda item for any radiologic facility. For instance, do patients who are recumbent need to be on a bed or gurney placing them three feet above the ground when they await a procedure? In some Indian hospitals, recumbent patients are placed just above the floor. Perhaps it is not esthetically pleasing, but those patients who fall cannot fall far. An appealing design can make a lower position esthetically acceptable.

Well, these notions are just starters. In fact, as we move ahead to formalize what I think is a "discipline in gestation," if I may mix metaphors, I welcome any and all thoughts about what the dimensions of both the discipline and the policies of geriatric radiology and gerontologic radiology should entail.

Reference

1. Guglielmi G. Imaging of the geriatric patient. Philadelphia: Saunders; 2008.

Self-Referral Remedies

In a previous essay we considered the matter of increasing utilization of diagnostic imaging from the point-of-view of threats to radiology hegemony by physicians in other specialties. Much concern has been raised about self-referral by non-radiologists and its effect on healthcare costs, radiation exposure for those tests using ionizing radiation, and overall a balkanization of radiology into many self-contained and hence poorly regulated pockets of imaging initiatives. This is, of course, a very big problem, but before proceeding to remedies one must recognize that it is not the whole issue. In a debate several years ago held at a meeting of the American College of Radiology, one did not hear anything about non-radiologist self-referral. The absence of discussion about this phenomenon does not mean that our adversaries will not discuss it when the debate starts to rage. They will for sure consider that point, at least to counter the proposals organized Radiology offers, which will have the effect of regulating or removing competition. That story needs to be recited and debated if we are to retain credibility in the matter at hand i.e. how do we limit or stop the unfettered self promotion of imaging by non-radiologists?

MedPAC is a panel that advises Congress on Medicare reimbursement issues. On its agenda generically is the rapidly increasing costs of diagnostic imaging, which are rising faster than even pharmaceutical charges. Stark regulations were imposed over a decade ago to prevent physicians from referring patients to their own practice except (and I must emphasize EXCEPT)

some important outliers. The exceptions have now become a mile wide in the guise of the ancillary service provision which allows cardiologists, orthopedists and gastroenterologists to self-refer to their own facilities. Within this exception orthopedists are buying MRs, cardiologists angiography facilities and gastroenterologists CTs. An outright repeal of the ancillary service agreement would face stiff opposition.

Thus, other strategies for utilization control are now being considered. Most importantly, MedPAC's new thrust has been to improve quality as the touchstone enabling the recognition of sites of poor quality and thus either take corrective action or terminate their function as provider. Submitted data to Medicare, based on quality indices, would serve to identify sites of overutilization. MedPAC also proposes coding improvements to enable the uncovering of abuses that accrue to the imaging of multiple body sites. MedPAC, furthermore, will consider recommending the setting of standards for imaging. This notion will be complementary to ACR initiatives to translate current credentialing patterns for hospital-based physicians to private offices as well.

These proposals sound good, but will they result in decreased tests, improved interpretation, fewer repeats and lower costs? Maybe yes, but I am skeptical. There is no promising initiative that cannot be gamed so that the untoward and unexpected effects may outweigh beneficial consequences.

But the last of the MedPAC proposals to narrow the ancillary service loophole may have an immediate effect until it, too, is circumvented.

S.R. Baker, *Notes of a Radiology Watcher*,
DOI 10.1007/978-3-319-01677-1_52, © Springer International Publishing Switzerland 2014

As you can sense, I wish these quality initiatives to be successful, but I am from Missouri, at least metaphorically. Show me.

Until then, we will continue to bemoan the adverse consequences of physician self-referral and its effect on patient safety, patient care, health services, costs and a further dehumanization of imaging. But genuine overarching reform, I believe, must apply to imaging done by everybody, out-patient and in-patient, non-radiologist and radiologist alike. Yet, as I have said the denouement will only appear in the scenario when all those who are apt to lose are players. The current drama, I believe, is only a rehearsal.

Self-referral by other physicians is a major problem, inhibiting improvements in a rational use of diagnostic imaging. Recent proposals by MedPAC to tie reimbursable radiology studies to quality indices is a promising initiative but attacks only one part, albeit a major one, of the problem. Radiologists should also acknowledge and move to correct radiologists' self-referral, which engenders mistrust among referring physicians but also induces increased costs, even as it does not resolve uncertainty [1].

Reference

1. Weixel N. With budget, Obama takes MedPAC's advice Bloomberg BNA. Bloomberg BNA; 10 Apr 2013. http://www.bna.com/budget-obama-takes-b17179873292/.

Part X

The Challenges Facing American Radiologists

The challenges facing American radiology are serious and diverse. Some are hypothetical at present, others are about to emerge, and still others confront us now. Considered here are the impetuses from non-radiologists to perform imaging examinations, the threat of computer-determined diagnoses, the spectre of trade liberalization with respect to services across national borders, the scarcity of commodities needed for radiology devices such as rare earth metals, the intrusions of the press, and the general economic outlook in this time of decelerating demand.

The Radiologist Assistant: Do We Need This Job Title?

The Radiology Assistant is a job title whose time has come, but the need for it may not be here anymore. Central to the tasks of this job category is the performance but not the interpretation of fluoroscopic procedures. However, the record of the past several years indicates a decline in such studies nationally, and an acceleration of that decline most recently. Thus, the increase in compensation demanded by Radiology Assistants by the mandate of their B.A. or M.A. degrees may not be justified by the paucity of the volume allotted to their enhanced responsibilities.

All of you know that Radiology is undergoing profound changes, at least with respect to the provision of personnel. The radiologist glut is upon us. At the same time a shortage of technologists has come to the fore as a major issue. One of the ways in which to respond to the decreased number of applicants per available position is to upgrade the status of the radiology technologists making them radiology assistants with expanded training and skills. This issue, controversial of course, was embraced several years ago by the American College of Radiology who, with the American Society of Radiology Technologists, has devised a curriculum for an enhancement of the technologist's responsibilities. Training guidelines encompassing a range of characteristics under the rubric of upgrading the capabilities of the technologist have been devised, and now approximately 15–20 programs have been initiated to train radiology assistants. The American College of Radiology has felt compelled to address this issue because state governments by themselves were going to approve both the concept and the specifics of radiology assistants, education and certification. So now we have the official imprimatur of the radiology establishment fostering the development of this new job title and its new capabilities. I am here to offer a criticism of the concept. I will endeavor to do that with data derived from a range of sources to try to demonstrate that the radiology assistant position does not really enhance quality very much, but certainly increases the cost of care for radiologists and ultimately for society.

Let me state that I am not against radiology extenders. In fact, we have used interventional radiology PAs for the last several years and are very pleased with their performance. Moreover, at first, I was not hostile to the concept of the radiology assistant. In fact, I have devised a curriculum for radiology assistants, and this year will give several 90-min lectures to our first year class of radiology assistants matriculating in our adjacent school of allied health. I will continue to pursue this project with determination, if not with gusto, but also with the knowledge that the positions we are creating may have untoward consequences for the practice of medicine. I was not initially aware of these negative features because, like many other initiatives, the unintended results take a while to declare themselves.

Now, why are there radiology assistants? Why has this notion become popular? Of course, as I mentioned before, the overabundance of radiologists is becoming widespread in the U.S. We now have enough radiologists to do all the procedures that can be scheduled for them. But there is also a shortage of radiological technologists with a current 15.3 % vacancy rate which, by the way, is the worst among all healthcare workers. Moreover, the average age of technologists is leaning toward the geriatric, since half of the technologists are over 41. In 2010, it was estimated that there will be a need for 75,000 more technologists. Presently, the technologist's position does not leave much room for advancement, and many consider it to be a career dead end.

Also, we have noticed the growth of non-physician advanced practice positions in other specialties. For instance, nurse practitioners and, especially nurse anesthetists, have shown that even without an MD degree they can take on much responsibility.

The adoption of the concept of the RAs was the subject of a consensus paper approved by the ACR in 2002 in hopes of managing then current shortage of radiologists. The stated expectation was that RAs would make radiologists more efficient, but no further elaboration of what efficiency meant was included. It was also stated that the radiology assistant would not interpret images. The need to codify the responsibilities of RAs nationally was in part a response to an avid interest in some states, especially in Kentucky, Washington and Montana, for the establishment of the job category of R.A.s. Moreover, the impress of marketplace considerations portended that this title would become a reality whether the ACR would approve it or not. Nonetheless, many radiologists were concerned, particularly in view of the eventual prospect that the radiologist assistant would bring power unto himself like the nurse anesthetist and take away some of our responsibilities, business and income.

The ACR was concerned that the RA programs should maintain patient safety, that supervision would also be vouchsafed, and that there would be one standard of practice throughout the nation, because they did not want 50 different scopes of responsibility, each mandated by one state. Now, one of the compelling urges from the technologist community regarding upgrading the tech's position takes impetus from the distinction between a vocation and a profession. Webster's

Third New International Dictionary states that a profession is a calling requiring specialized knowledge and often long and intensive preparation, including instruction in skills and methods, as well as in the scientific, historical and/or scholarly basis underlying such skills and methods, maintaining by force of organization or concerted opinion high standards of achievement and conduct, and committing its members to continued study and to a kind of work which has for its prime purpose the rendering of a public service. The curriculum for radiology assistant programs certainly encompasses all of the aspects of this definition, and certainly indicates that the job is much more than a vocation, which was also defined by Webster as the work in which a person is regularly employed, usually for pay, for the special function of an individual or group within a larger order. Notice the difference, a corpus of study is required, standards need to be met and a public service is rendered. All of these desiderata can be incorporated into a curriculum for a baccalaureate or even a master's degree for radiology assistants. No wonder this would be something greeted with glee by the American Society of Radiology Technologists. Yet, with this advanced training what do we as radiologists get clinically?

Specific roles were devised for radiology assistants. They would (1) obtain consent for procedures, (2) obtain a clinical history (3) perform procedure and postprocedure evaluations of invasive studies (4) assist radiologists with invasive procedures. These four, by the way, can be encompassed now by physician assistants in interventional radiology. They do not need a separate job category among all technologists.

The defining role of the RA centers on performing fluoroscopy for non-invasive procedures, with the radiologist providing direct supervision (which means incidentally that the physician is on-site and immediately available but not necessarily in the room). Let us look in some detail at fluoroscopy volume. Medicare data over a 5-year period from 1997 to 2002 showed that GIs with no KUB have decreased in this period, GIs with a KUB have also decreased, while GIs with a small bowel follow-through have maintained the same numbers over that 5-year span. When we look at double contrast GIs we see that for those with no KUB and for those with a KUB, the volume had been about the same over that 5-year period. In fact, double GIs plus small bowel follow-through increased in the early part of this century. Fluoroscopy declined for single contrast studies yet maintained stability, by and large, for double contrast studies. But now, too, it is declining as well. And, with barium enemas, there has been a marked and continuing decrease. Over the same 5-year period, the average for a single contrast BE was 259,000 studies registered with Medicare, but in 2002 it was 184,000. Similarly, for double contrast BE the 5-year average was 178,000 but in 2002 it was 121,000. More than a decade later, the decline has continued to a point where we should conclude that this examination is merely moribund. If we put these two examinations together using combined GI and BE volume numbers, we find that considering there were 30,000 active radiologists in 2002, a typical imaging physician performed less than 20 single contrast GIs and 25 double contrast GIs per year. Considering there are ten radiologists per group on average who would perform such studies, in a total year at one hospital facility, less than 500 GIs, both single and double contrast, would be performed, that is ten a week or two per day at most places.

Hence with this volume, on average, no more than 50 min a day will be spent in fluoroscopy in a typical hospital with a 10 man group of physician fluoroscopists. The average time a trained RA will have spent per day in fluoroscopy is 50 min out of a total working day of 500 min.

Is three studies per day valid or an overstatement? The data I have listed here includes all studies even though they are done by non-radiologists. For example, some upper GIs and BEs are performed by gastroenterologists. So, what does it mean to have a radiology assistant perform fluoroscopy? How much are we gaining from three or less studies per day taking one tenth of the RA's time?

The ACR accreditation criteria for general radiology and fluoroscopy first required that 50 double contrast BEs be done per year to enable a group to apply for accreditation. Because the number of BEs has decreased it was changed to 50 double contrast BEs recommended. Yet, of 91 applications received so far only 56 supplied a BE for evaluation. Actually, eight of them dropped out because they could not find an example of their best work barium enema and of the 10 best work barium enemas I have seen, only two are adequate.

Most RA training programs as currently being set up are not necessarily medical school-based. So, there is a further question about fluoroscopy teaching quality. Moreover, what will the radiology assistant do for the other 90 % of the day? They will be able to perform, under general but not immediate supervision, fistulograms, which are not common routine studies, hysterosalpinography, which is declining, arthrograms which have become uncommon, PICC lines which can be done by IR/PAs, and lumbar punctures which are also uncommon. The RA can also monitor IVUs, CT urograms, VCUGs and retrograde urethrograms. Again, outside of pediatric facilities, VCUGs are very uncommon and their total volume, I imagine, would be even less than fluoroscopy.

It is recommended that RAs do CT and MR post-processing. However, no advanced degree should be needed for this function. One could certainly train techs without those techs getting an equivalent of a college degree in a formal curriculum. It all boils down to the fact that, aside from maybe one hour a day, most RAs will probably function as before as techs but with increased pay and benefits.

RAs will also have an effect on academic practice. They will impinge on residency training, and occasion attending expenditure of time and effort for RA education itself.

Taking a look at double contrast BEs again, considering radiology residencies in general, for all programs, the number of annual barium enemas at the primary hospital was 268 but the median was only 201, indicating that there were few outliers that do much fluoroscopy still, but most places do very few of them compared with the past. If we consider the data for places with 16–19 residents, an average of 126 barium enemas are done per annum, which means that with 18 residents, seven barium enemas will be done per trainee per year and 28 would be done over the 4 years if there were no radiology assistants. Yet, if radiology assistants are integrated into the training program and they are expected to do ten BEs then a resident will complete the program with only four per year or a total of 16. So, both the RA and the resident will have too few fluoro procedures through their training period. Who, therefore, will become their teachers? It is unlikely the junior radiologist will gain or retain such expertise in fluoroscopy. In 5 years radiologist's capabilities in this area will atrophy. Moreover, the radiology assistant will have little training yet they will be expected to be the educators.

A paper in JACR by Smith and Applegate stated that the radiology graduate will become the instructor of fluoroscopy, freeing up faculty time. They will be able to perform better than residents. Yet, there have no studies of surveys specific to radiology extenders and radiology residents. Smith and Applegate then stated that in an academic setting it is important that individuals selected as RAs be oriented toward teaching as part of their duties, and that these individuals be given time and resources necessary to establish programs to teach residents and fellows in their expertise. But we have no assurance that the people we bring into radiology assistant programs will be good teachers. Yet, they will be the only teachers because radiologists will have lost this capability. Do we want this to happen? I suggest we don't.

Currently, for our RA training program, I will give 5 to 10, 90-min lectures and my staff will give 80, 90-min lectures for the first year trainees, and then in the second year of training we will be preceptors working one-on-one with RA trainees. Who will pay for the time and effort of radiologists as faculty members to teach RAs? Is it a free good? The nearly inevitable financial calculus of a BA or MA degree in medicine is that you pay your tuition now, therefore, enriching the schools of allied health, but you regain it in multiples as salary over a career. A radiology tech today makes between 60 and $80,000 but radiology assistants, completing a master's degree will make between 80 and 120,000 per year. Yet, reimbursement through Medicare for studies performed by radiology assistants will only be 85 % of what will be given to radiologists. Moreover, we must pay malpractice for RAs, which is an additional cost. And if we examine barium enemas once again, we see that in RRC data there are 7,500 breast imaging studies per year in a typical hospital and 200 barium enemas. We did a study of malpractice suits among 4,600 radiologists who had a total of 2,600 suits. Of those, 250 were mammo related and 18 were barium enemas related. Therefore, if we take a look at the index of risk as the number of suits per lifetime versus the number of studies per year, in mammo it is 0.03 but in barium enemas it is 0.09. In fact, barium enemas are probably the most risk prone studies in all of radiology in terms of the likelihood of malpractice suits per case. Therefore, we will have to contend with the fact that the now more enriched radiology technologist may be sued and the plaintiff's attorney may go after them too. Yet, they will be our employees, at least for a while until they gain independence.

So, the facts do not look pleasant for the consequences of the implementation of radiology assistants, either for academic practice or general practice. For those wishing to hire these individuals I repeat the age-old phrase, *caveat emptor*.

The radiology assistant is a job category whose time has come. But should it? Devised to ease the radiologist shortage, which no longer exists, and provide opportunities for advancement for radiology technologists, the key component of training for this position is instruction in fluoroscopy. All other parts of the job description can be done by PAs. Fluoroscopy procedures are declining rapidly in the U.S. Thus, the radiology assistant could be trained to provide a chimera as BE volume continues to shrink. Moreover, like other extenders, a likely eventual outcome will be autonomy for them and restrictions on a radiologist's range of responsibilities [1].

Reference

1. Baker SR, Merkulov A. Radiology assistants: a contrarian view. Emerg Radiol. 2005;11:187–92.

Challenges to Radiology From Below, Astride and Afar

A famous quote goes something like this "I am condemned to live in interesting times". Well, that condemnation applies to all of us because the times certainly are interesting as they are characterized by uncertainty, perhaps even foreboding, too. I am sure when you read these words the uncertainty in the economy will still be persisting. I need not go into detail about that. Uncertainty in the political arena will also continue to bedevil us or excite us but it will definitely challenge us. We as a nation must confront compelling domestic issues and try to reestablish or redefine our place in the world. Our once secure position as the global hegemon has now been buffeted by events and by increasingly hostile attitudes towards us from Europe, Asia, Africa, and Latin America. We also must contend with uncertainty in the United States in the social arena. Our population is changing in its ethnic makeup. Immigration has continued to increase, both for people of limited education attainments and for professionals. Moreover, these trends have been accompanied by modification in our collective assumptions of value, in our consumption patterns and in our regard for the importance of preserving the environment. At the same time we are now undergoing profound reassessment in our most highly valued institutions, specifically, the profession of medicine, and precisely the specialty of Radiology.

The beginning of the twenty-first century stands out along with the end of the 19th, with respect to medicine. One was and the other will be disorienting eras. They can be considered together as bookends of disorder which temporally flank the relative stability of the twentieth century. Remember, the Flexner report was written before World War I. It did a lot to dispel the anarchy and lack of professionalism that had pervaded medical education back then. The public demanded more accountability and expertise from physicians, which led to the imposition of more vigorous standards in licensure, and further regulations in the 1920s, 1930s and 1940s, including the introduction of the specialty board certification. This was followed in the latter half of the century by the codification of requirements for medical education, then for graduate medical education and finally for continuing medical education. These rules, as well as board certification requirements, are now in flux. In fact, the regulations which have molded the reach and the obligations of medicine through the creation of a reliable superstructure of organizations were implemented and monitored according to the prerequisites of a guild. From their origin in medieval times, guilds have acted to maintain the aims and the processes of their carefully chosen constituents. A standard dictionary definition for a guild is an association of merchants or artisans, organized to maintain standards and to protect the interests of its members, to enable them to be recognized as a local, or today, a national governing body.

Yes, we, in medicine, are in fact a guild, with sub guilds superintending the various specialties. We function through such organizations to foster the members' privileges and responsibilities. By so doing, sometimes we incur increased costs for the general population. Yet at the same time guilds profess standards to be pursued and met so that the public's trust then can be repaid by good works under the rules imposed by the guild and by accepted notions of integrity which we deem to be the proper attitude of guild members.

Nonetheless, anarchy and uncertainty are seeping into the heart of our master guild, the American house of medicine in general, as well as infiltrating the parenchyma of its other viscera including the specialty of Radiology. Such physiologic dysfunctions threaten to disrupt the parameters and paradigms of guild structure operationally, tactically and even strategically. They are attacking the equanimity of the status quo from below, as a result of the aggressiveness of seemingly lesser occupations, from alongside us in turf wars among specialties and now, with the advent of telemedicine and medical tourism, from afar as well.

Before there were physicians and nurses there used to be midwives and barbers who performed medical and surgical procedures. Now midwives have reappeared as an accepted category of health care worker. Alongside of them are myriad allied health occupations, ranging from social workers to respiratory technologists. Numerous titles abound filled by people trained in administration, in risk management, and as technical assistants such as phlebotomists. We have on staff play therapists, nutritionists and grief counselors. The top of the pyramid is still the preserve of physicians but this formerly solid structure formulated for everyone to have a place and everyone in its place is now revealing cracks on its sides and rumblings from below.

It seems that leaders in every lesser occupation want to make theirs a profession. Over the course of time initiatives to elevate the responsibilities and rewards of various job categories have generally borne fruit, although the process has been stow and halting. For example, until recently dental hygienists could not practice independently but had to be employed by a dentist. Today, in several states, they have now become independent contractors, thereby increasing their sphere of action and their income. The ascent of the nurse anesthetist is another example of the value of establishing and following a well-worn pathway for professionalization, enabling these non-physicians to become sanctioned to administer anesthetic drugs. In many respects nurse anesthetists are equal in responsibility if not in remuneration to anesthesiologists.

Furthermore a very important step was taken recently by the nursing establishment in a frontal assault on the primacy of physicians. Once a limitation but now an opportunity for nurses rests in the fact that the corpus of knowledge they must accumulate is not dissimilar from what physicians have to learn. They had been stymied by the exclusivity of physician management. Their intellectual advancement, on the other hand, rose only to the level of a completed master's degree. Now they have broken through the curricular glass ceiling. Today, a doctorate of nursing practice can be earned. Some proudly proclaim themselves as RN-DNP or doctor of nursing practice. Furthermore, the National Board of Medical Examiners has permitted appropriately qualified nurses to sit for an examination nearly identical in control and scope to Step Three of the USMLE examination. By this action the gauntlet has been thrown down in front of the family physician. The granting of such a degree to nurses, which may cause patient misinterpretation of the distinctions between a nurse and a doctor, is a complaint of the besieged family physician. Furthermore, the examinations such nurses will take and pass are comparable in format, measure similar competence, and apply similar performance standards to the physicians, akin to the Step Three of the USMLE. Consequently, family practitioners perceived that as a threat. The AMA issued a statement opposing the diffusion of the doctorate of nursing practice degree because it may make the nurse into a healthcare leader, predictably replacing the MD. Accordingly, the nurses objected to this criticism, stating it is no more appropriate for the American Medical Association (AMA) to regulate nursing practice than it would be for the American Nursing Association (ANA) to regulate medical practice [1].

The rumblings from below are also heard among radiologists. The establishment of the Radiology Assistant program was a means of professionalizing technologists, placing them in a new role as "super techs". Earning such a distinction requires an advanced degree beyond the B.A, or B.S. as a prerequisite but with it and with the gaining of the title after a formal program of study commands a relatively higher salary as a concomitant. The American College of Radiology embraced this concept somewhat hurriedly, in its present form, constituted as a national job title, because the ACR feared, among other things, that the various states would set up different terms for radiology assistants, creating disorder and perhaps stimulating impingements on radiologists' freedom of action.

The key point in the description of duties of the radiology assistant, as I related in detail in another essay, is that they would become more independent in the performance of fluoroscopic procedures. New programs have been set up to train radiology assistants, some of them have already graduated individuals to assume this role. However, it appears to me to be more of a tempest in a teapot because the major focus of their increased training is in fluoroscopy. Unfortunately for radiology assistants, fluoroscopy is decreasing and neither radiology residents nor radiology assistants will be able to obtain the requisite patient load to be able to perform barium studies to the same degree of competence that older radiologists have learned and practiced.

In Radiology the disruption of our guild is coming not so much from below as from alongside. The actions, attitudes and intrusions of cardiologists are the prime example. Because imaging is so interesting and has expanded so much and has been rewarded to such a degree by third party payers, many specialties besides radiologists want to get into the act. We are all aware of the highly organized, detail-oriented approach of the cardiologist. We await the same type of initiatives from the gastroenterologist once they see that virtual colonoscopy may take off to become a valuable modality. The neurosurgeons have adapted their training programs to allow a year of training in neuroimaging, and the neurologists have become eager to enter into residencies in endoscopic surgical neuroradiology, most of which are in non-ACGME approved programs. So we will have to fight harder to protect the traditional primacy of radiologists in imaging, especially to maintain control of newer modalities, which by their expansion have increased our productivity and our income.

However, I daresay radiologists as a group are asleep at the switch in this regard. The key point in maintaining our turf is to become specialized and, for that, the changes in the board examination will work to our advantage. Yet, that is necessary but not sufficient to meet the challenge that will confront us. In addition, we have to convince hospitals and insurance companies that we have the credentials to provide specialized imaging to the exclusion of other physicians whose training we deem less intense, less concerned with quality and less directed to patient safety.

In pediatric radiology, interventional radiology and neuroradiology we have three fellowships that meet specific ACGME guidelines primarily because a certificate of added qualification is offered to establish the detailed and concentrated pursuit of specific curricular goals. This involves meeting caseload requirements, maintaining program comprehensiveness and formulating specific competencies objectively and often quantitatively. Yet, as I have outlined elsewhere in this book, the leadership of many of these specialty programs needs to improve. And much more important, nearly all the other fellowship possibilities do not manifest the same rigorousness. In fact, only 45 % of graduating senior residents choose the three ACGME fellowships with CAQ possibilities. Ten percent go directly into practice, a number which will most likely decrease as the board examination scheduling changes take place.

Equally popular as neuroradiology as a specialty choice is body imaging, and emerging now as a highly popular subspecialty is breast imaging (or women's' imaging). Moreover, while there are ACGME programs in abdominal radiology and musculoskeletal radiology, more than 90 % of those choosing such specialties opt for programs outside ACGME overview. As a result the only thing that a young radiologist who completed a fellowship in them can show for his or her time in that period of advanced learning is completion of a term. They may compile a log of completed cases but there is no demand for it from a national accrediting body. Consequently, when their credentials are placed in front of a hospital or insurance company, the fellowship experience is incompletely delineated, in stark contrast with the detailed listing of cases that can be provided by the cardiologist. In order for Radiology to succeed as a relevant service we must increase the number of subspecialists. Yet we must also tighten the credentialing process or we will find ourselves having to share responsibility with other services or be excluded from them altogether. So the problems from "astride" are real. They can be remedied, but today there seems to be little impetus among the leaders in radiology to address them expeditiously and forthrightly.

Now for the future. Well, actually the future is now in relation to medical tourism. This example of the conflation of globalization and commodization is growing rapidly now. It will be a very significant activity in the future, and the future will be soon. Two recent analyses by well-respected consulting firms, McKinsey and Deloitte and Touche, differed in specifics but were similar in indicating the prospect for accelerated expansion of medical tourism, especially for outbound experiences involving the travel of American patients abroad. Currently the number of individuals partaking of such an experience is relatively small, less than 100,000 a year according to McKinsey. However, they did not include outpatient procedures or cosmetic surgery. When all medical trips are taken together the figure of 750,000 Americans traveling abroad as listed in the Deloitte and Touche study seems a more reasonable assessment. In many of the facilities it is not merely lower costs that attract patients, it is also the perception that quality is as good. If not better at a place beyond our borders.

Many such inpatient facilities have been evaluated and approved by the Joint Commission International, a branch of JCAHO, which since 1999 has been accrediting premier foreign facilities. Moreover, ten highly respected institutions including the University of Pittsburgh, Sloan-Kettering and Harvard Medical School have opened facilities or otherwise made arrangements with foreign treatment centers. Several countries have upgraded their services and have directed hospitals and clinics to cater to foreign patients almost exclusively. Although issues of malpractice and liability remain, insurers have become increasingly interested in covering foreign medical trips. For example, a bill was introduced in the West Virginia legislature to allow state employees to seek foreign services for medical care for which payment would be allocated.

There is no doubt that medical tourism is here to stay and will continue to grow apace, perhaps even explosively. Inherent in this process will be a realization that the radiology care given at these facilities will be at least adequate to what can be received in the U.S. Training of radiologists in various countries differs considerably from what is provided in our country, but there have been no widespread allegations that the interpretive capabilities of foreign radiologists for patients seeking medical treatment elsewhere have been inferior. And with the transformation of the radiology board examination to a computer based test it seems likely, if not inevitable, that as American insurers become more convinced of the value of medical tourism there will be a further attempts to standardize practice and certification. Inasmuch as teleradiology continues to lead in the application of telemedicine, it also seems likely that there will be a movement for universal licensure which will be guaranteed by the implementation of the new American board examination in radiology, because it can be given anywhere and it does not require an onsite evaluator.

Now, such a prospect may seem scary, raising possibilities that could make your hair stand on end. On the other hand, universal licensure would be a reciprocal process when it occurs. And I suggest that the opportunities for American radiologists to interpret studies from abroad will be enhanced by a universal licensure as well.

Well, that is, just the beginning of the subject. In the next essay I will try to explore medical tourism and medical licensure in more detail, not as an advocate although perhaps as a Cassandra. I do this because it is better to prepare for a likely event then to rail about its bad karma or unkind fate and then dismiss it categorically, hoping it will go away.

Reference

1. Baker SR, Merkulov A. Radiology assistants—a contrarian view. Emerg Radiol. 2005;11:187–92.

The Coming Revolution in Radiology: Beware and Prepare

Thomas Watson should be a familiar name to those interested in technology. In fact, it ought to be evocative of major changes in how we transfer information and ultimately organize work by dint of its identification with two individuals having that name. The first Thomas Watson was the assistant summoned by Alexander Graham Bell in the first telephone call. The second one was a long time CEO of IBM whose name was affixed to the computer that beat the star human performers in several games of Jeopardy.

The telephone call Watson #1 received heralded the transformation of medical care in many ways. Along with the coincident development of the elevator it made possible the modern hospital enabling it to be situated in a large edifice. The elevator made feasible vertical transportation and therefore stacking wards, operating suites and radiology departments in multiple stories with Radiology usually on the bottom. The telephone made possible efficient horizontal (and vertical) communication.

What has been revealed with Watson #2. It is but the latest manifestation of the astounding reordering of knowledge made manifest by the development of the computer harnessed to the internet. First the telegraph and the telephone enabled the rapid transmission of words beyond the delimited space extending from eye to eye and within the extent of the range of articulated speech. Next radio and television revealed that words and then images could be sent to many people at great distances from one source. First the fax machine and subsequently the Internet have

expanded the ease of bilateral word communication, or more precisely real time consultations, and added to it equally facile image transmission. As applied to radiographic displays it allowed the creation of the multi-billion dollar teleradiology industry. Watson #2 revealed that not just words and pictures were both ubiquitously deployable but that the whole of the universe factual knowledge, too, was readily retrievable and deployable too. It demonstrated that anything that had been archived can be retrieved in less than the time the human brain could recall it from memory.

So what is now to follow? Is every step ahead part of the irresistible march of the information juggernaut? For radiology I believe we have participated in a misstep-small though it may be-but one by the act of stumbling has distracted us from the inevitable eventuality of the transformation of work that we do and the value we add. I refer here to the application of the computer to the interpretation of images. We in Radiology have made the error of trying to use computer assisted detection first to aid in solving a more difficult set of questions when the easier ones have been at hand yet hitherto neglected. We have applied Computer Assisted Detection (C.A.D.) primarily to the evaluation of breast cancer. Indeed, I believe this may be definitively beyond the current limits of capability of computerization, and thus we are trying to pick the high hanging fruit and have not looked at the fecund lower branches of the tree.

Why? For one, mammography is a type of plain radiography. With regard to the spectrum of information it provides, plain films by possessing

S.R. Baker, *Notes of a Radiology Watcher*,
DOI 10.1007/978-3-319-01677-1_55, © Springer International Publishing Switzerland 2014

more subtlety and more range in their shades of gray, they are more electronically rich and diverse than cross-sectional images derived from CT or MR. Excluding mammography, plain films may not be as diagnostically incisive as CT or MR sections. And in the dense breast, lesions are hard to recognize with the eye alone and only slightly better at detected and discerned with computer assistance.

And that is not all. The purpose of mammography is not only to find a lesion but also to characterize it with, the expectation that an inference about its histology can be gleaned. More specifically and hopefully, computer assistance offered the prospect that it could differentiate malignancy from non-malignancy by assessing the presence of calcification, the pattern of that calcification, the contour of the lesion and the presence of ancillary findings in the dense breast. But judging from the literature on the subject, it has not been an unmitigated success.

Another application of computer-assistance has been to characterize small lung nodules seen on CT. Well, one half of the problem here is ameliorated. The electronic spectrum of CT is narrower than plain films yet a spatial characterization by computer assistance must still come up against the same major hurdle. You are demanding that the radiologist with his eye or his computer must make a microscopic diagnosis with macroscopic means.

The problem in the breast and in the lung, the two organs for which computer assistance has been most frequently applied, is that the computer is not as good at pathologic assessment of tissue. Incidentally, histology itself is not so foolproof for predicting tumor enlargement when the lesion is still small because the growth rate of these tiny abnormalities is still not known for each specific case.

Nonetheless there are now diagnostic questions in which emerging research has shown that an algorithmic approach to spatial analysis of CT sections, for one, promises to be not an example of computer-assisted diagnosis but rather of computer-determined diagnosis. For example, I refer to an estimation of the appearance of liver lesions as assessed by computer analysis. Work on this subject has been undertaken with promising results in Japan and at the Mayo Clinic, where radiologists are working closely with researchers from IBM-the same company that created Watson #2. These investigators are posing and answering the right questions computers today can answer. They seek answers to questions only of macroscopic distinction. The challenges they address are realizable. Is the lesion growing and are there now more of them? In the evaluation of the hepatic contours and substance by radiographic imaging means, there are only a few things to consider. What is the lesion size and what is its shape? Is it more or less radiodense than expected? What is its density at specific times after the injection of contrast material? Does it contain calcium and if so in what pattern? And are there lucencies in the liver? If so, what are their size, margins and multiplicity? These are more straightforward investigative matters for the creation of an algorithm that a computer could answer than they would be for the diagnosis of breast or lung cancer. These questions do not require a leap from macroscopy to microscopy. They all involve measurement characterizable from the computed images which are directly determinable.

If computer-determined diagnosis is possible in the liver, could it be applied to the kidney to the brain? Here is how it might be employed for tumor or vascular hepatic abnormalities. The initial diagnosis of metastases to liver is made by the radiologist who renders a report and is paid for the insightfulness of his expertise. But subsequent CT's are really seeking only two answers. Are the lesions shrinking, staying the same size or enlarging and are there more or fewer of them? The computer can now provide those answers without the radiologists even looking at the images if the algorithm is reliable. Moreover, unlike in the breast reliability is no longer a formidable theoretic or developmental problem.

Which bring us to the most important implication of this innovation. It is not merely a small step but rather a long stride in the progress of the aforementioned technology juggernaut. If the follow up CTs are computer-determined not just computer-assisted for liver metastases or in other organs, can we charge the same fee for what the computer does by itself compared to what we have done initially or previously before the follow-up studies are done? Assuming the widespread utilization of computer-determination, can we charge for successive CT's or MR's of the brain after a stroke or a bleed? Fundamentally what then will be the intellectual work of the radiologist? Is it image detection when we now have or soon will have an electronic competitor? Or do we in fact, or should we for that matter, do more in accord with our training as physicians to become more clinically involved caregivers which will demand a different paradigm about how we interact with referrers and their patients.

In other words as presently constituted will we become obsolete? Let me alarm you with a quote from an essay by the columnist Schumpeter in a recent editorial in the Economist "A university education (and a medical school education-my word) is still a requisite for entering some of the great fields such as medicine that provide secure and well-paying jobs. Over the twentieth century, academic guilds did a wonderful job of raising barriers to entry-sometimes for good reasons and sometimes for self-interested ones. But these guilds are beginning to buckle. Newspapers are fighting a losing battle with the blogosphere. Universities are replacing tenured tract professors with non-tenured staff. Even doctors are threatened as patients find advice online." And we may be the most threatened because we do not have patients to stay with us as the coordinators of practice change. Faced with this formidable threat, the ACR and other defenders of Radiological hegemony may not be the most effective advocates.

Teleradiology and GATS-An-800 lb Gorilla Down the Hall

In early February 2004 President Bush's chief economic advisor, N. Gregory Mankiw, who was once Harvard's youngest tenured professor, made a comment that attracted a firestorm of political invective. He told Congress that if a service could be rendered more cheaply by foreigners abroad than by Americans in the US, we were better off importing it than producing it at home. According to an article on his testimony which appeared in The Economist magazine, to prove his point Mankiw used the example of radiologists in India analyzing studies of American patients' images sent via the internet. This pronouncement elicited two types of responses [1]. Inasmuch as it was the beginning of the presidential election season, the remark was seized upon by populists in either party who rained abuse on Mr. Mankiw for such a statement. A common retort "how dare we talk about exporting jobs and in this case, the jobs are radiologists." Yet professional economists on both sides of the aisle agreed with him, understanding that this was a typical consequence of globalization. In the aggregate it benefits many, even though it may dislocate a few in the beginning, until those negatively affected relocate and redirect their employment. In fact, the increased liberalization of service provision spanning national borders under the rubric of free trade continues to be policy government.

Well, Mankiw was right about the effects of globalization and prospects for trade in commodities and services. However, he was wrong about radiology. In 2004 there were attempts to outsource radiology examinations to physicians in other countries who were not licensed in the state for which the images originated, and had not graduated from an American or Canadian medical school, nor had they completed their residency here. Furthermore, they had not achieved American Board of Radiology diplomate status.

Why does their expertise not count whereas for engineers, for example, foreign training is not a disqualification? The reason is because physicians have been very successful in regulating themselves by setting up barriers to the internationalization of their work product. Although it is possible and even likely that radiologists elsewhere may be as adept at reading images as American radiologists and that, presently, the mechanisms for the transmission of images results in no loss of quality, nevertheless the requirements of licensure, board certification, and training in an accredited program have all effectively prevented foreign nationals without American credentials from performing teleradiology, the exception being the significant although perhaps not very well publicized reviewing of radiographs and CTs on either side of the Canadian border by radiologists who are citizens of either country [1].

On the other hand, the politically and regulatory acceptable model for preliminary readings—the night hawk model—has developed into a very robust business in which American-trained radiologists, situated abroad who have secured licenses in each state they reviewed originated, render preliminary readings for Medicare. Such a protocol does not run afoul of federal regulations. However, despite Mankiw's proclamation, the free trade of radiologic images across national boundaries, and across continental and intercontinental spaces has not occurred. I imagine that most of you believe, too, that teleradiology arrangements, with reading done alone by foreign nationals in their home country, will not take place for U.S. patients.

But you may be wrong. In the nineteenth century, the U.S. erected rather high tariff walls to prevent free trade and yet the country grew. The reason was that there was so much infrastructure to be developed here and the population of the country was burgeoning, so our country's economy, the cotton trade aside, was insular. International capital outflows and inflows were a minor constituent of economic activity. Moreover, limitations in communication and transportation prevented all but the most stable and least heavy commodities to be traded abroad.

In the twentieth century, things changed. The response to the stock market crash of 1929 taken by congress and President Hoover was to erect restrictive trade barriers through the imposition of the Smoot-Hawley act. This resulted in a worldwide depression, the most severe in our country's history and probably the most severe in the world. Thus, after WWII there was a collective effort by the victors, particularly the North Atlantic countries, to lower tariff barriers through the continued collective efforts of trade representatives within the context of the general agreement on trade and tariffs known as GATT. Since its inception GATT has gained credibility and strength. Initially it was to be organized under the International Trade Organization, an entity which died in its infancy. Yet GATT agreements continued to be concluded and implemented. It took approximately 40 years of trade discussion and decision through GATT to formally establish the World Trade Organization which manages further negotiations regarding international trade for its 120 member nations. In the Uruguay round of trade negotiations which occurred in the mid 1990S GATS—the General Agreement on Trade and Services was established. This is a second treaty, if you will, and it refers to the international trade in services which has now become an accompaniment to the efforts to reduce trade and tariffs for goods. Since WWII our global economy has become more and more concerned with services as well as trade. GATS therefore provides another mechanism for trade agreements that abet globalization.

Bear in mind that teleradiology is a service that can extend across borders with no friction of distance or time. And thus it could be accommodated within the framework of GATS. Should you be concerned about GATS? Well, maybe not this year or next, but with 17 % of our GNP going for healthcare, further increases in this portion of the national economy may engender significantly more strident calls for reduction in costs. And what is the service most congenial to a reduction in costs through commodification and globalization? It is teleradiology of course.

So let's look at the details of GATS, to foresee how it might be applied and how it might be prevented from applying. Any application of the General Agreement on Trade in Services (GATS) can be directed to any or all of the 120 signatories to the World Trade Organization charter, if they wish to be involved. Trade in health services can fit under the rubric of GATS just like other services that are amenable to commodification including e-banking, distance learning, and remote gambling. All of them are readily integratable for internet communication.

The areas in healthcare that could be included under GATS are 1—health insurance, 2—hospital services, 3—medical treatment abroad, and for radiologists 4—telemedicine. GATS is organized under four modes of supply. Mode 1 is the cross border provision of services delivered in the country of nation one from the territory of nation two for patients in nation two. Teleradiology is the exemplar. Mode 2 is service delivered outside the territory of nation one in the territory of another nation to serve consumers of nation one. This is medical tourism, and even without GATS, medical tourism is beginning to become more popular. Mode 3—refers to health service delivered within the territory of nation one by the commercial presence of a company from another nation. Examples are foreign health insurance companies and hospital system doing business on US soil and vice versa. This is the one area of GATS which now has US participation. Finally Mode 4 the presence of nationals from another country, providing service in the second country, both of which are members of WTO. In essence, this requires the harmonizing of licensure across national border. For example, a Filipino doctor wishing to work in the US by virtue of GATS could achieve that goal if he met universal qualifications of competence. He is currently restricted to practice here by the dictates of demand, but through GATS his eligibility would be independent of demand. Currently Filipino nurses are recruited to the US because of job shortages here, but Filipino physicians are excluded unless they pass a series of tests more extensive than required by a US physician graduating from an American Medical School. Under GATS and GATT most favored nation status can be extended to any country that is a signatory of the WTO. Also there must be transparency of agreements and those agreements must make it possible for individuals meeting certain non-biased tests to practice in the US.

If teleradiology is the issue, we cannot set up examinations or qualifications that are so restrictive that we really exclude physicians from elsewhere from doing remote image interpretation. For some radiologists this point may be hard to swallow but that is what free trade is all about. Furthermore, there should be progressively higher levels of liberalization so that once you liberalize your laws, you cannot go back. And if you try to do that, there will be trade sanctions and other severe penalties to the country that restricts entry after it first liberalized its rules of engagement. GATS requires that no additional requirements should be imposed on others if not imposed on those in the US. In essence, foreign competitors should be treated as equal to American providers. There can be some need-based limitations but the principle still applies. If we decide to open access by radiologists at all hours from other countries to our X-rays, then those radiologists can be foreign trained and situated abroad. In essence, what is good for the goose is good for the gander. And in essence each

agreement under GATS can create a ricochet effect allowing US radiologists to do teleradiology for others.

Please understand that GATS operates under the philosophy that regulations are barriers. GATS agreements would trump existing regulations like state licensure. Hence GATS can work to effect governance as much as it modulates trade. Two or more nations can arrange conditional or unconditional involvement of GATS in their health sectors.

In an unconditional application of GATS all of a country's health services are open to all rules negotiated bilaterally by virtue of being a GATS signatory. For conditional acceptance of GATS, if there is a formal and explicit commitment to maintaining openness in one segment, for instance if that segment is teleradiology, then there would be no need to obtain separate state licenses to perform the service. In fact, radiologists in other countries could participate directly and bill for their services. Now that the Radiology board exam will be computer based, under GATS it is conceivable that anyone completing a residency program in any country will be eligible to sit for that exam at a convenient location and, if they pass it, they could work at their home base and interpret images from America and be paid for that service.

If you are interested in vouchsafing that GATS, when and if approved for teleradiology, does not hurt you too much as a radiologist, you must make that known to the ACR. In my conversations with representatives of the ACR, they are aware that GATS is out there but they do not have specifics about possible timetables for implementation or even if it will be implemented. Of course there are objections to GATS and other free trade agreements. Remember the riots in Seattle, where the protests mostly involved intellectual property and its relation to AIDS. Also note that GATS may not apply to public hospitals or the VA unless those hospitals compete with private facilities which, in many cases, they do. And, as one author has stated, GATS implementation with respect to the US healthcare system will be largely determined by the way in which the agreement is further specified. Health policy makers can play an active role in shaping those further commitments. Thus we need to be aware of it.

Could GATS happen here? It depends upon health care costs borne directly by consumers. It is likely there will be consumer vs. provider wars, and the consumers in the aggregate may have more clout than do radiologists. There will be malpractice issues, of course, and therefore under the circumstances of GATS, which allows physicians elsewhere to read images definitively, the home hospital or the imaging center must bear most of the protection from tort issues.

So, as you see, this is indeed an 800 lb gorilla. You may not observe it in the room just yet, but if we keep the door open it may amble in. When it does we should recognize it and learn that if we have to live with the GATS gorilla, it will mess up the furniture. Ultimately the result of GATS and teleradiology may be damaging to some practices, as will occasion cost lowering. Or perhaps we can find a way to live together tolerably, but certainly not you and him, perfect together.

Reference

1. Baker S. Teleradiology: from the confines of place to the freedom of space. Emerg Radiol. 2005;11(3):125–6. doi:10.1007/s10140-004-0399-3.

Within Radiology, the word commodity is becoming heard with increasing frequency. The customary definition of commodity is a physical good, something useful in commerce. Recently its meaning has been extended to individual services and often, specifically, the services rendered by a radiologist. One of the bugbears causing consternation in our specialty is the so-called commodification of radiology, a process in which the service we provide is no longer considered by the consumers of our consultative expertise as a distinctive, avidly sought manifestation of special competence, but rather as a standardized product that could be offered by anyone with a modicum of training who can be situated either nearby or at some remote distance from the site of clinical encounters.

But while the specter of the commodification of our capabilities is perhaps a real threat, we face and have faced threats also with regard to the traditional meaning of commodity—that now relates to the withholding of actual physical "stuff" crucial to our work. Radiology services are beholden to very sophisticated machines, devices and medicaments consisting of materials rendered through intricate processes into special, often ingenious products that we may use routinely, even as they are really at the cutting edge of technology. And many of the ingredients that comprise these goods are expensive, exotic and limited in supply. Moreover as we have entered into the era in which science and engineering are now globalized, we depend for our livelihood on the availability of these substances extracted from remote locations and mined and/or fabricated in only a few places, mostly outside the United States. Yet the realization of such international extractive and manufacturing preparation is subject to the whims of unanticipated political considerations as well as the machinations of global markets, sometimes manipulated by greedy souls inimical to patient needs in particular, and to the provision of healthcare in the United States in general.

We in Radiology may think we only deal with a few equipment purveyors. We might assume that innovation and availability depend on their policies alone. But in actuality, in many instances, our famous corporate suppliers are in a sense only middlemen subject to the motivation of the owners and extractors of commodities which are vital components of the machines that may bear the name of GE, Siemens or their competitors.

In this discussion, I wish to relate four instances in which radiologists were bamboozled by commodity restrictions. Two are historical, one began to be a problem 2 years ago, and the most recent one is still playing itself out today. For this last example the longstanding implications are the most wide ranging.

Commodity Problem One: The Danes, the Nazis and Contrast Material

In the late 1920s Egas Moniz, a Portuguese neurologist and renaissance man, developed Thorotrast as a radiographic contrast agent.

S.R. Baker, *Notes of a Radiology Watcher*,
DOI 10.1007/978-3-319-01677-1_57, © Springer International Publishing Switzerland 2014

Incidentally, Moniz had several other distinguished careers. He was for a time the foreign minister of Portugal and he was also the prime initiator of the lobotomy operation. For this he received the 1949 Nobel Prize in Medicine, an award perhaps for which the Nobel committee might have lingering regrets. Anyway, Thorotrast had many virtues. Its clarity and incisiveness of enhancement of hollow structures that contain it was due to Thorium's high atomic number of 90. That was its main ingredient. It was a colloidal preparation, which means it could reveal both a parenchymal pattern in the liver and vascular distribution in the portal system. It was also used to opacity the ureters and the maxillary sinuses. But it had one drawback. Thorium is radioactive. It is an alpha emitter with a half-life of 22 years. Early on its carcinogenic effect was recognized and after the early 1950s it was no longer administered anywhere. It is reckoned, though, that several thousand people still harbor Thorotrast in their liver, spleen and peri-pancreatic nodes.

In World War II Germany had to husband its industrial resources which became increasingly scarce after 1943. The Nazi government decided to restrict the supply of conventional iodinated contrast material to the fatherland, depriving conquered nations like Denmark from the use of it. So physicians in Denmark resorted to Thorotrast even though the knowledge of its oncological ill effects were by then widely known. Several decades after the war, the surgeons who administered the compound were sued by patients who had received it but now had become cancer sufferers from it.

Fast forward now to the 1970s. The fabulously wealthy Texas-based Hunt family whose paterfamilias had made his fortune in oil devised a way to make their money make even more money. I am referring to two of the Hunt brothers, William Herbert and Nelson Bunker Hunt who began to buy up supplies of silver which cost $1.50 an ounce in the early 1970s when they started to try to corner the market. By 1974 they had possessed 200,000 ounces of the metal or 60 % of the world's supply. Six years later, they continued to hoard their stash, causing global prices to reach $50 an ounce. This raised the cost

of X-ray films and led to an increase in criminal activity whereby X-ray film libraries were illegally raided by unscrupulous individuals looking for a fast buck, some of them radiology department employees. They then melted down the silver from their sequestered, stolen films and sold the silver. Remember in those pre-PACS days a film was simultaneously, diagnostic, financial and archival material. Their silver bubble then came crashing down on the Hunts leading to a felony conviction for each. Eventually the silver market was restored to sanity. But during this episode of commodity control by two greedy men, the cost of healthcare was artificially increased.

Several years ago, another commodity crunch afflicted diagnostic imaging—this time because of withdrawal of a commodity from the market, not for nefarious reasons, but because its major manufacturing source closed down [1]. Technetium 99m is derived from molybdenum. Tc99m is the workhorse substance in nuclear diagnosis. Hence a steady uninterrupted supply is needed. Of course, because of its short half-life it could not be accumulated and stored for future use.

The parent compound Molybdenum 99 is itself a fission product. Its production is limited to nuclear reactors and in 2007 industrial production occurred in only five sites worldwide. By far the largest supplier was the National Research Universal Reactor in Chalk River, Ontario which was the source of between 50 and 67 % of global supply. The reactor shut down abruptly in November 2007 because of a cooling pump problem and reopened several weeks later. But 12 months after that in December 2008 a heavy water leak closed the plant down again. Then for most of the next 2 years it was non-operative. Part of the deficiency in supply has been made up by increased supplies from a fabricating plant in South Africa. Currently plans for new facilities are being pursued in Russia and Canada. Yet at the height of the crisis, a GE subsidiary reported that its stocks were reduced by 50 %. The shortage affected 85 % of American hospitals and clinics that used Technetium 99m. Some sites decided to use an imperfect substitute, Thallium 201 for myocardial perfusion studies but the long half-life of this isotope (3 days versus 6 h for technetium99m) makes it less efficacious and imperils the patient by the deposition of more dose.

The effect of this commodity squeeze led to calls in Congress for legislation to stimulate American production sites, but the resultant bill, while passed by the House, died in committee in the Senate.

Thus a precipitous cut off in supply of a commodity critical to radiology can have a variety of causes from deprivation of a scarce resource to a conquered nation and population, to the malevolent manipulation of a few individuals and to a failure of a production by only a few sources from which the world depended to an inordinate degree.

Yet the most profound supply problem is now still with us. Here the reason is not conquest, greed or mechanical failure but the aggressive action of a powerful nation seeking to direct economic and political objectives through a policy of withholding a vital resource only it maintains. I am referring to the events of 2010 and 2011 characterized by the self-centered and self-aggrandizing decision of the Chinese government to limit the distribution of rare earth metals beyond its borders.

Before proceeding with a recitation of these events let me detail what are the uses of rare earth metals as a class of elements and why a continuing supply is necessary for radiology. The rare earths encompass 17 elements including scandium (atomic number 21) and Yttrium (atomic number 39) and the lanthanides—15 elements ranging sequentially from atomic number 57 through 71. First of all, by and large these elements are not rare, just widely distributed but with only a few sites at which one or more of them is particularly concentrated. Most of the rare earths were discovered in the nineteenth century yet for nearly all, their special uses were only appreciated and developed in the latter part of the twentieth century. Many are useful for medicine as they have been incorporated in a wide variety of products. It is in diagnostic imaging where they have been most broadly utilized.

Here are some examples. Favorable magnetic properties are possessed by Yttrium, Praseodymium, Scandium, Neodymium, Samarium, Terbium, Dysprosium, and Holmium. Hence they are components of both superconducting and permanent magnets, which are components of MRI machines. The closeness of the K edge of Iodine and Cerium is the basis for the incorporation of Cerium into angio units, enabling a more perceptive demonstration by X-ray at vascular anatomy. For the last 30 years the phosphor enhancing capabilities of Yttrium, Lanthanum, Europium and Terbium has made possible more effective radiography screens. Gadolinium, of course, is a well-known contrast agent but Lanthanum too has advantageous properties and may become a commercially viable contrast agent as well. The isotopic properties of Promethium, Thulium and Yttrium offer the prospect of the creation of self-energizing portable X-ray machines. Lasers composed of Neodymium Yttrium Aluminum and garnet (the ND.YAG laser) are widely deployed. Finally many rare earths aid communication as they are components of cell phones and other electronic devices. Their heat reducing properties are in large measure responsible for the shrinking in size of these devices.

The United States, at one facility in California, the Mountain Pass Mine, used to be by far the world's major supplier of rare earth elements. But environmental concerns and price competition from China led to the closing of the mine in 2002, thereby devolving to China a near monopoly on global production of these commodities. In the Fall of 2010, China announced that it was reducing the export of rare earths because of increasing domestic demand as well as for environmental considerations. Many of the mines in Southern China were illegal and the techniques employed there were damaging groundwater and inducing other spoliations of the countryside. But that was not all.

In the eastern East China Sea just north of Taiwan sits the Senkaku Islands, small specks whose sovereignty is disputed between several nations although it is occupied by Japan. Several Chinese fishing boats or vessels outfitted to look like fishing boats got too close to the islands and the crews were arrested and sequestered for a while by the Japanese. The Chinese responded by cutting off all rare earth supplies to Japan. After several weeks the crisis was defused with the release of the Chinese sailors. This episode was in effect a shot across the bow not only to Japan but also to the rest of the world. The Chinese demonstrated that they were not reluctant to "play hardball", so to speak, with the allocation of resources they control.

As a result prices of rare earth have risen markedly especially with regard to those with magnetizing-enhancing properties.

The Mountain Pass Mine, according to its owner, Molycorp Inc. will open again but it will take 2 years to be ready. Other countries are seeking to begin production. A bioleaching process is being developed which promises to improve extraction efficiency.

But still today, we must deal with, for example, Samarium prices which have risen from $18.50 a kilogram in 2010 to $146 a kilogram in 2011 and Neodymium prices which in the same interval have gone from $42 a kilogram to $283 a kilogram. China has reduced export quotas to all countries. It increased export taxes on some rare earth.

From 15 to 25 %, and has raised taxes sixteen fold on its domestic mining companies for some refined products. Furthermore, Chinese rare earths are to a greater percentage composed of the high value, relatively uncommon rare-earth elements whereas the Mountain Pass Mines rare earths' deposits contain the more common, lower priced elements.

Echoes of the OPEC oil crisis of the early 1970s resound here. Only with rare earth the tones of discord and deprivation regarding needed resources may be louder and more deafening for radiology than was the scarcity of oil for the world as a whole. These days if one can get the stuff it will cost more to fabricate it into useful commodities. Perhaps those costs will be passed along to the purchasers of imaging equipment but it will be more difficult to pass them further along to the consumer.

Reference

1. Humphries M. Rare earth elements: the global supply chain. Collingdale: DIANE Publishing; 2010.

I am sure the range of opinions of the press that each of you holds as residents or citizens of the United States and as physicians and radiologists varies considerably. Some of you, myself included, believe that you should only be mentioned in newspapers three times in your life, and two of those times you would not know it. There are others who relish the fact that they could be quoted in press reports or in magazines reaching the general public. In my career, and especially in recent months, I have become aware that one must be extremely wary of presenting yourself to the press at large. The hazards are great and many of them are hidden from you initially. So in the next few paragraphs I would like to talk about some of the things I have learned in my recent dealings with the journalistic profession.

Our institution, now part of Rutgers University, had been under siege several years ago. With a steady stream of allegations of Medicaid fraud. In the past few years that is not unique to our institution as it has been the bane of several other medical complexes throughout our nation. One might say somewhat cynically, perhaps, that these claims result from a misinterpretation of complicated federally-generated reimbursement rules which are apt to affect all medical facilities at some time or other. In fact, judgments for compensation might be considered an adventitious but inevitable tax to be paid from time to time. What has made the situation at New Jersey Medical School more difficult is that there have been claims of outright criminal activity, not accidental but purposive. Thus, the press has been all over us finding large issues and, at the same time, looking to exploit minimal or small ones.

In my capacities both as Chairman of Radiology and Associate Dean for Graduate Medical Education at a state-owned and, therefore, very public institution I am on the firing line. The press has scrutinized almost every activity we have engaged in, even the seemingly most mundane. So my experiences with reporters from our regional newspapers, whom I believe were on a campaign to discredit our institution, have been frequent and somewhat insistent.

The first amendment of the Constitution of the United States that "Congress shall make no law respecting an establishment of religion, or prohibiting the free exercise thereof; or abridging the freedom of speech, or of the press or the right of the people peaceably to assemble and to petition the government for redress of grievances". Freedom of the press is a hallowed tradition in the United States. It has helped make our country great because the press serves an essential function to expose those who try to cheat us or rule us inappropriately. Among the champions of freedom of the press is the press itself, whose representatives and touts in both print and electronic media and in the cinema, present frequent assertions of the right of reporters and investigators to find the truth. The responsibility to inform the public cannot be gainsaid but rights and abuses of those rights sometimes work together.

You might think that as a radiologist the press would never bother you if you work in a small

S.R. Baker, *Notes of a Radiology Watcher*,
DOI 10.1007/978-3-319-01677-1_58, © Springer International Publishing Switzerland 2014

to medium-sized hospital. However, you should remember that much of what you do is compensated by state and federal agencies. Thus, even though you maintain that your practice is private, in the main it is really comprehensively public. Many states have what we have in New Jersey, a variation of the Open Public Record Act, which mandates that the press may have access to any files that you have, and contracts you have made and other records you have if they seek to investigate you in the service of the public good. You as physicians present a potentially fat target because even today as individuals you retain much prestige as a profession. Hence, we are under scrutiny and often under attack, liable to be brought down if an irregularity is found and trumpeted in the press. So, if you have never been engaged in this process it does not mean you never will.

What are your rights with respect to press attention? A qualification; here I am talking about the public press, not the specialized press in medical journals, where a more dignified attitude is taken with regard to your testimony and your opinion. In the public press you may be called by a reporter at any time about nearly any issue. It is my view that you should be reluctant to speak to the press unless it is a matter that irresistibly and without question demands their attention and therefore, your attention. If you give your opinion in the press in an offhand way, bear in mind you may be quoted correctly or you may be partially quoted and therefore incorrectly. The import and subtlety of your statements in matters of medicine and science may not come through in the written synopses and the sound bites that appear in the media. So, unless you have a clear and resolute opinion you will adhere to without fear of misrepresentation I would be reluctant to volunteer it after a chance phone call by a representative of the press who seeks more information. That refers also to requests for your expertise when you are not the focus of the story but merely supplementing it.

What happens if there is an allegation made against you or your institution? In this instance the press tends to be edgy about any response. It has the right to find out as much information as possible and may solicit records from you that

you initially may deem private. Some of them may be deemed private by your lawyers but others may have to be divulged.

Here is a likely scenario. A case is being made against the institution and perhaps you in some way. The press is seeking a statement from you. Here is what I suggest. Remember the ax the reporters are grinding may be inimical to your reputation. Do not speak off the cuff. You should secure the evidence you need before you provide an opinion. Say, at first, either no comment or call me back in several hours. In that interval you should acquire and check the facts so that you do not make a misstatement. Say also, I want to be certain of my facts before I respond. That will usually put them off for a while. Furthermore, in a telephone interview or a face-to-face interview make sure that the institution's press officer is with you on the phone or in person. Furthermore, tape the conversation. There is no law preventing you from taping your own words. Consequently, in any press interview, make sure those two things are with you, the press officer and the tape recorder because if you are quoted incorrectly you have a witness and you have a record. Never, never, never say "this is off the record". How would you know how scrupulous the reporter may be about what you say next? Moreover, what you may say off the record may give the reporter a chance to find others who would refute you or are hostile to you.

A statement has been made in the press or on television or radio which you feel is incorrect. It may even be libelous. You wish to respond so you write a letter to the editor. Do not assume because you are in high dudgeon that that letter would be published. Furthermore, do not assume that that letter will be published soon after the offending story appears in the paper. Most likely, if the press finds that your letter is contrary to what they have said they will publish the letter but later in a back page. Furthermore, they have the opportunity to edit your letter. You have very little recourse by saying that this was an expurgated version which maligns the truth as you presented it. You have very little appellate rights here. How do you prove libel? It is extremely difficult. When you think that a newspaper or television reporter has misrepresented, there also has to be evidence of malice. How do you prove that? There has to be evidence of reckless negligence. How do you prove that? For the most part when you are the object of a story related to your position as a radiologist or a chief of radiology or some other officer of a medical institution, you have to put yourself in the public eye. Putting yourself in the public eye results in much less protection for you.

By way of analogy remember that other dreaded institution, the law and its relationship to what you do. I am speaking specifically of malpractice litigation. There is a great difference between the press and the law in relation to your protection. In legal proceedings discovery must be transparent and rule based. In journalistic procedures discovery is opaque and sources are protected, not revealed. Note the journalistic heroes who go to jail because they protect their sources. You cannot do that in the law. You must reveal them. Getting out the story is opportunity-based and there is no real accountability to the evidence-gathering process. Throughout the proceedings there are no appeals you can make against the press. In a judgment made in a court of law there is always at least a glimmer of the possibility of redress, through the appellate process. In the press it is a process of, let us say "undress". You are left exposed. Your reputation is placed under question. Further discussion (even if you try to exonerate yourself for the inappropriate comments made against you in the press) will only raise further questions in the eye of the public. We all wonder and worry about malpractice, which happens to about a third of us at some time or other at least in relation to the filing of a claim. I say some of you should worry even more about the press even when you have done nothing wrong but you have come under their gaze. Words to the wise, be careful, be circumspect, be sure of your evidence, have a press officer with you and tape your conversations. And finally, do not expect that after a comment is made about you in the paper that everything will come out right in the end. The movies are not a reliable guide to dealing with the press. In REEL life the good guys always win. In REAL life, the bad guys sometimes get caught but the good guys sometimes get snared [1].

Reference

1. Baker SR. Radiology and the press: an often immiscible interface. Emerg Radiol. 2006;12:147–9.

I doubt many of you have not heard by now that the job market for Radiologists-both newly minted ones and those already in practice-is very tight. Tales of woe abound, told by those finishing their fellowship and now in the hunt. They relate their angst to more junior trainees who in turn pass theirs along to senior and junior medical students. And some of them who have expressed an interest in our specialty are being put off by a fear of being unemployable after 6 years of post-graduate preparation. It is likely they may decide to pursue another specialty for this reason. This past year the number of allopathic American medical school graduates accepted to Radiology residencies declined by 27 % from the previous year. This decline does not take into account those dissuaded from seeking a residency in the first place. Much of the discrepancy between offered positions and filled positions was taken up by foreign medical graduates, which an immediately substantial supply accommodates. But, if present trends continue, it will change the complexion of residencies in terms of homegrown talent. This will deflect us from our present resemblance to Dermatology, which many accomplished students choose, and we will become more akin to Pathology, in which in many programs American-trained residents are a distinct minority. Of course, brains do not stop at the border, but even those bright, productive foreign-born residents may experience the same dearth of jobs when they finish that our allopathic fellows perceive they will contend with when they finish training.

So what of the job market? Is it a temporary imbalance between openings and applicants, soon to right itself, as has happened several times before in the 40 year history of Radiology's stupendous and continual growth from 1970 to 2010? Over those two score of years it was actually a cyclical event, reflecting the ebb and flow natural to any economic situation across time. Or is it a structural metamorphosis, a signal of Radiology's inevitable and soon to be protracted contraction as forces conspire to limit our growth and even reduce the volume of studies we will be allowed to perform and interpret?

First let us consider how this latent imbalance occurred. This is important because it can give us clues about the consequences to be anticipated in the near and medium term.

In the 1990s, as you may remember, Clinton proposed his ill-fated omnibus health care bill. The political atmosphere was suffused by notions of gatekeepers, the need to enhance the role of primary care etc. It was projected back then that health care expenses or at least those more directed to imaging would decline by a fourth to a third. As we celebrated the centennial anniversary of Radiology in 1995, many thought that Radiology must adjust to the projected decline, and consequently residency positions were reduced by more than 15 % nationally from 1992 to 1998, declining in number each year. At the end of 1996, the Medicare cap on residency positions became law and it remains in place today. So if a program wished to increase the number of residency lines and have Medicare pay all or part of the salary and benefits for each of them, then the Radiology department could only secure lines from some other specialty with residents in the institution that wanted to give some positions away.

Clinton's health care initiatives did not pass. Significant advances in the capability of CT and MR came on stream by 1997, and in 2000 began the rapid increase in residency positions that has continued until last year. The expanded clinical applications of the latest generations of CT and MR led to increased volume, which in turn financed the hiring of more residents and the expansion of fellowship opportunities. Permission to expand teaching programs rested with the Radiology RRC of the Accreditation Committee for Graduate Medical Education. I was a member of the Radiology RRC from 2005 to 2012. The only criteria we could use to accept or reject a request to expand a residency complement was whether there were enough cases to support an expanded contingent and whether there were enough teachers to teach them. Demographic and economic projections could not inform this calculation. The result almost always was to approve the plea for more. And many of such requests were not just for an additional resident but for, say, two a year for each of 4 years expanding a cadre of 24 trainees to 32 four years later, an increase of 33 %. So radiology residencies grew and thus so has the number of radiologists at the end of the pipeline. This was all well and good as volume increased. In fact in the early to mid-years of the first decade of this century, we thought we did not have enough people to do the work, thus justifying the relatively inexpensive labor provided by senior residents and fellows.

A typical title in a radiology journal commentary on manpower needs was "Coping With the Radiologist Shortage," Radiology Management 2004:26 pp 91–97 and "Too Few Radiologists," AJR 2002:178 pp 291–301. During the past 13 years, the number of residents in Pediatrics, Internal Medicine, OBGYN, and Surgery has stayed the same, Family Medicine declined by 10 % but Radiology increased by nearly 20 %. Only Emergency Medicine and Anesthesiology grew faster, the former as numerous standalone walk in clinics proliferated and continue to do so, and the latter because free standing surgical centers and GI centers, each growth poles, need anesthesiologists on site.

But Radiology manpower growth was tied until 2006 to volume increases. From 1998 to 2005 Medicare utilization rates for all high-tech modalities of diagnostic imaging grew by an average of 4.7 % per year while the national radiology residency pool increased by 2.78 % per annum. But CT growth slowed after 2006, MR utilization actually declined even as residency numbers continued to increase as multiyear approved accretions filled in. Now, finally, residency expansion has stopped and is stable, but imaging volume decline in numbers continues.

A relevant article that appeared in "Diagnostic Imaging" was entitled, "Radiology Job Numbers Will Improve, Eventually" the article followed promptly on the heels of a news report of the precipitant closure of an osteopathic radiology residency program at St. Barnabas Hospital in the Bronx which appeared in late March 2013 in the New York Times.

Was the point of this article, "an assertion of reassurance", something on which hopes could rest, or was it whistling in the dark? The author, Dr. Samuah Jha, stated "So fret not trainees. Referrers will still demand imaging". But how much? No specific prediction was offered by Dr. Jha. He further states "uncertainty is temporary, Radiologists will start retiring, soon more of them than in past years".

Other arguments raised for this roseate view are, it has happened before and things got better, it always will. The baby boomers are aging, they will flood the market and then there will be more imaging. Likewise The Affordable Care Act will bring 40 million more people into the health care system, and new uses for radiology will inevitably be found. And anyway, don't complain, we are a wonderful specialty. Don't talk negatively. It will scare people away. Let us examine each of these nostrums in turn.

The past is the prologue fallacy. Just because there have been cyclical changes before, why does that make this downturn in employment opportunities one that will be like all the others? In each situation of a temporary tight market, the problem occurred in a period of growth in imaging. It lasted for 40 years—a long time but not for all time. In fact Radiology's Golden Age, now ended, was about 40 years and is about as long as other Golden Ages like the Augustan Age in Rome, the high renaissance in Italy, the Age of Dutch painting in the 1600s, the apex of the Broadway Musical from 1935 to 1970. By the way the public no longer regards imaging as an unalloyed good. We now worry about radiation dose, insurance companies place ever more restrictions on utilization, government regulations will increasingly limit testing, at least some of those radiologic studies now uncritically requested and performed by routinized protocols. Moreover, public criticism by influential critics like the Avoiding Avoidable Care movement will gain adherents, and new computer techniques will move in to take away our reading of follow up liver scans or even head CT and MR studies. Even mammography for these 40 years to 50 years old has become increasingly questioned by the policy makers, as evidenced by an article in the New York Times Magazine. There are no new energy sources on the horizon or even below it to provide a quantum leap increase in imaging, as did the introduction and the upgrades in CT, MR, Nuclear and Ultrasonography.

Moreover, not all job titles remain forever. The telegraph supplanted the town crier, the telephone operator is no longer an actual person in the US or is one offshore. Other modes of diagnosis besides imaging could supplant Radiology. And aside from IR and mammography we don't "own" patients. So I think we should fret.

Now why should one suppose that the pace of retirements will quicken. I am at the age to consider this life-changing decision. But I am not assured that the benefits of social security and Medicare will be there for me so abundantly as it has been for my older colleagues. After all, other segments of society want a piece of the redistribution of wealth, and they could secure the votes to get it. Moreover, people retire in the expectation that the money they worked for should now work for them. But at interest rates below 1 %, your safe investments actually lose money. So many will keep working to maintain their estate when later on, if they lived long enough, they can live on what they earned now by the sweat of their brow, not their deposits in a CD.

Obamacare will bring a lot of people under its umbrella. But many of them already go to ERs and are charity cases. Most others are young and often poor and they have rationalized that their age protects them from incurring medical costs. Now with insurance backing they will still be considering themselves nearly immortal, and for the most healthy, will not be the carriers of the hoped for imagining bonanza that the Pollyanna's are banking on.

So really I am not a curmudgeon nor an unconstructed naysayer, but the tea leaves don't look good to me. It is always best to prepare for bad news as you hope for good news. I believe this downturn is a game changer for radiologists. So do many of the best and brightest who used to be attracted to Radiology. But no longer—maybe I and them are both right [1].

Reference

1. Baker SR. Job prospects for radiologists in the United States. Imaging Mange. 2013;13(1):12–4.

American Radiologists at a Crossroad

60

This essay is another in a series of challenges to Radiology as a specialty, specifically as a challenge to the prospective employment characteristics of American radiologists. I think that because of a conjunction of compelling if seemingly disparate events, the moment is now so unique with engaging prospects but also with foreboding, that I need to comment about it in a summative way. But I will assume the role of Cassandra in this forum (for the last time, at least for awhile) before once again paying attention to more pleasant radiology-related matters.

But, as I said, I must acquaint you with some inferences about the near future, as if you did not know about some of these trends already. A long record of success in any venture (or should I say adventure) can inure us from inherent risks that exist for sure but are submerged below our consciousness. A protracted skein of good results is the pre-requisite for overconfidence and under preparedness for when things turn negative. Unlike all other specialists who are engaged in the care of individual patients (with the exception of Pathologists) we do not have face time with them, save for interventional procedures and breast imaging. By and large, the subjects we provide expertise for are not patients that we "own" in a caregiving sense. Instead, our connection with them is mediated by the technology we employ, not the trust and camaraderie we engender. In essence, our currency is embedded in the machines over which we have gained dominion. Thus, as the record of the past 40 years has shown, the more and the better image creating devices under our purview, the better we do. Moreover by dint of our specialized training and also by the long history of effective politics pursued by the organizations that represents us, we have become for many conditions the arbiter of diagnosis and, in an increasing array of illnesses, the conveyor of therapy. We have been riding the growth curve for a long time. Mostly it has been a smooth ride. But all growth lines reach a terminus eventually and we are almost there now. It is folly to assume that the journey would be never ending. Here are some golden rules we should acknowledge and obey as we come to the end of the ascendency pathway and seek to make our way under an array of restraints.

All innovations run a course. If such a novelty is found to incur an advantage, after an initial period of ambivalence, it then gains acceptance and soon enthusiastic adherence as the procedures and insights of the pioneers and early adopters are improved upon and expanded by the rank and file. But, after a while and inevitably, the benefits revealed early on must be considered in concert with the risks and drawbacks which appear in force in the medium term. I challenge you to nominate one discovery that has been both transformative and error and risk free at any time beyond its initial adaption. Moreover, once a new development matures and becomes established, it is bound to be subject to criticism about its faults and limitations which were not recognized initially. And nearly always it is also apt to be replaced by another wave of creative destruction resulting in novel paradigms.

S.R. Baker, *Notes of a Radiology Watcher*,
DOI 10.1007/978-3-319-01677-1_60, © Springer International Publishing Switzerland 2014

So, the technological breakthrough in image generation and communication of the last 20 years have spawned further advances beyond our constraints. CT has enabled enhanced detection of tiny hepatic metastases by the radiologist, but the organization of CT patterns can be, and already has been, rendered by algorithms that cannot just assist but actually distinguish the size and multiplicity of lesions on subsequent studies. In this regard, for that particular problem, technology has advanced beyond us. If it can be done for liver lesions, and it has been achieved in some centers, it is theoretically possible and really nearly actually achievable to render diagnosis by computer programs without the radiologists intercession in neuroradiological examinations using cross sectional imaging [1].

1. I have no doubt that computer-determined not just computer-assisted diagnosis is achievable and will be widespread within a decade. The rising costs of health care have turned the public at large, their electoral representatives and their appointed regulators to all cast discerning eyes at imaging as a source of expenses that need to be reduced. If the computer becomes as good as or better than a radiologist for a particular set of diagnoses, who is then expendable? Hence our traditional scope of works as we currently define it will be constricted.

2. Another negative effect caused by the devices we use is their potential toxic inducement of radiation related damage. Today, we are sort of nibbling at the edges of this problem. We know that radiation leads to cancer as evidenced by studies of A-bomb survivors. We have a record of increased thyroid cancer cases in young women downwind from the Chernobyl meltdown. We have extrapolation studies that predict that CT is now the source of more than 50 % of radiation received by individuals worldwide from all radiation sources. Consequently we may be soon seeing more cancers as a result. And with the advent of the electronic medical record we may create a global radiation reporting system, so that at our disposal will be not just small samples, but a massive database to definitively determine

the magnitude of the risk, of say, recurrent CT in young patients for a range of malignancies. The prudent course at present is to husband radiation exposure, to have carefully drawn limitations on CT use, to provide substitution protocols using non-irradiating imaging, or to avoid imaging entirely for situations in which we now use it liberally. Each of these stratagems will further retard the growth of radiology generally.

What is more, these ruminations ignore another inevitability. That is, all macroscopic detection mandated through MR, CT, PET, etc are in one sense rather crude means for recognizing cellular derangements and biochemical disruptions that are elaborated as diseases or as disease precursors. For a range of abnormalities today, analysis by microscopic or chemical determination is definitive. We should expect that more diseases will be recognized by their cellular or laboratory test profile and so will the therapy to control or eradicate them. Here is another broad area which will serve to end the imaging growth curve under the hegemony of the radiologist.

Now, added to this roster of impingement, is the demographic imposition resulting from our myopia about the size of the American Radiology contingent which our supposed success has paradoxically brought into clear view. Frankly our greed to foster further our rapidly expanding volume of CT and MR by recruiting the cheap labor of more and more residents and fellows comes with a price that must now be repaid. The cadre of trainees we brought on board in the first decade of the twenty first century will be in practice for 30 and 40 years more, competing (if they get jobs at all) with older radiologists for a likely shrinking imaging pie of which all want a piece. And training programs are not yet getting smaller, so the next decade will bring more Radiologists into the crowding pool. We have already seen a decline in radiologists starting salary. If present trends continue, perhaps the income of established radiologists will be reduced and, for sure, some will be let go.

Persistence of the current constraints in the economy may make senior radiologists delay retirement. Moreover, unlike every other specialty whose percentage of women has risen in accord with the increasing percentage of women as medical students, only in radiology has the percentage of female radiology trainees remained constant at about 27 %. Inasmuch as women more than men are inclined to work part time, do not expect that the offsetting trend of part-time work will become more important without the cultural insistence to stimulate it.

The only way (and a small way at best) to affect a countervailing tactic, is for radiologists in hospitals to assume the function of consultants. Now this term, as recounted again and again in the radiologic literature, has been a cop out, in a sense a chimera that sounds good but means little. So let me redefine that notion so that it in my sense at least it has substance. A radiologist as consultant should be no different from a gastroenterologist as consultant or an oncologist as consultant. They are each called upon to assess a patient for a G.I. or tumor problem. They review the chart, they speak to the referring physician, they visit the patient and after that they write a report which enters the patients chart. For that demonstration of expertise they get paid a fee. It is time consuming but can also be rewarding. The radiologist too is the expert in decision support. Traditionally such advice is given as a free good. But it can be crucial to the patient's care, and by tailoring imaging choices to the individual, instead of to a complaint or a symptom, as is done when so-called appropriateness designations are used, it can reduce cost, discomfort, dose and hospital stay.

I see no other option to expand our book of business in this emerging period of constraining forces, the problem is ours. Yet to some little extent we have some choices to make.

Reference

1. Baker SR. Job prospects for radiologists in the United States. Imaging Manage. 2013;13(1):12–4.

Part XI

Research

Research in radiology should certainly be positioned within the gaze of a radiology watcher. The continued validity of peer review is a fit subject for investigation with respect to biases and ethical issues, not only in conventional publishing, but also in electronic publishing. Presumptuousness and tendentiousness are frequent but unwelcome concomitants of research activity and they must be brought to light as they are in the last essay.

61

Peer Review-Peering Over Its Shoulder

Unless you are over 90 you probably cannot recall a time when peer review was not regarded as an essential qualitative process in the evaluation of manuscripts for inclusion in medical journals. It was and is still believed that peer review ensures that presentations of putative scientific merit will be carefully assessed by disinterested yet committed and qualified experts whose judgments enhance the quality of published papers.

Inasmuch as these review exercises have become so well entrenched as a standard of investigative rigor and the consensus about its pros (seemingly many) and its cons, (relatively few except for the transitory disappointment of rejected authors) so well accepted that critical evaluations of its merits and drawbacks have until recently received scant attention. Yet today the established patterns of publication of scientific articles are being challenged by several developments, (1) the rapid diffusion of electronic open access protocols and journals, (2) the effect on journal reading patterns with the increasing subspecialization of content and (3) the multiple modes available for the rapid transmission of information both to subscribers and to the general public. These developments have elicited the cracking if not the total breaking of conventional models for the delivery of discovery and revisions, the two stocks in trade of basic scientists and clinical investigators.

Everything is now on the table open for inspection in the ongoing ferment about how new knowledge in medicine is announced and deployed. The once hallowed rules and rituals of peer review are now under particular scrutiny. Yet this should be of no surprise to us, for in times of disruption occasioned by advances in communication, periodic assessment is required to ascertain contemporary relevance and possibly the need to renovate, revamp or eliminate traditional assumptions, attitudes and algorithms that govern behavior.

Peer review today is still applied with similar tenacity to journal submission and grant applications. The history of its deployment in both spheres has not been smooth over the 150 year period between its introduction at the end of the Napoleonic era and its general acceptance after World War II. Its gradual penetration into the schedules of scientific publications has been characterized as haphazard at first; originally it was the domain of enthusiasts only. But by fits and starts, generally without formal concerted effort, it eventually permeated the mindset of editors and publishers of medical journals. After the war the expansion of medical studies in general and the coincident increases in the specialization of investigations not only spawned new journals but also stimulated the establishment of vigorous standards of quality. Hence, peer review conducted by individuals of akin credentials to investigators offered a means for the sustenance of scientific excellence. Currently, medical periodicals professing to become prominently regarded by present and potential contributors and readers alike as a source of new knowledge cannot be so regarded without having peer review as a standard method of manuscript evaluation.

S.R. Baker, *Notes of a Radiology Watcher*,
DOI 10.1007/978-3-319-01677-1_61, © Springer International Publishing Switzerland 2014

Now, what are the presumptions of peer review specifically? What are the traits that for the most part still are essential for the establishment and maintenance of esteem for both journals and their authors? A manuscript is submitted to an editor who then distributes it to two or more so-called experts for their careful analysis of its scientific content including, often today, an analysis of the statistical means used to test the significance of the data, an assessment of the validity of the hypothesis presented and examined by the authors, the import of the study with respect to its novelty, its relevance in conjunction with general topics within the purview of the journal, and for some investigations, its application for the improvement of patient care. As part of their charge, peer reviewers often check references, critique the quality of images and legends and comment upon the pertinence and skillfulness of the narrative.

The insights these experts bring to the process can improve the paper. Moreover, the citations they offer can lead to revisions which make it more acceptable for publication. Furthermore, negative comments made without rancor and invidiousness can serve to stimulate the authors to seek more data, to sharpen their narrative focus and concentrate more pertinently on careful substantiation of their hypothesis. Even outright rejection can be salutary, not just for the sake of truth, but also because it will stimulate the investigators to be more careful in their next submission.

Nonetheless, despite its virtues and proven value, peer review is now under stress. Doubt has arisen by the many developments which together are comprising a metamorphosis in information transfer and data display. Some of these concerns about peer reviews' enduring worth are timeless, independent of technological changes in publishing, and intrinsic to the presumption of the nature of colleague review. They may have always been there but somehow seem more acute and nettlesome today. Other concerns about peer review are novel ones which have risen to the fore even though only a few years ago, they were perhaps not even contemplated. The remainder of this discussion will give consideration to each of these types of concerns.

I wish now to ponder on the permanent controversies inherent in peer review. Is it really a form of censorship? That is a question that many have asked, especially those disconcerted by the process. Does it prohibit fair treatment of unpopular views? Does the choice of reviewers and the assumptions they hold, and the sensibilities by which they render opinions, offer nothing more than the acting out of predictable biases? Is peer review merely a routinized function of a guild with all its members like-minded and hidebound, inevitably prejudiced against dissenting notions or radical reinterpretations of data? As scientists we claim to maintain at least formally a liberal (small l) reading of the history of science. Also, we remember that many fundamental breakthroughs were often not accepted at first. The heliocentric theory of Copernicus and Darwin's revolutionary research in evolution both received at best a skeptical consideration at first and even a hostile one by the entrenched establishment. Yet in past centuries their notions were provocative and ultimately persuasive among those learned in the field. Their science ultimately won out by the strength of their discoveries after their insights were tested and validated. Yet, under peer review discharged by a hostile coterie of supposed colleagues, perhaps the truth of the enlightened outsider may never gain entry into the corpus of accepted knowledge and, even more important, never become part of the public consciousness about a particular subject.

Therefore, perhaps peer review has restricted to obscurity potentially valuable discoveries which have never seen the light of day because the manuscripts that announced them were rejected. This is certainly a valid criticism, perhaps, and, at times, very true. From my experience as a former editor-in-chief of a peer-reviewed radiology journal, as a member of the editorial boards of three journals, as a reviewer for three more, and as a diligent investigator who has often experienced rejection, I realize that controversial subjects, even when they are data-driven, are apt to raise hackles. I realize that some of the peer reviewers of my submissions did not read my articles carefully. Others raised peripheral issues, sometimes merely to display to the editor his or her erudition on a subject not germane and sometimes even distant and distinct from the topic of my paper. With other so-called peer reviewers, in my experience as a recipient of their criticism, I have found that their comments were grossly misinformed, and some were egregiously hostile for no apparent reason. So there have been and/or continue to be lazy reviewers, ignorant reviewers and angry reviewers.

But their incompetence or inappropriateness should not be an indictment asserting that the system of peer reviewer is fundamentally flawed. It is up to the editor to counsel peer reviewers, to educate them or eliminate them if they are not up to the job. And sometimes, too, the author is at fault for the choice of journal for which his or her work was sent for judgment. If the topic is multidisciplinary in nature, the reviewers may not understand, for example, that the subject requires reviewers who know about both radiology and demography if the focus is radiology manpower. Or a journal may be delineated to such an extent by a particular ideology that an hypothesis could be rejected not because of inadequacies of description, data presentation and exposition but rather because it is seemingly heretical.

These ideological currents are most often operating subterraneously and quietly if you will. But at other times they may roar like a fast flowing stream full of white water. A classic example of their phenomenon has been termed the Duesberg Phenomenon. An article in Science in the early 1990s related that Peter Duesberg, a world renowned retrovirologist at the University of California, Berkeley in 1987 published a paper arguing that HIV infection was really harmless. Duesberg's position was that HIV did not cause AIDS but that illicit drug use and AZT, an anti-HIV compound, actually induced its signs and symptoms. Back then Duesberg's notions were condemned by the scientific establishment. Yet before that for more than 20 years Duesberg had had a stellar career, filled with rewards and admiration. When, with seemingly some scientific buttressing, he propounded his notion of the harmlessness of HIV, his views were met with scorn, and his ability to publish subsequent material reduced. In this instance was the proper use of peer review to prohibit publication of arguments that were unpopular or even distasteful to prevailing opinion? As the Science article relates, Duesberg went from notable to notorious. Yet, was it the function of the reviewers to criticize his opinion because of their inimical social significance, or was it the obligation of the publishers to present a range of opinions as most newspapers, do with the establishment and support of op-ed pages?

Some maintain that the peer review function is to analyze the methodology of the science per se, not the conclusions or the presumptions of the investigators. With such a philosophy a medical journal may become a more lively forum for discussion of new ideas, bringing to public awareness both mainstream concepts that are expected as incremental advancements, as well as radical, sometimes disruptive theories for which there is some data to provide support. On its face this is an important issue for the future of peer review. It is important not only in itself, but because of the advancing and broadening import of subspecialization that may make peer review less attractive for journal editors as electronic publications proliferate. For the most part copy in e-journals is harder to read when displayed on a video screen than in print. Although there may be an adjustment period for which this difficulty will no longer apply for young scientists and physicians, yet for older investigators it is an enduring problem. Note the slow adoption of e-books for example. Nonetheless, e-journalism in science will encourage more and more specialized issues with shorter articles and a narrowing spectrum of tables of contents. Thus, there is the implicit danger that the peer review process may become less relevant and that very specialized journals will become nothing more than blogs in which the readers and investigators share the same perceptions and the data they consider becomes more insular in focus.

Yet, an argument can be made on utilitarian grounds alone that the reaction to Duesberg's radical ideas was helpful to science and society because it was not believed by so many and if believed would do harm to patients specifically and generally, which is indeed what happened.

Policy planners in several parts of the world found that the separation of HIV from AIDS was congenial to their notion of statecraft. This was especially true in southern Africa where the president of the country, Mr. Thabo Mbeki, rejected the idea that there is a relationship between HIV infection and AIDS. As a result HIV has proliferated in South Africa and in nearby countries. When I was there in 2006, it was still widely believed by intelligent lay people that the way to treat AIDS was to eat your vegetables. This idea stemmed from the currency given the Duesberg phenomenon, at least among health officials in that country. Only recently has the South African government come to the realization that Mbeki's policies were a disaster. With H1V present in over 40 % of adults, the life expectancy has decreased in the countries of southern Africa, even in otherwise successful ones like Botswana.

Hence, perhaps radical ideas even presented with some scientific support but which are at variance and even in conflict with mainstream ideologies should not get a hearing. And in this context peer review has worked. Yet, utilitarian arguments alone are dangerous, too, because if other "Duesbergs" warnings are in fact correct, perhaps by not publishing them we have made fundamental mistakes in the other direction.

Well, so much for ruminations on these larger issues. The next essay considers peer review in specialized areas where change has been called for, including responses to such questions as should authors pick the reviewers, should their reviews also be published with the accepted article, and should some articles be peer reviewed while others not?

Peer review is a key element ensuring scientific integrity in medial publishing of original research. It has not always been so, its adoption only becoming universal after World War II. While seemingly well-established, receiving a broad consensus of approval until recently, it is now undergoing increasing scrutiny for two reasons. One, is it really an unbiased, dispassionate process conducted by well-informed disinterested but committed reviewers who are largely unpaid and unrecognized for their efforts or is it subject to biases, petty, jealousies and incompetence? Two, are the developments of internet journalism, the desire for rapid dissemination by scientists held back by the strictures of conventional peer review? In this two part discussion each of these issues will be given consideration [1].

Reference

1. Mahgerefteh S, Kruskal JB, Yam CS, Blachar A, Sosna J. Peer review in diagnostic radiology: current state and a vision for the future. Radiographics. 2009;29(5):1221–31.

Peer Review-Innovations and Ethical Issues

62

In the previous essay I introduced the topic of peer review, presenting in abbreviated form its history, its enduring virtues, its problematic considerations presently and some implications for its future given the impact of electronic information flows and the consequent emergence of e-journals.

Now I have two objectives: (1) a discussion of proposed changes to the dynamics of the peer review process and (2) to expose some of the tyrannies that continue to infect peer reviews. For this I will try to relate how to recognize institutionalized dishonesties and how perhaps to change them.

Let us begin by considering a newly initiated policy established by one journal with which I am familiar and which may be followed in other publications today. That is the editorial practice of asking the authors to suggest possible reviewers for their manuscripts [1].

Now upon first becoming aware of such a notion, I was taken aback. My immediate reaction was positive. I could identify individuals who would know my work. I could then direct the editor to the small subset of fellow radiologists who could understand that generally my offerings are multidisciplinary. Those I thought to be suitable for such a review were also apt to appreciate contributions to the journal that bridge differing subjects and thereby will be congenial to my presentations. Moreover, I thought that my recommendations would be of acquaintances or friends of mine who would be able by content and experience to recognize that I was the author of the accompanying manuscript that they would be chosen to review. As a relationship between me and each of them had been established beforehand based upon our professional interactions, I presumed at first that they would be predisposed to regard my contributions affirmatively. So I was in like Flynn, so to speak.

But then reservations set in. I was only to make suggestions to the editor, not to direct the appointment of reviewers. I would not know if my recommendations would be heeded. Also my circle of acquaintances vastly exceeds my circle of true-blue, bosom buddies. How could I come to conclude that none of those acquaintances harbored a secret animus towards me that he or she wanted to discharge through a devastating review?

And most importantly, the innovation of suggesting your reviewer really calls into question the integrity of the peer review process. If, in fact, one or several of the suggested peer reviewers are chosen, does the likelihood of acquaintanceship impart a bias that had not existed before? Does it not impinge on the validity of the process itself? By analogy, do plaintiffs or defendants in civil suits choose their jurors? Their lawyers can seek to disqualify prospective panel members but they cannot offer up friends or acquaintances tied to their clients. Well, of course, the peer review process is not by nature fervently adversarial. Nonetheless, reviewers sit in judgment. Would not the process be sullied by linkage to relationships with authors? I think that the tendency is there.

S.R. Baker, *Notes of a Radiology Watcher*,
DOI 10.1007/978-3-319-01677-1_62, © Springer International Publishing Switzerland 2014

Another suggestion made by authors, editors and reviewers is to publish the review along with the article. A reviewer would be known by his or her byline being listed along with the review. The purpose here would be to minimize the irrelevancies and other inappropriateness that sometimes inform reviews. Could not this attempt at transparency be a further effort to reduce antagonism because the review would be available for everyone to observe? What could be wrong with such candor?

Well, here again, problems arise. Knowing that his or her reviews will be published, assuming of course, that the editor chooses to publish the article itself, ad hominem comments would be restricted as the identity of the reviewer is displayed. But that also means that pertinent, trenchant comments appropriate to the scientific content of the paper could also be curtailed, modified or eliminated to the detriment of the pursuit of truth. Would not this desire for fairness scare away both prospective and long-term reviewers, who do their work anonymously and usually without compensation because they believe in the process of peer reviews and do not want or seek public awareness of their selfless, devoted commitment?

Moreover, publicizing the reviewer means that the accepted articles and their appending peer-reviewed analyses by previously anonymous reviewers will take up more space than before. Can the publisher afford such an expense? Perhaps it would be helpful for journals with optimistic page expectations but heretofore not enough copy to fill them? But for more successful and hence more widely read journals, it means good contributions may not be accepted or if accepted its publication may be delayed because previously chosen articles have ballooned in length as the reviews are included in the total package.

An enduring problem, one that continually threatens peer review and given the anticipation in Radiology that reimbursement will be cut, is the issue of payment for this activity. Mostly, peer review is a free good, performed with no compensation as an obligation in the service of science. But how long can that attitude persist in an era of revenue constriction? The journal benefits from the labor of reviewers, and perhaps their altruism makes possible the diversity of scientific publications and the large roster of journals. Yet free work is always granted on contingency. Many might decide it is no longer worth the time and effort to pursue it if not balanced by a reward. In academic practice, the lack of financial compensation is merely one problem. Another issue is that many medical school evaluation systems accord little or no weight to peer reviewing as a manifestation of productive activity as it is not really clinical work, nor is it teaching, research or service to a hospital or the medical school itself. In many evaluation schemes, there is no place to consider it. So for many, why do it? And this denigration of peer review applies not only to work product but also to promotion criteria. Most committees of appointment and promotions, including the ones I have served on, give little weight to peer review. Hence the threat to it is real and may become profound as circumstances change with regard to revenue generation.

Now I would like to talk about two tyrannies. The first relates to the words author and authority. They are cognates etymologically but have vastly different meaning with respect to peer review allocation. An author should be one who contributes materially to the intellectual effort to create a paper. In Radiology, just by supplying a case which by happenstance you have interpreted should not be a criterion for membership as a coauthor on a scientific manuscript. And merely by being the section chief or chief of service or chairman should not automatically be the criterion granting that you have the right or the eligibility for inclusion on a paper for which you have done no specific work. You may have authority over a section or a department but that should not mean that the exercise of that authority extends automatically to inclusion as a co-author on anything associated with the paper.

The policy of some journals demanding the intellectual contributions of each putative co-author is admirable. Equally valid is a limit on the number of co-authors because it codifies to the degree that authorship relates to effort. Authorship should not be perceived as an honorific or a manifestation of authority.

The second tyranny relates to the inordinate demands made by a national or international authority who is situated on one or more than one editorial board. Some such individuals who have established their reputation as having expertise in a specialized area of knowledge can manage to gain membership on the editorial board of competing journals- becoming recognized by each as the pre-eminent expert in one narrow field or niche subject. In such a fashion they become the arbiters of taste, so to speak. No contributions on the subject can avoid their oversight. Such a situation can stifle innovation. Moreover the "gatekeeper" expert can demand that the terms of acceptance requires that you cite his work in your article in case you have forgotten his eminence. Failure to do so may lead to rejection. And inclusion of the "authority's" authored references will improve his or her impact factor. Such demands are an abuse of power yet they are not always well understood by the medical reading public or by junior authors. There is a need then to limit simultaneous multiple editorial board membership. Such an injunction should be on the agenda of meetings of editors as it is potentially an important ethics issue. For most subjects in Radiology there still are enough knowledgeable people in every niche area, and enough of them still do peer reviews so that this problem when it exists can be ameliorated or eliminated or, if not considered strongly, allowed to fester.

Reference

1. Leek JT, Taub MA, Pineda FJ. Cooperation between referees and authors increases peer review accuracy. PLoS One. 2011;6(11):e26895.

Electronic Publishing: A Boon or a Bugbear

63

An abruptly imposed technological change is almost always both liberating and unsettling. Invariably, it is accompanied by the emergence of at least four stereotypical mindsets that inform positions taken during public debates about the value of the innovation. Inevitably, such discussions are characterized by confusion, discord and disagreement, often displayed with rancor. In essence, the impress of rapid and profound technological initiatives frequently induces the same roiling controversy that Thomas Kuhn described in his analysis of scientific revolutions [1]. When the presumption of "normal" is disrupted by a major discovery, uncertainty and discontent emerge until a new paradigm is established. That paradigm in turn holds sway until the next revolution.

Among the actors in this drama are the pioneers, the drum majors of the new technology, who understand the mechanistic reordering of work a profound technological change engenders. They are also aware of the behavioral modification such innovation induces. But at the same time, the euphoric pronouncements of the pioneers never really come true because, imprisoned by their enthusiasm, they fail to recognize the "yin-yang" effect; i.e., everything new and good brings with it unintended consequences, which are often bad and as enduring as the good. On the opposite side of the spectrum are the persistent deniers. One hundred years ago they yelled "get a horse" as a model T rolled by. They are blinded by the comfortable past no one will return to except within a museum or in idle moments of nostalgic reflection. The early adopters do not possess the same fervor as the pioneers. They can wait for the tumult to die down before more carefully assessing what the new technology can and cannot do. Before there is widespread decision opportunities and constraints imparted by a new procedure, method or machine, societal adjustment has begun to take hold and the technology's real advantages and limitations have become more apparent. The late adopters are more skeptical and that reserve may be a disadvantage. Yet, it may place them in good stead, because the third generation of a new implement or service may be the first one for which all the bugs have been removed inasmuch as by the time the later adopters come on board, purpose and function have become aligned.

Medical publishing is no different than any other industry confronting the imposition of a technological revolution. Now that pictures can be manipulated electronically as easily as words and writing does not require putting pen to paper, the traditional journal is becoming a thing of the past, not so much because the actual bound document has been foresworn by readers in favor of the computer screen. Rather, the retrieval of information is no longer limited by the physical bulk of "Gutenberg" artifacts. Hence, almost instantaneously, one can now call up all references on an obscure subject when even in the very recent past such an activity would require the learner to partake of the joyful but laborious task of rooting around in the stacks of a library much like, if you will, a trained sow sniffing the ground for the exquisite truffle lying beneath her feet but hidden from view.

S.R. Baker, *Notes of a Radiology Watcher*, DOI 10.1007/978-3-319-01677-1_63, © Springer International Publishing Switzerland 2014

I predict the immediate availability of electronically retrievable, focused databases will do the following. We will not read journals in the pleasurable, somewhat aleatory way we do now, scanning the table of contents for the subjects we know will be there and at the same time becoming surprised and intrigued by other reports, the context of which resides within our specialty but perhaps outside our particular area of expertise. Traditionally, the avid journal reader would follow a buffet line approach at the table of contents, reading some of this and some of that according to what delectable at the moment his appetite dictates he consume. As a result he (or she) could maintain a general currency across the broad expanse of his field even while concentrating on specific interests.

But now with the advent of electronically available literature collections, offered complete and current, the specialist will tend to be more narrowly directed but less generally informed. Such a limited menu will eventually tend to restrict communication among the various branches of medicine and even to a great degree to reduce knowledge and interaction within a specialty. Most likely jargon will become thicker among the cognoscenti yet more opaque to those outside the constricting boundaries reserved for a coterie of super specialists. Eventually this will lead to intellectual disenfranchisement as those positioned beyond the ken of the recondite will become progressively ignorant of the advances in one or more of these micro-disciplines. For example, we now have a society of biliary radiology. It is not too farfetched to posit the establishment of a spinoff, the cholecystic duct society, for which communication about its fascinations and intricacies would be confined to an electric journal dedicated to it. This arrangement may persist for a while to be supplanted, perhaps, by a blog so that those recurrently informed and interested can learn from each other in real time no matter where they are, thereby bypassing the formalities of structure and deliberation inherent in the publishing process. And in that setting, will the time-consuming rigor of peer review be set aside for the sake of promptness of reportage? Perish such thoughts, yet they will not die unless we give additional consideration to how we can keep communication of new knowledge open to a wide audience, even as we gain the capability to generate customized dissemination through cyberspace. I am pessimistic but perhaps that is the natural response of a chronic late adopter [2].

References

1. Kuhn T. The structure of scientific revolutions. Chicago: University of Chicago Press; 1962.
2. Baker SR. Electronic publishing, boon or bugbear. Emerg Radiol. 2005;12:1–2.

The Tendentious Tendency in Radiology Clinical Research

64

For many, tendentious is a fancy, unfamiliar word used by academics in an attempt to impress you with their erudition and confuse you about their purposes. But it should be employed more in common speech and writing because it is apt as a label for which no other word is as good. According to Webster's New Universal Unabridged Dictionary, it is defined as having or showing a definite tendency or bias. In clinical investigations, we should recognize it, because tendentiousness is imbued to some degree in a host of articles in radiology which, without reading the abstract, one can guess at the conclusions presented in the introduction. After perusing the imaging literature, an innocent may think he is clairvoyant by predicting outcome just from the title of the article. In such reports, there will almost always be one statistically significant lesson to be presented and confirmed (I did not say learned), and the results will almost always be in line with the authors' preconceptions, even if the upshot of the premise is revisionism of a previous widely held view.

Tendentiousness perhaps cannot be avoided because often the validity of a cherished theory requires one to make the results come out right. And thus when an initial evaluation of the facts allows one to draw no conclusions, the tendentious temptation lures and entreats the investigators to change the premise and the terms of the study.

Often, such bias-laden investigations follow in the wake of an initially unpopular or at least disconcerting mandate alter existing arrangements that have been comfortable for most parties for a long time.

Several years ago, the radiology RRC outlawed independent participation by first residents in after-hours cases. The reasons for the proscription were that these very junior trainees were not capable of avoiding mistakes which were a result of their inexperience. The outcry stemmed from trainees from the fact that if first year residents could not read by themselves, their senior colleagues, especially fourth year residents would have to take call. However, tradition required that these very advanced residents retire from such an onerous task by virtue of their seniority and by the need to prepare for the Oral Board Examination, a herculean labor as formidable as cleaning out the Augean stables. "Surely no intrusion into the schedule should be permitted" was the common response to the policy change. Such a rancorous reaction needed legitimacy via a tendentious display of questionable science, Yet, every attending whose job it is to review the ER knows that residents do indeed make mistakes, and do it often the more eager they are in their training. So one would have to question any interpretation which revealed either that they fare by themselves no less adequately than a fully certified radiologist who reads in the ER a lot, or that the discrepancy rate between the two was small.

So how to manipulate the measurement. Let's look at radiology demography for the answer. Since 1980 we have added 70 million people in this country. Let us assume that, in the aggregate, contemporary individuals are no sicker nor more

S.R. Baker, *Notes of a Radiology Watcher*,
DOI 10.1007/978-3-319-01677-1_64, © Springer International Publishing Switzerland 2014

well now than before. We did two million CTs in 1980 and about 70 million in 2007, almost no MR's in 1980 and 35 million 30 years later. The age structure of the population is roughly the same over the past 27 years. So imaging utilization has outstripped population. Hence, ER radiology sections are busier because they are doing more normal studies. In fact, if my ER is like others in safety net hospitals, more or nearly all of the x-rays we do for mild chest pain and all of the CT's we do for headache and syncope are negative.

Hence when an investigation of error rate purports to show that residents missed only 1.8 % of significant findings whereas attendings missed 1 %—a data set which represents the collective conclusions of five recent studies on the subject- it looks really good at first. But at 30,000 exams per year a 0.8 % discrepancy rate is 240 missed diagnoses of a serious nature, almost one a day. Now it looks really bad. Hence prevalence manipulation is a major tool of the tendentious. Watch for it. As you read the literature, examine the premise and the data critically. Rare things rarely occur, that is why they are rare, but equally correct, a low percentage of a very common phenomenon still affects a lot of people. The ER population is better off by not having first year residents read alone and fourth year residents ultimately are better off learning to exercise the responsibility they have gained even if it means rationing time, especially if they are reimbursed through Medicare for clinical work performed. Moreover, the board schedule has changed and fourth year residents have passed the qualifying exam, and have a long time to go before taking the certifying exam. Then the notion of having had first year residents as first readers will occasion the comment `how could that have been allowed to happen?

Let us consider another tendentiousness ploy. A radiology benefit management company named Med Solutions in Nashville came up with a neat idea. They set up a new company called Premerus to correct what they claim is a "real

problem, perhaps even an epidemic". Wow that is scary. What is it? The pathogen, if you will, is the general radiologist. That is, many like you and me. Premerus asserts, but does not provide data, that generalists had a very high error rate, but their subspecialist radiologists had a negligible rate of misses. Can you believe it? In mammography a negligible rate of misses by some super radiologists. Astounding.

Moreover, they claim to have more data which revealed that so called at-large radiologists missed many MR and CT findings which is at great variance with the superior results of some specialists, incidentally employed by Premerus. They also claim a non-convergence rate of between 38 and 45 % comparing the two groups. They further state that they will share these results with potential clients but they are not ready to submit it to a peer-reviewed journal. Hmmm! Now how could you detect such a high lack of concordance between diagnostically poor yet presumably board certified general radiologists versus their very qualified other radiologists. You could not do it just by reading a stack of studies in a typical out-patient practice or a general hospital because once again, you would have to omit the vast number of negative studies overall, because of the increase in utilization that comprises the majority of examinations except in very specialized hospitals. There, too, a supposedly general radiologist would *be* aware of a panoply of subtle observations because those are the cases he or she inspects daily. But, if you can manipulate the terms of the comparison in a tendentious way, you can get data to support your position even if it is spurious and the means to it are specious. In this case, the attempt by Premerus is to gain employment for their doctors and profits for themselves, whereas with the senior residents in the other example the objective was to avoid work. In either case, if you wish to become adept at tendentiousness, load the terms of the investigation to guarantee that there will be confirmation of your perceptions and you will go on to gain fame and influence for your insights. Caveat emptor.

We must be aware of the measurement of dose, especially in CT. Specific considerations of the implications of dose depositions in particular and with respect to thyroid radiation are subjects for which all radiologists should gain awareness. MR issues, too, need to be addressed in specifics as they are in the concluding essay.

Radiation Dose: A Primer of Units and Limits

65

The increasing use of CT, especially in the last decade, has forced us to look at the issue of dose. A recent study from the National Academy of Sciences, examining a wealth of data accumulated over 10 years, announced that there is no threshold below which radiation is safe. Several months ago a governmental report indicated that radiation was a toxin. Whether you accept these two statements is probably beside the point. Despite disclaimers by several leaders in our specialty, the issue has now been raised to public consciousness. Increasing CT use will undoubtedly be accompanied by increasing surveillance of the possible ill effects of that use with respect to the induction of genetic damage, the instigation of cancers and the elaboration of vascular changes [1].

The debate has already been joined and the stakes are high. We can deny the issue at our peril; to claim that radiation has no ill effects will probably be reckless, to not change protocols and practice will be foolhardy, and to ignore the whole issue will open the door perhaps to later malpractice claims. So to be engaged in a discussion about dose means we have to talk the talk and learn the basic facts of the effects of radiation on human tissue and its relation to health. Most of you have been through this territory preparing for the physics part of the boards. You may have remembered everything from that time but even so things have changed. New units have gained popularity and new information has been generated about the deleterious effects of radiation along a range of doses.

So allow me to begin a mini-refresher course. There are two sets of units for nearly each measurement of radiation and its interaction with biologic tissue-the traditional units most of us learned the first time and System International or SI units which in most of the world have supplanted the old labels to which incidentally they are still related. The primary unit of exposure has been and remains the roentgen, which is the amount of ionization per mass in air due to X-rays and gamma rays. It is measured as a quantity of unit of charge per mass and is otherwise denoted as coulombs per kilogram. Measurements of exposure are very important, especially in rating the characteristics of an X-ray machine. Ionization can be measured directly. Since the composite atomic numbers of elements in soft tissues for all biologic specimens are roughly the same, exposure is nearly proportional to absorbed dose in soft tissue over the range of energies commonly used in radiology. However, such units of exposure have limits to their usefulness because they are derived from a calculation of ionizing photons in air. There is a more complex relationship between the ionization in air and absorbed dose for each photon energy and for structures containing elements not found in soft tissue normally- for example calcium—a major constituent of bone.

I now introduce the concept of absorbed dose which is the amount of energy imparted by radiation per mass for each unit of biologic tissue. It was traditionally measured as the rad which equals 0.01 J/kg. The SI units employ the gray

S.R. Baker, *Notes of a Radiology Watcher*,
DOI 10.1007/978-3-319-01677-1_65, © Springer International Publishing Switzerland 2014

which equals 100 rads and, correspondingly, one rad is equal to 10 milligrays. Rads and roentgens vary being approximately one to one for soft tissue in the diagnostic energy range but approaches four to one for bone when the energy is below 100 kev. Hence, in relating radiation to biological effects, the roentgen is less valuable than the rad or the gray.

Radiation imparts energy but not every type of radiation causes the same biologic damage per unit dose along the path the energy traverses- a notion incorporated as the Linear Energy Transfer factor or LET. For example, high LET energies such as alpha particles or neutrons are more potent breakers of DNA bonds. Thus, a radiation weighting factor was introduced to produce the equivalent dose which relates to absorbed dose times a coefficient for the LET of each type of radiation. The equivalent dose can be measured traditionally as the rem which has its corresponding SI unit, the sievert. One rem equals 10 millisieverts while 100 rems equals one sievert. These are the units that are most often considered in looking at radiation dose for particular organs.

Various structures have different weighting factors. For example, the bone surface weighting factor is merely 1,120 of that for the gonads and 1,112 of the bone marrow. Thus, when assessing total body radiation we need to compute the sum of weighting factors to measure effective dose. For the most part for X-rays in the diagnostic range for gamma rays there is a close approximation of sieverts or reins and grays and rads.

On average individuals occupying some place on the surface of the earth are exposed to background radiation which averages globally at 2.4 millisieverts per year. At least half of that is due to exposure to radon which is a high LET form of radiation. Of course, radon presence varies widely from place to place. Cosmic radiation supplies 4 % of background, again, varying with altitude and latitude. The remainder is low LET radiation from ingestion of substances containing some radioactive element initially present on the surface of the earth. Now the total radiation one may receive throughout the world consists of both natural background radiation, which accounts for 82 % of the radiation received globally, and man-made radiation which accounts for 18 %. Of manmade radiation, nuclear medicine imparts 21 %, consumer products 16 % are by-products of the nuclear fuel cycle 3 %, occupational 2 % and 58–60 % are from medical X-rays. But the percentages have not taken into consideration the phenomenal growth of CT which is discussed in the next essay.

Now let us consider what the radiation absorbed dose may be from various medical diagnostic tests. A single chest X-ray is generally associated with an absorbed dose of 0.1 millisieverts, a dental oral exam is 16 times more intense depositing 1.6 millisieverts, a mammogram imparts 2.5 millisieverts, a lumbosacral spine study 3.2, a PET scan 3.7, a bone scan using technetium 99 m, 4.4 millisieverts, a cardiac nuclear scan 7.5 millisieverts, a cranial CT 50 millisieverts, a barium contrast GI with 2 min of fluoroscopy 85 millisieverts and a spiral or multidetector CT 30–100 millisieverts. For those who receive radiation therapy as total body radiation between 10 and 20 sieverts will cause acute GI destruction, acute lung damage and severe cognitive dysfunction with death certain in 5–12 days. Hence, total body radiation as therapy must not exceed 3 sieverts. Most radiation therapy protocols imparting a larger dose are limited to ports encompassing only a section of the body.

Yet, a multidetector CT for trauma, for example is in essence total body radiation. Typically, if a spiral or multidetector imparts 100 millisieverts, then 10 of them will produce an accumulation of one sievert and 100 will impart a dose equivalent to lethal total body radiation. Bear in mind, however, that the radiation received from the theoretical 100 multidetector CTs will be given over time, which may have some sparing effect compared to one unit of whole body radiation. What that effect is in quantitative terms is not known.

A round-trip plane voyage from New York to London will impart 0.1 millisieverts, a thousand times less than the multidetector CT. The dose limit for the public is one millisievert per year, the dose limit for workers in the environment of low LET radiation is 50 millisieverts per year or 5 reins per year. Thus, the maximum dose for radiation workers per annum is one half of a conventional multidetector CT of the whole body. Now, while it is true that one multidetector CT may not impart much damage to adults, it is not clear that that same dose to children will be as ineffective. Individuals receiving recurrent X-ray studies, assuming the absence of a safe threshold for each study, may be subject to considerable risk. That risk may be small in total but averaged over the population of the United States, 300,000,000 people, it will not be insignificant as a public health problem, especially as CT use continues to expand. One estimate is that CT use today will induce 20,000 and 40,000 new cancer cases per year within 2 decades. Of course, this is a "guestimate" and further information must be provided to determine if such a number of cases will correspond to actuality.

Where will those cancers occur? In my next presentation I will focus on the thyroid gland as the likely place where we will observe cancer incidence to increase rapidly in relation to previous, persistent or recurrent CT use.

Reference

1. Brenner DJ. Exploring two two-edged swords. Radiat Res. 2012;178(1):7–16.

CT-ER-Dose and Cost and What to Do About It

66

It had to happen. First there was the CT revolution. We are still in it. It started in the mid-1990s when CT was then thought to be at the end of its developmental skein with its limits seemingly defined and appreciated, especially when compared with exciting advances disclosed with regularity in MR. But unanticipated yet substantiated advances in CT, particularly the advent of multidetector units, revitalized CT, putting it at the forefront of radiology with respect to clinical versatility and widespread adoption. MDCT generated faster scans which enabled studies to be done on the young, the enfeebled and the injured. Not only anatomy could be discerned. Now physiological processes could be assessed and even quantitatively evaluated. Moreover, vascular investigations could be accomplished with venous infusions producing information as relevant as could be done intrusively, arterially with conventional interventional procedures.

Even today, the widening deployment of CT remains unbounded. However as I said it had to happen. With every technological resolution comes a critical reaction, with an agenda that almost always focuses on the dangerous and wasteful effects of the innovation, initially hidden when its virtues were proclaimed. For the very popularity of CT by now has brought with it questions about whether its use has become abuse by dint of excessive application. Recently there was a feature on the evening news with the title "Too many CTs". Hence the issue has come to the fore as a natural, inevitable consequence of the national healthcare debate which has focused mostly on access, to a lesser extent on cost, and until recently only peripherally on quality. But as the debate became more focused, quality and cost have appeared together with risk as a new triumvirate of concerns centered directly on CT.

Facts abound regarding CT utilization while fears about its deleterious effects swirl in a maelstrom of projection and speculation. Before delving into the implications for individual health, here are some hard facts. Background radiation in the United States has doubled in the past 25 years. Almost all of that increase to reach an average level of 6 millisieverts annually comes from medical imaging. Today, radiography, which still constitutes three quarters of all imaging tests, imparts only 11 % of total medical radiation. Interventional procedures comprise only 4 % of imaging but are responsible for 14 % of exposure to the population. Nuclear medicine studies, predominantly for cardiac assessment, comprise 5 % of procedures but generate 25 % of exposure. And with merely 17 % of procedures, CT alone contributes 50 % of the radiation burden [1].

In 1980, CT examinations in the U.S. totaled less than five million in a population of 250 million. In 2010, 69 million CT studies were performed with some seven million done on children. CT slices in 1980 were generally 1 cm apart. Now they can be done in millimeter intervals. One half of CTs are centered on the abdomen and pelvis and about 113 of the patients' studies are middle aged, approximately equally divided on either side of 40.

S.R. Baker, *Notes of a Radiology Watcher*,
DOI 10.1007/978-3-319-01677-1_66, © Springer International Publishing Switzerland 2014

The risk of one CT for the development of cancer later in life is age-dependent. Dose susceptibility is greatest in children and young adults. The typical exposure of 6–20 millisieverts may be damaging to a relatively small percentage of individuals after one examination. It has been estimated that one CT may result in 1–2 cancers per 1,000. Obviously, the risk if real, is slight for any one exam in any one patient. But 1 per 1,000 in a country of 300 million people translates into 300,000 putative, eventual cancer cases, placing radiation among the top four or five causes of death. Again, this is speculation based on a hypothesis, which is reasonable but as yet unverified. Because the cancers induced by radiation are biologically and histologically indistinguishable from cancers not induced by radiation, the true measure of risk from CT will not be known with any degree of certainty for another generation or more.

Until then, should we go on according to the theme of business as usual, or should we become more wary of the future ill effects of CT? Should we become less exuberant, more cautious in its utilization? And should we modify protocols to gain information prudently, not expansively? Well, we should start off by identifying those who have had many CTs, because inasmuch as cancer induction is a stochastic process, it is likely that the larger the dose overall and possibly the more frequent receipt of dose, the greater the risk. Many have had and will have multiple CTs. By one estimate, 250,000 patients in the U.S. will have had 40 plus CTs in their lifetime. At 12 millisieverts per study they will receive a total dose of nearly one half sievert, a dose received by survivors of the A-bomb blasts in Japan. Those people have had a significantly high cancer rate than others similar in all other characteristics who were situated outside the environs of Hiroshima and Nagasaki when the bomb exploded.

Surely, most repetitive CT patients do not need every study. How do we prevent or minimize the exposure? First, we should know a CT history before deciding to do the next CT. Yet in many ERs, no one asks. Histories are often truncated to the needs or urgency of the moment. This practice represents an administrative failure. Surely no police department would accept such deficient detective work, failing to seek out and obtain crucial information. Why do we let E.R.'s operate so callously? Where is comprehensive history taking an important function? Probably in only a few places.

The issue of managing CT use and the ultimate risks of imaging radiation was the subject of a National Council of Radiation Protection in Bethesda which I attended and contributed some thoughts to. The focus was on CT in the ER, and the workshop had meaningful contribution from radiologists, ER physicians, physicists and government officials. Although consensus was achieved on many matters, differences remained between the scientific focus of the radiologists and the legal, regulatory and customer relation impingements considered very real by the ER physicians. The value of ACR appropriateness criteria was discussed as an ultimately valuable tool for education, but presently as merely a nonutilized construct not readily applicable on a case by case basis. Nonetheless some agreements were reached about tailoring examinations and about questioning the automatic repetition of CT.

Perhaps accumulating a CT history will be a concomitant of every admission, and some yardstick will be put into place to either restrict further studies by CT, or submit the need to a judgment panel before agreeing to proceed.

Computed Tomography like any test should only be done when the results will affect patient management. Thus a CT to "better characterize a pneumonia" when clearly seen on chest x-ray does not meet this standard. Likewise a CT of the abdomen in a patient who has experienced recurrent intestinal obstruction due to adhesions is unnecessary if the plain film reveals obstruction.

To me a classic overenthusiastic use of CT which has become established as a pillar of urologic practice is the computed tomography exam for ureteral stones. Yes, CT will find big and small stones, but it will not reveal if the calculus is obstructing unless the obstruction is prolonged.

And the charting of stone passage by repetitive CT's is unnecessary unless there is a compelling clinical reason for each study. Plain films and ultrasonography are probably equal to CT for relevant information for surveillance. And yes the forgotten, discredited IVP should be rescued from the dustbin of out-of-date procedures. My most satisfying night of ER radiology duty was when at 12:00 midnight, then 2:00 am and at 4:30 am three individuals each with renal colic came in. Each had an IVP, each had an obstructing stone and each passed the stone as the contrast material in the ureter provided both diagnostic insight and the solute load to recognize the calculus and propel it down and out of the urinary tract. In truth CT of the abdomen for renal stone provides an opportunity for urologists to add another visit to their stone therapy ritual. They now manage therapy in entirety, whereas in the past in selected cases, immediate resolution of symptoms for some patients was within the purview of the radiologist. Perhaps we should not forget this subtle redirection of management, or perhaps we have been too dazzled by the virtuosity of CT to realize how its therapeutic limitations have changed the protocols of therapy in stone disease.

We need to tailor CT to the part of the body under interrogation and not be overly inclusive. For example a CT to assess for appendicitis may be confined to the lower abdomen, not all of the abdomen. And we don't need to overlap when evaluating contiguous body parts. I have queried members of the American Society of Emergency Radiology about their technique for total body CT for trauma patients. More than three fourths acknowledged that the lower margin of their neck scan was below the upper margin of their chest scan-the overlap occurring at the level of the radiosensitive thyroid gland-thereby routinely giving this organ a gratuitous extra radiation dose.

The roster of inappropriate CT exams/techniques is long. My examples only skim the surface. We must be smarter about CT use because that is our intrinsic responsibility, which is all the more crucial today, because now the public is watching, and with increasing frequency demanding that we do good without doing harm. Consequently, we must face the certainty that posterity will judge us. The verdict will rest on not only what we can do but also what we have anticipated we should not do even if we have the capability to do it.

Reference

1. Baker S, Hsieh Y-H, Maldjian P, Scanlan M. Inadvertent thyroid irradiation in protocol-driven trauma CT: a survey of hospital ERs. Emerg Radiol. 2009;16(3):203–7. doi:10.1007/s10140-008-0784-4.

Radiation Dose Redux

67

Recently, major developments have occurred involving organized radiology and the public with respect to the topic of radiation. This renewed interest has stemmed from general awareness of the putative effects of dose. A report issued at the National Council of Radiation Protection and Measurements, which met in Arlington, VA in April of 2007, has fueled the discussion. The author of the report, Dr. Fred Mettler, emeritus professor of Nuclear Medicine at the University of New Mexico made the pronouncement that the estimated collective dose the US population receives from diagnostic imaging procedures in 1980 was 0.54 mSv per capita. However, 26 years later, that total has increased to 3.2 mSv per annum per capita, a more than sixfold increase [1].

This report was directed by a National Council of Radiation Protection scientific committee that compiled estimates on radiation exposure of the US population both from background radiation and from medical imaging equipment. Data for this study includes records of imaging modalities that did not make it to the last such comprehensive evaluation in 1987. In that year, CT fluoroscopy, Nuclear Medicine studies like PET and hybrid scans such as PET/CT were not included. The contemporary data was gathered from public and private sources including information from Medicare and the Veteran's Administration hospitals. The medical radiation sources encompass radiography, CT, dental x-rays, Nuclear Medicine, Radiotherapy, and Interventional Radiology.

The assessment of the committee, as announced by Mettler, was that CT and nuclear medicine studies account for the largest increase in dose with CT, representing 12 % of all procedures but 45 % of collective dose received. Nuclear medicine is responsible for merely 3 % of the total number of medical imaging exams but deposited 23 % of the effective dose. The growth of CT has been greater than 10 % per year and I am sure that it was accelerated in the last 5 years with the advent of multi-detector CT. In comparison, the US population has grown only 1 % per year.

As I have stated before we went from less than five million CT's in 1980 to more than 60 million in 2006. Similarly, nuclear medicine has grown steadily, about 5 % per year, since the 1980s. In 2005 there were almost 20 million nuclear procedures performed. Cardiac nuclear examinations accounts for 57 % of all nuclear medicine studies and 85 % of the dose derived from them. By the way, most cardiac studies are now done by cardiologists, not radiologists.

The most recent increase in studies under the purview of radiologists and nuclear medicine physicians has been from PET. Whereas over the past 20 years, there has been a steady rise in nuclear imaging studies done by radiologists and nuclear physicians, it has been PET scanning that has shown the marked increase most recently.

S.R. Baker, *Notes of a Radiology Watcher*,
DOI 10.1007/978-3-319-01677-1_67, © Springer International Publishing Switzerland 2014

Mettler stated that the Chernobyl nuclear power plant accident in 1986 produced a global collective dose of 600,000 per person/sv. Although the estimated collective dose of 930,000 per person/sv in the US population today seems impressive by comparison, it is too early to extrapolate figures to make meaningful predictions. The conclusion of this study was that dose has increased markedly yet physicians do not understand the magnitude of this increase even though the largest collective source of radiation exposure is medical imaging. Nevertheless, imaging remains unregulated, a circumstance perhaps initially to the benefit of radiologists. Yet ultimately, it will most likely induce a health problem which radiologists must now attend to or be blamed for.

In that regard, and in anticipation of the NRCP report, the ACR convened a blue ribbon panel which met for several months and recommended a raft of changes governing the tracking and physician management of radiation exposure. This committee was chaired by Dr. Steve Amis, and consisted of radiologists and physicists. It offered 33 recommendations which were announced to coincide with the revelations announced by the NRCP which I have just referred to.

I would like to go through some of those recommendations and then later provide some comment as to what was included, what will work and what was not included. The deliberations and conclusions of the American College of Radiology panel represent a sea change in the ACR's attention to dose issues. In the past, and in fact the very recent past, the notion that radiation is a toxin and that there are ultimate deleterious effects from excessive deposition of radiation was regarded in a word as "stonewalling" by some of the leaders of the ACR. Now the evidence is overwhelming. Dose has increased; the implications of that increase, while not conclusive, are worrisome. So these recommendations reflect a new attitude by the ACR which underscores that the college now shares with other segments of the population concern about the long term consequences of added dose deposition through medical imaging.

From the report, I would like to quote from its abstract. "The benefits of diagnostic imaging are immense and have revolutionized the practice of medicine, the increasing sophistication and clinical efficacy of imaging has resulted in strong growth over the past quarter century. While data derived from the atom bomb survivors and other events suggest that the expanded use of imaging modalities using ionizing radiation may eventually result in an increased incidence of cancer in the exposed population, this problem can likely be minimized by preventing the inappropriate use of such imaging, and optimizing studies which are performed to obtain the best image quality with the lowest radiation dose."

Let's examine that statement critically. The abstract states that "problems" can likely be minimized by preventing the inappropriate use of such imaging and by optimizing studies to obtain the best image quality with the lowest radiation dose. I certainly agree with the second part of that statement that we can optimize studies and reduce dose, but there is no effective means presently of reducing the inappropriate use of such imaging, as the growth of CT and nuclear medicine procedures have revealed. It is undoubtedly true that a large percentage of those studies are not indicated. To me the real solution would be to have more stringent requirements for initial and recurrent imaging. The recommendations of the report in essence do not address this issue. The authors of the ACR report state that in 1987, medical x-rays and nuclear medicine studies contributed less than 15 % of the average yearly raised exposure received by the American population. Two decades later they claim that this percent has most assuredly increased. That is a tentative statement at best. Of course it has increased, we all know that. The blue ribbon panel suggests that the ACR should adopt a policy of expressing quantitative radiation dose values as dose estimates, and replace such terms as dose with dose estimates. This is an important recommendation because as best as we can determine, we deal with dose estimates and not actually absorbed dose in most of the measurements we undertake in this issue.

Furthermore, the panel recommended that the ACR should work to convince the LCME and AAMC of the need for development of methodology to introduce medical students to the realities of radiation exposure and medical imaging. They offered to prepare learning materials in support of this initiative. I certainly could not agree more. The danger of radiation dose is one that most medical students are only dimly aware of. The panel goes on to recommend that CMSS, which is the Council of Medical Specialty Societies, and the AMA likewise distribute information in the form of further education to physicians about radiation dose. Moreover, they stated that the ACR should sponsor a summit meeting with leaders from emergency medicine to discuss developing consensus guidelines for imaging conditions where CT may be overutilized. This is very important, too, because the ER is a place where excessive dose is administered through inappropriate utilization.

We have shown in another study recently presented, that even with ACR appropriateness criteria available, ER test ordering behaviors, in many respects, is out of control. If CT is available it will be obtained by imaging physicians even though indications for its use may be available but not enforced.

The ACR panel recommended that multi organizational efforts should be undertaken to improve radiology resident training in medical physics. In fact, an independent panel of physicists and radiologists has recommended reordering of the curriculum for such teaching. They have concluded that radiation safety and patient dose should be part of the annual in training examination. Again, we have here another excellent recommendation. Also they offer that the American Board of Radiology should consider requiring at least one SAM on patient safety to include radiation dose every 10 years as an integral part of maintenance of certification requirements. Moreover, they recommend that CT accreditation programs sponsored by the ACR should examine the use of appropriate scanning protocols. In JACR there should be a monthly patient safety column to include radiation exposure issues. The panel encourages radiology practices to record all fluoroscopy times and compare them to benchmarks, as well as evaluate outliers, as part of an ongoing QA program. All of these measures are sound, and should be implemented with mechanisms to ensure that they are put in place and faithfully followed in every institution.

It was proposed that the ACR should encourage radiology practices to provide in-service training on radiation safety for technologists on a regular basis. Actually, "encourages" sounds too soft. It really should be mandatory as part of ACR accreditation requirements. Recommendations were offered for the ACR to improve effective teaching of medical physics and medical physicists. The most important recommendation would be that the ACR should work with NEMA in pursuit of the principle of ALARA, which is to say devices should be optimized to achieve as low as reasonably attainable patient doses. Furthermore, the ACR should encourage third party payers to develop a process for identifying patients who receive frequent imaging exams utilizing ionized radiation, and provide feedback regarding those patients to the referring physicians. Again, a baby step in the right direction. The greatest risk from radiation will be to those who receive many studies, not those who receive just one or several CT's in their lifetime. For example, opting for recurring CT's for placement of intraventricular shunts, or numerous follow-ups for the evaluation of ureteral calculi, are clinical situations in which dose accumulation can occur rapidly. Another egregious example is excessive use of radiation in sickle cell patients who routinely get repetitive chest x-rays, usually on average of once a month, and frequent chest CT's to rule out pulmonary emboli. Most of the time these studies are negative, but over the course of decades the accumulated dose can approach the oncogenic range. Most importantly, the panel recommended a system of dose accountability so that an individual's radiation dose accumulation record will be a part of patient history, which will be as available and portable as the rest of the medical record.

Now, here are a few things that I believe the authors left out. In their preamble, the authors state that medical exposure might be responsible for approximately 1 % of all cancers in the US. This rate can be expected to increase, based upon the higher number of exams performed today and even greater numbers in future years. On the other hand, as the use of medical radiation has increased, the incidence of some cancers has actually decreased. Lung cancer is actually decreasing in men because of smoking cessation, and breast cancer is leveling off. This rosier picture requires further elaboration.

The decrease in breast cancer rate seen recently may be due to a decrease in utilization of mammography, so if patients do not have mammography, their cancers will not be detected. But most importantly, the authors forgot one important cancer. There is only one malignancy that is increasing rapidly in the US. That is thyroid cancer, especially in women. It seems that the medical community has blinders on in terms of this amazing statistic of a 5 % increase per year. That increase has occurred in the last 10 years, coincident with the increase in use of rapid multi-detector CT. The authors of this report have failed to indicate that they are aware of this important association of cancer and radiation dose in time and in space in the US [2].

The panel acknowledges special patient populations, notably children, pregnant females and potentially pregnant females, which radiology departments and organizations should provide with additional radiation protection. Yet, the authors have failed to mention that there are other populations at risk. For example, radiation sensitivity is not the same in every individual. Those who are recessive for ataxia-telangiectasia are at greater risk for radiation damage per unit of dose received. The authors of the report do not mention that it may be important, in fact crucial, that we do radiation risk testing of individuals for genetic susceptibility by developing different protocols for those who are inherently at greater risk than others.

I regard the alarm registered by the NRCP and the response by the ACR panel to be positive steps in protecting the public from the oncogenic consequences of increased radiation dose from diagnostic procedures. The idea of a dose registry is important conceptually, I think the devil will be in the details however. Yet, there are other issues not fully addressed by this report that need further publicity and awareness. Thyroid cancer and inherent genetic susceptibility are just two of them. Unfortunately, the problem will probably not be resolved in the near future, unless incentives for appropriate use are modified to prevent the situation which frequently occurs today, occasioned by promiscuous radiation which is still essentially unregulated. Until that happens, little will be done to change things, and the next generation will wonder why we were not up to the task.

References

1. Brenner DJ. We can do better than effective dose for estimating or comparing low-dose radiation risks. Ann ICRP. 2012;41(3–4):124–8.
2. Baker SR, Bhatti W. Cancer of the thyroid gland—is it the dark side of the ct revolution? Eur J Radiol. 2006;60:67–9.

CT Techniques: Risk and Challenges—Who Will Control Radiology

68

Radiologists by obligation and by predilection are avid to be informed about new developments in diagnostic imaging. Yet a recurrent caveat in any promotion of a new technique is ever present, the intrusion of unintended consequences which in actuality often become more profound and deleterious than the good they seek to invoke. I feel compelled to jump into the warning business. I must alert you to the harbingers of a gathering storm, or more appropriately, gathering storms, each of which will shower us with the insistent pressure of teeming rain, or even the destructive power of small hailstones.

What am I hyping here? Nothing less than a thunderous assault on the prestige of our specialty and its continued control of territory which is now being invaded both insidiously and directly by aggressive practitioners in cardiology and gastroenterology.

All of us know that too much of a good thing is bad. That goes for radiation as much as milkshakes. We enter the specialty with the foreknowledge that our pioneering forebears suffered grievously from the harmful effects of photons and radioactive isotopes on unprotected eyes, thyroid glands, limbs and lungs. Yet, today, as innovations using radiation have enlarged our capabilities, we tend to get caught up in the enthusiasm for their virtues, neglecting at the same time a careful accounting of their risks. Hence, we have enjoyed a generation- long explosion of CT use and only recently paid some heed to dose issues [1].

We also know that at least two steps in the general education of the public with respect to threats to their health must occur to galvanize change. Initially, and for a long time, there is often an awareness of scientific data which functions, apparently, like background noise within our collective consciousness. Except for the strident alarms of enthusiasts who warn us about the dire consequences of uncontained toxins and deviant policies, behavior and attitude are usually not affected. It is only when the press and government join together to impute either an emotional and/or a moral value to a particular carcinogen or irritant that public opinion is mobilized. Everyone knew in the 1950s that smoking caused cancer, but it took the Surgeon General's report of 1964 to transmute the science into a reassessment of mores. More recently, throughout 1998 every baseball fan had learned by September that Mark McGuire was taking steroid supplements. It was only his appearance before a senate committee, convened in consequence of a collective sense of moral outrage about the unfair advantages of performance-enhancing pharmaceuticals, that his reluctance to acknowledge what everyone knew tainted his reputation and sullied his record.

A recent announcement by the United States government that x-rays and gamma rays are cancer inducing agents has brought to us the latest manifestation of an escalation of the moral consequences of risk. One should now expect closer surveillance with regard not just to radiation

S.R. Baker, *Notes of a Radiology Watcher*,
DOI 10.1007/978-3-319-01677-1_68, © Springer International Publishing Switzerland 2014

protection but also to radiation use. The American College of Radiology reacted to the raising of the stakes through the assumption of the counter-productive posture of qualified denial. I believe this was a mistake. It will not serve our purpose to fail to accommodate to what is an irrefutable fact which has now acquired a patina of public concern.

One might have taken comfort in the supposition that, since there seemingly has not been an increase in cancer incidence since the CT revolution began in earnest in 1980, there never will be a realization of supposed scary consequences of cancer inducement, despite what the purveyors of "Chicken Little" profess. But carcinogenesis from radiation has a latency period of 2–3 decades. Nonetheless, when storm clouds are accumulating beyond the horizon one might still believe they are not coming our way. In that regard, one could look at Japan to see if radiation is really as dangerous as the doomsayers profess. The Japanese have nearly 5 times as many CT machines per capita as the United States. Generally, adult patients there are thinner and hence more subject to radiation damage per exposure than their American counterparts. We should watch Japanese data closely because it is always best to prepare for a possible eventuality before it happens, even if the danger is remote and not necessarily inevitable. For example, the cost of a tsunami warning system in the Indian Ocean would now in retrospect have been a good investment.

Yet, I must bring to your attention that any doubts about the uncertainty of radiation danger from diagnostic studies should now be dispelled because of a report I read recently in our local newspaper, the Newark Star-Ledger, which demonstrated clearly that thyroid cancer in women in the United States and especially in New Jersey has risen approximately fourfold in the last 5 years. A slight increase in men has also occurred.

What could be the reason for this precipitous rise in thyroid cancer cases? Well, a reasonable hypothesis is that the increase in radiation deposition in women via mammography, chest x-rays and CT use in the past 20 years must be playing a significant role in the heightening incidence of thyroid cancer in the last 5 years which, by the way, is still continuing to increase. Any debate about the dangers of diagnostic radiation, and that means mostly CT, must now deal with this disturbing reality. The government was right to announce that ionizing radiation is a carcinogen. It is up to the radiology community to adjust its practices and expectations now. That means not only reducing dose per case, but also minimizing unnecessary exposure by limiting utilization to only those situations for which competitive non-radiation inducing modalities are not available, and the information derived from the chosen CT study is crucial for diagnosis and management.

We are over the full-body screening bubble that appeared 10 years ago, resplendent as it was in hope and the prospect of profit. One thing we should have known beforehand from this misadventure in the application of technologies to the apparently well is that false positives are much more frequent than true positives when the prevalence is low. We also learned that the public does have only a limited quest for narcissism, a concomitant of which has been that many dedicated screening centers have shut down for lack of customers. Moreover, we have come to appreciate that, despite the screed shouted by touts, the scientific community was not fooled about it at all or for very long. Recent studies have proven that low-dose CT screening for detection of early lung cancer in smokers saves lives. Therefore, a cardiologist who performs cardiac CT in a smoker without scrutinizing the lungs may be jeopardizing the health of the patient, in addition to exposing him/herself medicolegally.

Manufacturers are now aggressively marketing fast multidetector CT scans with 64 (or even as many as 320) detector rows, which can demonstrate soft plaques in coronary arteries in a single breathhold. The introduction of 64 row multidetector CT may now enable physicians to detect soft plaques in coronary arteries. The visualization of these excrescences are much more important clinically than the recognition of calcium deposits in arterial walls because they are more apt to ulcerate thereby precipitously decreasing the caliber of the artery, severely reducing blood flow and initiating a cardiac event. Such an observation can be accomplished with a 64 multidetector CT through an intravenous injection, obviating the need for diagnostic catheterization through the traditional arterial route. Thus, the ongoing tussle between radiologists and cardiologists will now enter a new, more active phase. A bidding war for control of this modality has already begun. It has all the earmarks of an arms race, stimulated by weapons manufacturers avid for more sales and profits.

Compared with the physician interpreting the scan, the vendors have less to fear from an eventual class action suit against them by sufferers from an incurable malignancy or from their survivors, because recent federal legislation has removed such initiatives from state courts to place them within federal jurisdiction. This law was enacted with the express purpose of reducing the likelihood that class action suits could be successful because it is more difficult to define a class in federal versus state courts.

Yet, I see an even greater danger to radiology from the deployment of such equipment. If it is possible to exclude the rest of the thorax when viewing the heart then it would be equally possible to exclude the rest of the abdomen when viewing the colon. Hence, virtual colonoscopy (or CT colonography) could be accomplished by filtering out everything beyond the limits of the large intestine even though radiographic depiction of all other abdominal structures could be achieved. Remember that gastroenterologists are exempt from Stark regulations when they open up a free-standing diagnostic and treatment center. In that setting they can self-refer without impunity. The opportunity accorded to a CT vendor's marketing department is obvious. Offer gastroenterologists a visually-restricted, colon-specific CT scanner. The advantages to a gastroenterologist are equally obvious. Having this device means control of both CT colonography and optical colonography. The patient would no longer see a radiologist for colon cancer detection by virtual colonoscopy. Rather, he or she would go to the gastroenterologist for a complete colonoscopic evaluation. If anything suspicious would be seen (even if only a retained fecal fragment simulating a polyp) then an optical colonoscopy would be ordered and performed in the same center. The gastroenterologist would be able to corner the market on diagnostic procedures for the detection of large bowel cancer, as a separate CT colonography performed by a radiologist would no longer be so attractive to a patient. Then the gastroenterologist could hedge his bets and hire a radiologist to read his CT colonography studies. Inasmuch as the real income is in the technical fee and not the professional fee, the radiologist's income would be reduced at the same time that the gastroenterologist would be enriched.

It has been almost a Sisyphean adventure to get Medicare to reimburse for virtual colonoscopy. It would be disheartening at least to see that we got the proverbial rock to the top of the mountain, only to have the gastroenterologist steal it from us and as a concomitant put himself in charge of the radiation such a test dispenses.

Reference

1. Levine C, Hirschorn D, Baker S. Radiology coverage 24/7—what can we do, who can we call? Emerg Radiol. 2003;10(3):119–20. doi:10.1007/s10140-003-0307-2.

CT Utilization and Thyroid Cancer: Is There a Connection?

69

I do not need to tell you that the last 15 years have seen a revolution in how patients undergo diagnostic workups. That change had already begun about 35 years ago with the phenomenal growth of radiology, including the advent of ultrasound, CT, MR, nuclear medicine and interventional radiology. And from 1995 to 2009 these has been a precipitous rise in CT utilization occasioned by fantastic advances in that technique [1]. Growth has leveled off and declined a little, but more than 60 million CT exams are done each year in the U.S.A. This period of growth has caused not merely an increase in the number of cases but, in fact, a transformation, actually a metamorphosis, about how patients are evaluated. For many diseases diagnosis has been ceded to the radiologist. That change is not merely a modification of medical practice but a sociological transformation that has been accepted by the public as well as by other medical practitioners. Are there implications in this increasing reliance on CT that perhaps are not salutary? I am not only talking about economic issues but actually also issues of the induction of pathology.

In 1980 two million CTs were done nationally. Today on average nearly one in four American will have a CT exam every year. Some will have less or none but others will have them more frequently than annually. Not only has CT utilization increased, but the protocol of CT examinations has also changed. We now do much faster studies, which enable us to do more regions per exam, more slices per region, more doses per slice, and more studies of children. The National Academy of Sciences recent report has stated that there really is no threshold below which radiation causes no damage. Now that may still be debated, but when we do a study of the chest and abdomen with CT slices as close together as 1 mm, we are imparting a radiation dose much higher than any low threshold. For the purpose of this talk we need not get into specific dose numbers, but the point is that the doses we are giving for one CT and then repetitive CTs approach a level where we must give consideration to the fact that perhaps what we are doing has some ill effect as well as some good.

Recently, the manufacturers of CT units have responded, in several ways, to the emerging issue of dose. They have devised in their machines certain techniques to reduce the dose per slice. At the same time they have encouraged increasing use of CT with more slices. Several years ago one manufacturer even suggested that they could erase part of the area they irradiate to make it easier for other specialties to interpret studies specific for their organ of expertise. Witness the fact that one CT purveyor had been willing to sell a CT to be used for the heart, erasing coincident images of the lung so that only the cardiac contours and interior can be viewed. If permitted the same purveyors might seek to sell CTs with the capability of looking only at the colon, eliminating the rest of the abdomen. So what manufacturers are doing or plotting in this regard is at best a mixed bag. What the radiologists have not been doing is to consider that the dose per repetitive

S.R. Baker, *Notes of a Radiology Watcher*,
DOI 10.1007/978-3-319-01677-1_69, © Springer International Publishing Switzerland 2014

examinations may in fact be a problem. In other words, what have we done about utilization? Well, perhaps we need to do nothing about utilization except for this disturbing fact. The biological effects per dose of radiation received vary inversely with age. That is, younger patients are probably at greater risk for the deleterious effects of CT than older patients, with the inflection point at about 30 or 35 years of age. Although we are now able to do more CT examinations in children, we are imparting a danger perhaps to be expressed in a decade or two or three of adverse consequences to these children, to be realized when they are adults. Also, we fail to realize that individual radiosensitivity varies. Patients at risk for the ataxia-telangiectasia gene, which is perhaps 3–5 % of the population, and those with the BRCA 1 or 2 genes, are more susceptible to radiation damage. With completion of the human genome project it is likely other genes predisposing to radiation sensitivity may soon be identified. This might raise the question should we prescreen individuals before doing a CT as least collectively because of the inherent radiation risk whose results may be expressed 10–20 or 30 years from now?

Let us also look at current situations independent of genetic studies. Cancer of the thyroid gland is one of only a few malignancies that are really accelerating in incidence in the United States today. Thyroid malignancy is increasing 4.3 % per annum over the last 10 years. This is a fact that has been noted in the United States generally as well as in specific states where it has been studied, such as New Jersey and Iowa. Moreover, the increasing incidence of cancer of the thyroid is much more rapid in women than in men. Is this an isolated phenomenon? Unfortunately, it is not. Thyroid cancer is increasing, especially in women, in Finland, France, Slovenia, Spain, Australia and New Zealand. In fact, everywhere where it has been measured, thyroid cancer cases are up, especially since 1995. Traditionally at greater risk are Filipinos, Icelanders, Polynesians, other than Maoris and Alaskan native women. Yet, putting aside those particular populations, thyroid cancer is increasing everywhere. Is it a mystery? I think not. There

are no specific or focal risk factors to explain the global rise. Environmental issues such as volcanic eruptions and locally high iodine n the diet do not explain it. Family history, previous attack of Hashimoto's thyroiditis and the various MEN syndromes also are known risk factors, but do not explain the general incidence increase. Perhaps the augmenting popularity of ultrasonography and fine needle biopsy may be a partial answer as it has led to the detection of more cases. Yet, this impress of technology probably cannot explain all of the added cases worldwide.

Recent studies from Chernobyl indicate that the health effects of that accident have been minimal, except for a persistent increase in thyroid cancer. In fact, that malignancy has expressed itself with a higher incidence within 5 years of the accident, suggesting that if CT use is related to thyroid cancer, the deleterious effects would not be delayed to future decades. In actuality, a rise in CT use has been accompanied in lock step by the rise in thyroid cancer.

Why is the thyroid at risk from CT? Well, the thyroid is exposed in CTs of the head and neck and CTs of the chest. Sometimes these examinations are done together. There is also a relationship that has been established between the presence of iodine and thyroid dysfunction and perhaps thyroid cancer. Until the 1980s, some of you may remember, myelography was done with fat-soluble contrast material, which could never be completely removed. Gradually, the contrast agent, usually Pantopaque, leached into the general circulation and accumulated in the colloid of the thyroid gland. When patients were then given head and neck radiation for cancer therapy the likelihood of hypothyroidism was raised. Presumably this was due to the fact that the presence of high atomic number iodine molecules in excess within the thyroid thereby increased the focal linear energy transfer of received photons, so that much of the energy that would ordinarily pass through the gland was deposited locally. Now, when we give contrast material prior to CT of the face, neck or chest we are, for a few moments, converting that thyroid gland to a zone of iodine excess. If the incidence of thyroid cancer has been shown to be related to CT perhaps we should devise different protocols preventing accumulation of iodine in the moments just before CT slices are obtained.

In any event, we cannot deny the fact that thyroid cancer and CT use are going up nearly exponentially at the same time, at least for women. Technical modifications by manufacturers of CT scanners may result in a quantum leap decrease in dose. But do not bet on it. More likely, improvements in dose accumulation will be minimal or moderate. The key factor, to me at least, is that we must control utilization. That means, (1) we should only do CT examinations when the study is really indicated. For example, not everybody with minimal trauma to the head or neck needs a CT. We need to adopt something akin to the Ottawa rules (for ankle trauma) to subselect the patients who really need this examination, (2) it has been now routine that patients who have face trauma have an obligatory CT. However, if the plain films were negative it is unlikely that anything significant would be seen on a concurrent CT examination. Yet, that same CT examination results in significant thyroid radiation. We need to be careful when we do chest CTs because the thyroid is in the field of view. Need we do a CT for everybody with acute lung disease? Can some of those patients wait and see what the results of a repeat chest x-ray might show? Does everybody with chest pain now need to have a CT to look for a pulmonary embolus? I think not.

The consequences of taking no action will be serious if in fact a relationship is proven to exist between CT use and thyroid cancer. The data are strongly suggestive here but have not yet been established as indicating a causal relationship. CT use continues to expand and thyroid cancer continues to increase in incidence. If there is someone that society is going to pin this epidemic on, in a decade or two, it is going to be radiologists. Therefore, it is up to us to think about how to be more prudent in protocols utilizing CT from above the middle of the chest to the top of the head. We must accept the dictum that any innovation brings with it untoward consequences as well as salutary benefits. Multidetector CT is no exception.

Reference

1. Baker S, Hsieh Y-H, Maldjian P, Scanlan M. Inadvertent thyroid irradiation in protocol-driven trauma CT: a survey of hospital ERs. Emerg Radiol. 2009;16(3):203–7. doi:10.1007/s10140-008-0784-4.

MR is probably the most complex, diagnostically incisive and potentially dangerous implement in a hospital or outpatient center. Safety and safeguard surveillance must always be paramount and continually engaged for the protection of patients, the reputation and careers of the radiologists involved and for the protection of the machine itself.

The ACR has produced an excellent compendium of safety concerns and the means to minimize untoward events. A few of those concerns are underscored in this presentation.

All those who may be situated near the magnet must know the risks and how to avoid a bad event. This requirement applies not only to hospital personnel, patients and their families, but also to police and firemen who may be called to the unit in an emergency. The risk of bringing in metal-bearing individuals who are not trained in MR safety is considerable, perhaps even a second disaster waiting to happen if they are not schooled in the potential of an MR accident. We all should beware, too, of other rare but preventable events, such as a patient creating a closed electrical loop when in contrast with the bore, an unauthorized person presenting at the scan room, and an adventitious entry by a family member. Some of those opportunities for mayhem will be discussed here.

MR Safety Another Look

There is probably no implement in any hospital or any clinic potentially more dangerous than an MR machine. The diagnostic power of this novel technique has advanced radiology since its clinical introduction more than 30 years ago. Yet, one cannot deny the dangers inherent in placing a patient within a very strong magnetic field, an exercise which requires utmost consideration of safety by all of those individuals who come near it. Moreover, attention must be continually paid to safeguards so that the complex assemblage of parts that constitutes this implement is not damaged by its own magnetic capabilities.

In this discussion, I will refer liberally to the American College of Radiology's white paper on MR safety that was published in AJR in June 2002. I would also like to highlight some areas I believe are important and require renewed emphasis. I will disagree with the recommendations in some respects and underscore others most emphatically.

The MR white paper was a result of careful consideration by a range of individuals, all of whom are experts in either MR functionality or MR diagnosis, or who have special knowledge related to how to bring matters of safety to public awareness. The principal author was Dr. Emanuel

Kanal, probably the foremost expert on the subject of MR safety. I am sure many of you are familiar with the fact that MR accidents have happened, and there have been a few, well-publicized tragic events. There is no need to account in detail for about what occurred in those incidents, except to say that unless we maintain careful and continuous vigilance, anybody near the machine is potentially imperiled. Nearly as significant, perhaps, your reputation—if not your career in radiology-will be imperiled by the facts and also by your clientele's perception after one untoward incident. All the accidents that have been reported were preventable if care was directed to be compliant with comprehensive safety rules.

In addition to assuring uninterrupted maintenance of the machine, the most important task a director of MR at any facility must do is establish safety policies and procedures which then must be implemented, routinely reviewed and updated. For this reason there must be a designated director of MR safety who will schedule and conduct frequent meetings regarding safety issues. An analysis of every near-miss situation must be undertaken in order to learn from that error what systems problems caused it and how they can be eliminated. Just as in the air travel industry any potential error in safety and surveillance must be addressed and corrected, not swept under the rug.

Now, crucial to any safety program is the commandment that any health care worker who gets near the machine must have undergone a safety program. That means retesting every year if you are in an academic medical center. Each year a new cadre of anesthesiology residents comes on board. They should go through and pass an MR safety program at orientation or just after that. All patient transporters should undergo the same training. Moreover, all radiology residents and any other new hires, be it attending radiologist, technologist, staff person, file room individual or member of any job category in Radiology should go through an MR safety program, pass the test, and do the same at a refresher test annually, When at our facility we instituted a formal training program to all the aforementioned individuals, it took about 3 months to get everybody involved. Fortunately for us, no terrible thing

happened when untrained workers came close to our unit. But we were just lucky. MR safety training programs should be part and parcel of entry requirement of any new staff member, physician or employee when they come on board.

But MR safety goes further than that. Let us consider this scenario. A fire has been reported in or near your MR suite. The fire department is called. They come in to save people and property carrying their metallic equipment. Guess what could happen? Maybe they put the fire out or not, but their heavy metallic devices are attracted to the machine. Some may fly into it with a patient in there or not. What a horrific prospect. Or consider another scene. A patient has been acting up in or near the MR machine and your security force or the city police are called in to help. They bring with them their gear and other metal on their bodies. You can imagine what might ensue. How many of you have really tried to undertake a program of safety with the police or fire personnel in or near the hospital? I doubt few of you have. Nonetheless, it is only a matter of time before a tragedy will occur, unless we have the foresight and commitment to include among mandated training the complete roster one of potential MR interacters.

Another issue. Do you know how much insulation is in your machine? It is entirely possible, especially with high field magnets, that a patient may touch the inner part of the core, and by having their arms and legs in a certain position, they may induce a current, leading to a burn. There are specific guidelines to prevent this from happening, but do your technicians know that when a patient feels suddenly warm it may not be anxiety or contrast material that is causing it, but actual searing of their flesh? You should determine whether this unusual possibility could happen by checking the machine out for proper insulation, by providing guidelines about how patients should be configured when they are in the magnet, and by ascertaining how your technologists should respond to patient complaints. Often as a procedure nears completion and a patient starts getting uncomfortable, there is perhaps a tendency to tell them to endure it a little longer. But if what they are feeling is increasing warmth, having them stay in the machine for too long can result in a burn.

Another consideration. What rules and protocols do you have in place to prevent a wayward individual from entering the MR room? First of all, you must be diligent about enforcing the prescription that only certain persons can be in certain zones near and about the machine. Those who want to be close to their friends or loved ones during the procedure should be dissuaded from doing so, because you often do not know if they have metal within them. Moreover, how should you test them and what should you charge for it and who should pay, etc., etc. You do not know how they will respond when the patient starts to complain. For example, they could rush in to help before you can stop them or redirect them. Or you and your employees should be less than assiduous about inquiring about what metallic objects the patient has within themselves either in their eyes, in their brain, or affixed to vessels elsewhere in the body. Deviation or migration of any of these objects by the impress of the magnetic field could result in damage to nearby structures or worse. If you did not ask, they may not tell. If you did not ask, they may not stay well. So it is important that you have policies that cannot be circumvented, even if it means the patient may have to return for the test at a later date, or even if they cannot have it at all.

In our institution, we have a metal detector surrounding the opening to the MR machine. The device itself and its physical placement are not approved in the ACR committee recommendations. It could be averred with some urgency that one may get a false sense of security if a patient passes through a metal detection scanner registered by a handheld or framing metal detector. We agree. However, just seeing the metal detector so positioned might alert individuals who seek to enter the MR facility unexpectedly, without permission. We believe that situating a metal detector at the room's opening is one further psychological barrier to inappropriate entrance. Perhaps you may not share this view, but it has helped us stop intruders just in time.

I could go on and on about each of the issues pertinent to MR safety. Many of you know them quite well of course. Nonetheless, I was surprised that at a recent meeting of Chairs of Radiology, very few of the attendees realized the potential risk to police and fire personnel, if called upon emergently to perform their duties near the machine. Others of my colleagues expressed the view that they should do more to ensure prompt training of all health professionals who might enter the MR suite. What are you doing [1]?

Reference

1. Kanal E, Borgstede JP, Barkovich AJ, et al. American College of Radiology White Paper on MR Safety: 2004 update and revisions. AJR Am J Roentgenol. 2004;182(5):1111–4.

Part XIII

Nooks and Crannies in General Radiology Including Some Forgotten Observations

In this potpourri of "neat findings", the following subjects are discussed – nipple markers exclusion, bullet migration, phleboliths, pills, splenic findings, the workup of mild to moderate pancreatitis, eponymous abdominal hernias, illicit drug transport, and a group of things you've been told to know that ain't so.

From Nipple Shadows to Bullet Holes

71

Experience is a Janus-faced character which can both affect insight and expertise and be molded by them. For many situations, increasing familiarity breeds enhancing ability. Many of you are aware of Malcolm Gladwell's notion that virtuosity in a particular occupation requires 10,000 h of labor to learn its techniques superbly and master its unique corpus of knowledge. True enough when a questioning spirit keeps the mind alert to rare events and their management and repetitive tasks become imprinted in muscle memory or thought processes.

But not uncommonly, experience may not be enlightening when the encrustations of tradition, bias or unquestioning certainty compromise one's ability to appreciate variation or novelty. Distracted by other attentions, routine work may become so automatic that one becomes hidebound, unable to sense a new finding or welcome a new approach.

This double-edged sword now affects not only individuals but the whole domain of practitioners who mindlessly accept a dogma even when obvious facts come on the scene but are not recognized. The Emperor Who Has No Clothes may be appearing in a radiology department near you if you are not aware.

This long-winded introduction is a lead in to an observation so simple, so obvious, so deliciously trenchant that it was missed by all of Radiology for nearly 85 years, until recognized by one former resident of mine in the early 1980s. I refer to the recognition of a nipple shadow as being distinct from a lung nodule on conventional frontal radiography of the chest. The fact that that once new (now decades old) observation is still not part of the canon of pulmonary imaging teaching is emblematic of the persistence of a notion long held, even if it is clearly wrong.

The standard, hallowed paradigm of action after observing a rounded density overlying the lower lung fields is to obtain a lateral image. If it cannot be localized in the lungs then a request for a P-A film with nipple markers had been de rigueur. But what if the nodule is precisely behind the nipple marker? What then? Could you be sure of its location? No! So more tests including obliques or fluoroscopy in the old days or CT currently would be done.

But Dr. Moss, my former resident, simply suggested to raise the arms and repeat. That would move the nipple but not the nodule, and the answer would be achieved without any lingering ambiguity. So the nipple marker would by the adoption of this simple expedient become superfluous. And instead of keeping them in the radiology department, we should assign them instead to lie quietly in a time capsule.

Actually we have found that we do not even do the anus up film in most cases, because typically the nipple does not project straight forward in the path of the beam, but is actually oriented on a more sloping axis, so that the shadow imparted by it is not circumferentially sharp because it is not completely outlined by ambient air. Rather, it is distinct for only most of its border, but not where it merges with the subjacent chest wall.

S.R. Baker, *Notes of a Radiology Watcher*, DOI 10.1007/978-3-319-01677-1_71, © Springer International Publishing Switzerland 2014

Lung nodules, in contrast, are completely sharply demarcated by the air in the lungs that surround it. Hence by his observation, a stultifying misconception of tradition was broken by a lone radiologist who looked at the issue with fresh eyes and a novel vision that was disarmingly correct.

But what about the other side of the experiential coin? I would like to present to you two signs that only through long experience have I been able to identify. These two observations reflect insight gained not through scientific experiment but by repetitive, slowly- accreting recognition of recurring facts or tendencies which eventually I have found myself unable to ignore. Such cues are not always correct but I am not loath to resist their import as explanations when I see them. Much like about how an experienced trucker on non-paved thoroughfares gets the feel of the road, I have come to regard them as telltale signs, even if I have reached that realization without control groups to help me verify their validity [1].

The first of these observations is the necklace sign. Many patients wear a thin chain that hangs down from their neck to overlie their upper chest. For some, it is a mark of identity, something that is part of their everyday appearance. When thin in width, this item of jewelry does not generally intrude on our ability to recognize findings on a chest X-ray. Nonetheless, excellent technique requires that they be placed out of the way. For those patients who choose not to remove their necklace, a convenient maneuver is to place it in the mouth before and during the taking of the exposure. Typically, "anchoring" of the treasured necklace by the patient in the oral cavity is recognized with the metallic chain appearing as two arcs, each overlying one lung area as it rises out of the field of view in the midline when it is drawn into the mouth. Now this expedient works well for most individuals who are not in acute distress. But for dyspneic patients, there is great reluctance to place anything but food in the mouth and hold it there when a technologist is instructing them to hold their breath. That is something difficult or unpleasant to do by such patients even when the oral cavity is unoccupied. I have found, by experience, that a negative necklace sign i.e., the metal chain is not anchored in the mouth-is therefore a good sign of dyspnea. Conversely when it is present, then one can be assured that at that moment when the film is taken the patient is not acutely short of breath.

Observing I.C.U. films every day for decades has led me to realize that for women, there is a chest X-ray sign that almost always portends further clinical improvement. I.C.U. patients are of course acutely ill. They are placed in a dehumanizing environment with no privacy in most facilities and they are often tethered by tubes placed through the mouth and in the trachea. Many may also have tubes and other devices which enter their pleural space or abdominal cavity. Often they are monitored by chest X-rays done at least on a daily basis. A film every 24 h is a tradition whose efficacy has been questioned by several recent studies especially when it is obtained on stable patients. Moreover, a daily chest X-ray is not always closely cropped, so often the top of the image extends upwards to include a section of the face that includes the lower ears. So I often can see on such images earrings placed there by the patient. In fact when I do see those earrings, I am confident that the patient is getting better and will likely leave the I.C.U. alive and functioning. The earring sign is an indication that the woman is now mindful of her self image and wishes to ornament herself in a way that boosts her confidence as she can now care about her self image. The sign is not foolproof of course. The X-ray must include the ear lobes beneath its superior margin. But when seen it is a reliable marker of impending treatment success.

A few caveats. The earrings must be bilateral. And I do not know what it means if the wearer is a man. But otherwise, I am grateful when I see it.

So, experience by attentive regard and repetitive emphasis can create meaningful associations of clinical significance whose validity can be reinforced by recurring examples, even if the observation does not lend itself to careful scientific assessment. And yet, at other times, preconceptions can color understanding, leading to the perpetuation of error or the performance of less than optimal practice.

Well what about those nipple markers? Before we finally commit them to posterity, a new trauma surgeon came on board. He likes to denote the site of bullet holes radiographically before oper-ating. He had been partial to the marking of the entry or exit site with a paper clip. But clips are too big and can hide other findings. The solution: Mark each hole with—voila—a nipple marker!

Reference

1. Baker S, Cho K. Abdominal plain film with correla-tive imaging. 2nd ed. Radiology. 1999;212(3):724.

Pelvic Phleboliths

72

In this essay I would like to address a topic most of you have learned a little about during your training, and likely have not given much thought since then. And such abbreviated attention could be considered adequate for the establishment of competence. But with your indulgence, I will address my remarks about the lowly pelvic phlebolith, perhaps boosting its importance as a diagnostic marker, or at least, I will endeavor to supplement somewhat general knowledge about it. I will delve into history, putative pathogenesis, morphologic appearance, positional changes and differential diagnosis [1].

Phleboliths-stones in veins-were first recognized by Rokitansky in 1852. Thirty years later von Recklinghausen stated that they were harmless entities. Yet 20 years after that statement, some physicians maintained that they were actually the cause of pelvic pain. They were thought to be frequently associated with non-hemangiomatous tumors. Faced with this supposed risk, operations to remove them were fashionable at that time. Remember that in the early decades of the twentieth century, in Middle Europe at least, diverticula were rare, epiploic appendagitis was common, and sigmoid volvulus was a relatively frequent diagnosis in middle-aged individuals, even those lacking present-day risk factors for it.

Phleboliths were first described radiologically by Orton in 1908, and 1 year later Clark demonstrated that they were intact intravenous concretions, appearing at autopsy, as seen by x-ray after the pelvic veins were dissected.

Phleboliths are stones made up of thrombi attached to venous walls. They consist of closely congregated laminae of platelets within a netting of erythrocytes and fibrin. Calcium deposition takes place only after the clot has fully formed. Almost always their opacity is due to the accumulation of calcium carbonate, with lesser contributions made by ammonium phosphate and magnesium ammonium phosphate.

Why do they form and why especially in the pelvic veins when they are rare elsewhere in the body? In adults pelvic veins are valveless and poorly supported in loose connective tissue. It has been proposed that sudden, intermittent increases in intra-abdominal pressure, as with straining at defecation, can serve to damage the vessel wall and thereby predispose to thrombosis. From this notion, Burkitt found support in his grand theory of the pathogenesis of the so-called diseases of western civilization, all of them occasioned by the consumption of a low-fiber diet characteristic of developed countries in which residents shun cellulose-laden foods. This leads, he theorized, in addition to the precipitation of phleboliths, to the propensity for colonic diverticula whose formation is abetted by straining at stools and, by a similar mechanism, related to prolonged colonic transit time, to large intestinal polyps and colonic malignancies. Interestingly, phleboliths have not been described in veterinary radiology, presumably because horizontally-oriented four footed animals do not subject the pelvic veins to increased pressure with the passage of stool.

S.R. Baker, *Notes of a Radiology Watcher*,
DOI 10.1007/978-3-319-01677-1_72, © Springer International Publishing Switzerland 2014

The phlebolith-low fiber connection is at best a conjecture, not a fact. We charted the number and position of phleboliths in a cohort over age 40 who underwent a barium enema study. There was no correlation between the presence of calcified phleboliths and the occurrence of diverticula. There is, moreover, no relationship between phleboliths and a history of appendicitis, nor an association with urinary tract infection. So their development, or at least their propensity to form, remains a mystery.

Most investigations have found that phleboliths increase in prevalence through the fifth decade of life. The youngest patient in which we have seen one was 16 years old. But by the third decade of life they are not rare. Some reports have indicated that phleboliths continue to increase in number with age, but others have noted a cessation of increase by the sixth decade. Two studies from 1980 reported a female preponderance, but others have revealed similarities in prevalence between the genders.

Yet, whereas an appearance of at least one of them in the pelvis may be similar in men and women, females have a wider roster of pelvic veins in which calcified thrombi can form. In both sexes, phleboliths are apt to be found in the perirectal and perivesical veins. In women they also occur in the veins of the broad ligament. In any location, they tend to be sharply radiopaque, oval to round in configuration and have a completed, uninterrupted circumference of radiodensity. Hence they exhibit the characteristic morphology of calculi i.e., evidenced by no breaks in their opaque rims whereas their interiors may be laminated with concentric rings of opacity, or they may have a single central lucency, or they can even be homogeneously dense. None of the configurations are emblematic of examples of the three other morphologic classes of calcifications, to wit—conduits often have an irregular wide interrupted opaque margin, cyst walls are more thinly and incompletely calcified and describe a larger radius, and solid calcification tends to be patchy or fluffy in morphology. Phleboliths are usually differentiable from appendicoliths by location and their central lucency, and from ureteral stones by their smooth rounded margins, whereas ureteral calculi often have parallel, straight or jagged contours. Phleboliths by their tendency to be spherical have similar diameters and densities when seen frontally or in oblique projections, while disc-shaped iron pills differ in area and density depending on the orientation of their length and thickness to the radiographic beam.

Sometimes two or more phleboliths can be conjoined, giving the resultant density an oblong configuration oriented with their long axis aligned with the course of the vein in which they are housed.

In men, phleboliths are found in perirectal and perivesical veins. In women, they occur also in veins in the broad ligament where they are situated near the termination of the vein and, hence, are laterally positioned. Occasionally, phleboliths are located in a more medial position but are still off the midline. The great preponderance of phleboliths lie at or just below a line drawn from the ischial spine to the fourth sacral segment. When there are many phleboliths, the majority are below the line, when only a few, all are. Their course, proceeding caudally, is from lateral to medial. Often phleboliths are situated slightly below the superior margin of the symphysis pubis. In men, phleboliths can occasionally be present in scrotal veins, sometimes in large numbers.

Sometimes, a pelvic radiograph will reveal one or several concretions in the superior pelvis, often without phleboliths present inferiorly. If the concretion is outside the urinary tract, it may be a phlebolith located in a gonadal vein. These concretions tend to be multiple and are seen along the course of the vein as it ascends in the abdomen adjacent to the ureter. Gonadal phleboliths are almost exclusively seen in multiparous women, many of whom also have pelvic masses, so it is apt to call them ovarian vein phleboliths. Stasis in the ovarian veins during pregnancy has been suggested as a predisposing factor in the formation of these concretions.

It is often difficult to distinguish between a ureteral calculus and a phlebolith in the pelvis or in gonadal veins. Ureteral calculi often have angulated margins and usually lack a central lucency. However, their appearance can exactly mimic a phlebolith. One way of distinguishing between the two is to obtain serial films a few hours or a day apart. Uretetal calculi may move in either an antegrade or retrograde fashion, whereas phleboliths are usually fixed in position. If there is no movement of the ureteral stone, however, it may be impossible to distinguish the two types of concretions even on repeated plain films.

Careful attention to the position of phleboliths can be rewarding in determining the presence of pelvic masses or ascertaining the nature of previous surgery. Normally, phleboliths situated in perivesical veins can be displaced slightly interiorly and laterally if the bladder enlarges to a great degree. Occasionally, perirectal phleboliths are deviated laterally in the presence of rectal distention, however, these movements are usually minimal. Greater motion may be observed n the presence of masses. In fact, when a phlebolith is displaced, its migration may be all that is necessary to monitor the growth or shrinkage of tumefactions or hematomas.

Periurethral masses can elevate phleboliths as well as displace them to either side. Prolapse of the uterus moves phleboliths inferiorly, sometimes repositioning them below the superior margin of the pubic bone.

The veins of the pelvis are connected across the midline through the inferior vesical plexuses in both sexes, and the periprostatic plexus in men. However, crossing veins are usually small, and are not the site of radiographically visible phleboliths. Hence, a phlebolith in the midline should always be regarded as abnormal. It can be deviated by a mass and, in women, medial migration is often a consequence of hysterectomy. Abnormally sited venous stones are found in hemangiomas. Radiologically visible phleboliths have been noted in many abdominal locations within hemangiomas. Although an uncommon tumor in the pelvis, an hemangioma should be considered when phleboliths are seen at the midline in the absence of a previous operation, or when multiple phleboliths are seen on only one side of the midline. A spectacular appearance of phlebolith-type calcification can be found in the Klippel-Trenaunay Syndrome, which consists of bony abnormalities and large hemangiomas that occur in the abdominal wall or within solid organs.

Not all concretions with central lucencies in the pelvis are phleboliths. A spectrum of other densities simulating venous calculi may be mistaken for them. In addition to ureteral calculi, concretions such as appendicoliths in low-lying appendices can be positioned in the pelvis. Bladder stones, rectal stones, calcified appendices epiploicae, and calculi passing through the gastrointestinal tract may also be present in the pelvis. Ossification and tooth formation in ovarian dermoids can occasionally look like phleboliths. Bilateral clusters of discrete densities, suggestive of concretions, characterize calcification of ovarian corpora albicantia.

From time to time, foreign bodies can be mistaken for phleboliths. Radiopaque pills may ostensibly resemble venous calculi but their homogeneous density, absence of central lucency, and movement on sequential films are points of differentiation. Fallopian tube occlusion rings are implanted devices used in tubal ligations. They consist of siliconized synthetic rubber impregnated with barium sulfate, which makes them appear as annular opacities on plain radiographs. Often, they can closely simulate phleboliths but they are usually situated in the upper pelvis. Moreover, the marginal rims in these occlusive rings do not vary in width along their perimeter as do phleboliths.

Reference

1. Baker S, Cho K. Abdominal plain film with correlative imaging. 2nd ed. Radiology. 1999;212(3):724.

Eponyms abound among the roster of abdominal hernias. This report will discuss these pathologic protrusions, identifying their location and relating them to the physician and/or surgeon who discovered them. This first part of this two-part essay will be confined to the upper and middle regions of the abdominal cavity.

In order to master the incredible wealth of material a physician must know, one cannot succeed in this profession without a good memory. Often, retention is favored by the nomenclature of anatomy, physiology and pathology where the name of the entity relates to a salient feature of its identity. If forgotten it can often be deduced because it acquired the label it goes by through a logical process, related to form or function or both. Thus, a muscle that bends the wrist is the flexor carpi ulnaris-once you get attuned to the Greek or Latin etymology, the reason for its naming becomes clear.

Yet, also in Medicine we are sometimes bedeviled or at least burdened by eponyms, names honoring the discoverer of a process, site, dysfunction or disease. There is no rhyme or reason to help us retrieve such names, once we have forgotten them. However, bear in mind that the accumulation of knowledge has occurred along a time continuum. Hence, it is important to remember the brilliant observers of yesteryear because, if not for their insights, we might know less today about how to recognize and treat illnesses and injuries. So eponyms persist, lending a semblance of immortality to the investigators of past ages, helping us marvel at their cognitive breakthroughs.

One place where eponyms abound is in the abdomen, where anatomical structures and pathologic syndromes honor their discoverers [1]. The various hernias in this region are particularly eponymic, probably because most of them were recognized as peculiar bulges accessible to the discerning eye in the era before X-ray and other means of looking inside the body were developed. In fact, most abdominal hernias were first reported in the interval between 1600 (just after Paracelsus) and 1895, the year the first radiographic image was obtained.

The purpose of this discussion is twofold; to describe the various hernias and for some, their distinctive radiologic findings, and also to list a few of the accomplishments of the persons whose name is affixed to them. Stedman's Medical Dictionary lists 18 hernias identified by a surname and I have found two others. A description of all of them would be too exhaustive so I will limit my discussion to a select list.

Let us start our journey at the top. That is, at the junction of the thorax and the abdomen as delimited by the diaphragm. A Bochdalek hernia is the most common internal hernia in a newborn. The extrusion of abdominal contents through this posterior-lateral rent in the diaphragm occurs most often on the left side. The prevalent notion is that the liver protects the upward extrusion of bowel and omentum because it is situated just subjacent to the right hemidiaphragm. This hernia is caused by failure of closure of the pleuro-peritoneal canal which is a feature of embryonic life. Occasionally, we encounter Bochdalek

S.R. Baker, *Notes of a Radiology Watcher*,
DOI 10.1007/978-3-319-01677-1_73, © Springer International Publishing Switzerland 2014

hernias in adulthood, but mostly this is a child-hood phenomenon.

Who was Bochdalek? Vincent Alexander Bochdalek was a Czech anatomist who lived in the nineteenth century. His fame is substantiated by his name attached to many other things including Bochdalek's cyst, which is a congenital cyst at the root of the tongue, Bochdalek's flower basket, which is an arrangement of the choroid plexus within the fourth ventricle and Bochdalek's foramen which is an alias for the pleuroperitoneal canal. Also, there is the Bochdalek ganglion which refers to nerve tissue in the maxilla above the canine teeth. One could go on and on listing the contributions of this spectacular anatomist.

Equally important to medical knowledge was the contributions of Giovanni Morgagni who lived between 1682 and 1771. Yes, he died at 89. Morgagni's hernia, which is an anterior protrusion on both sides of the diaphragm, often first comes to attention in adulthood. A pitfall on plain radiography is to confuse the bowel that has migrated superiorly into the chest as a normal lucency or as a lung abscess. Morgagni is equally as prominent as Bochdalek, having had his name assigned to more structures than Donald Trump. There is the Morgagni foramen which is the right-sided diaphragmatic fissure between the sternum and anterior ribs through which this hernia passes. The Morgagni cyst is the appendix of the testes, and the Morgagni concha is synonymous with the superior nasal concha. Morgagni worked closely with his mentor Antonio Valsalva. Together they should be considered the progenitors of the science of pathologic anatomy. Morgagni was also the first one to identify what is now known as Laennec's cirrhosis. It is no wonder that Virchow called him the father of modern pathology.

Moving to the middle of the abdomen we come now to the Treitz hernia related by location to the ligament of Treitz. It is the most distinctive but not the most common internal hernia in the middle of the abdomen. Entrapment in the fossa lateral to the ligament allows the capture of loops of bowel in a sac adjacent to the fourth position of the duodenum. The sac usually contains much of the proximal jejunum. Venszel Treitz was a compatriot and a near contemporary of Bochdalek.

A distinctive hernia in the abdomen is named after Adrian Spigelius, a Flemish anatomist who lived in the 1600s and did most of his work in Padua, Italy. The caudate lobe of the liver was named after Spigelius, although that eponym is infrequently used today, Spigelius also produced a magnificent book called The Opera, in which are found probably the finest anatomical drawings of the seventeenth century. He was the popularizer of Harvey's insights into the circulation as evidenced by the illustrations in his book.

The Spigelian hernia is amenable to plain film diagnosis. The posterior sheath of the rectus abdominis muscle is formed by the fused medial aponeuroses of the transversalis and internal oblique muscles. A separate internal oblique aponeurosis becomes the anterior sheath. Below the fold of Douglas (a semicircular fibrous band that marks the halfway point between the umbilicus and the symphysis pubis), the posterior sheath is often thin or incomplete. Thus, at the lateral margin of the lower rectus, there are many potential points of weakness through which hernial sacs can protrude. Because the much stronger external oblique muscle prohibits passage of the hernia through the abdominal wall, Spigelian hernias are likely to extend peripherally within the space between the internal and external oblique muscles. For this reason, they are also known as interstitial or interparietal hernias. Most are small, contain only fat, and are easily reducible. However, some trap, obstruct and deviate small-bowel loops far laterally. Spigelian hernias can be recognized as peripheral air or fluid-filled structures that sometimes displace the peritoneal margin medially. They resemble extraperitoneal abscesses but until strangulation supervenes, affected individuals are not febrile, and the properitoneal and lateral intermuscular planes are usually preserved. The radiographic findings are not pathognomonic, being closely simulated on occasion by bowel in a laterally positioned incisional hernia.

I conclude the first part of this abdominal argosy with two other mid-abdominal protrusions; the superior and inferior lumbar hernia. The superior lumbar hernia is also known as Grynfeltt's hernia, named after a French surgeon of the nineteenth century. It refers to the extrusion of peritoneal and sometimes bowel contents through the superior lumbar triangle, which is bordered above by the end of the 12th rib and serratus anterior muscle, medially by the internal oblique muscle and posteriorly by the quadratus lumborum muscle. Almost always the Grynfeltt's, or superior lumbar hernia, occurs after surgery. In contradistinction, a spontaneous hernia occurs in the inferior lumbar triangle which has the appellation Petit hernia in memory of Jean Petit, a French surgeon who lived between 1674 and 1750. Petit's triangle is defined by the latissimus dorsi, the external oblique muscle and the iliac crest.

Well, we have gone halfway through the abdomen so far. As we move lower down we will get close to that area where the eponyms become exceedingly dense and cluttered. I refer here to the region around the inguinal canal. So, if you will bear with me we will proceed onward and downward.

Reference

1. Souba WW. ACS surgery: principles and practice. New York: Web MD Professional Publishing; 2006.

Eponymous Abdominal Hernias, Part II

Lower abdominal hernias comprise a wide range of protrusions, nearly each one affixed to an eponym. Above the lower pelvis can be found the Littre hernia of Meckel's diverticulum and the Littre-Richter hernia of a part of the bowel walls. In addition to the common inguinal hernias, both direct and indirect, there is also an inguinal hernia sac containing the appendix (Amyand hernia) the Holthouse hernia just under the skin, the subperitoneal hernia of Kronlein and the infantile Malgaigne hernia [1]. The differences may be slight, but the advent of CT now allows a preoperative diagnosis of each.

Eponymic femoral hernias include the Cooper-Hey protrusion and the Velpeau and Cloquet's hernia. Just below them is the Hesselbach hernia. We begin in the lower abdomen with the possibly confusing overlap of protrusion designated by the names of Littre and Richter.

Alexis Littre (1658–1726) was a French anatomist and surgeon who was a zealous prosector. He is known also for being the first to describe the small mucous glands of the male urethra. Littre identified two abdominal hernias which hear his name-the more obscure one is a hernia of Meckel's diverticulum into the inguinal region. That abnormality he owns alone, although now the definition of Littre's hernia has been expanded to include herniation of any intestinal diverticulum, not just Meckel's.

The more common hernia for which he is remembered is the parietal hernia named by him in 1700 and described in further detail by Richter 78 years later. August Richter, a German surgeon

who lived from 1742 to 1812, was a Professor of Medicine and Ophthalmology at various universities in Germany. Richter's line, you may remember, extends from the umbilicus to the anterior superior iliac spine and is well known to surgeons. Richter's hernia is a bowel entrapment in which only a part of the caliber of the gut is involved. Often the two proper names are joined together as the Richter-Littre hernia. Forget the rare intestinal diverticular hernia described before—you will probably never see it. It is perhaps best to honor these two eminent surgeons by referring to the parietal hernia by their names linked together.

Not that I want to avoid some rare protrusions, especially when a proper name is affixed to it. For that reason I present to you the Amyand hernia. Claudius Amyand in 1735 or 1736 removed an appendix containing a calcified mass surrounding a pin which had migrated to the inguinal region. The pin had perforated the tip of the appendix. Hence, Amyand's hernia is reserved specifically for an inguinal hernia with the protruding sac containing the appendix. The term is also applied to appendicitis with the vermiform appendix in the inguinal canal, even in the absence of a concomitant irreducible herniation. By the way, I have seen several cases where the occlusion of the appendix is due to a foreign body. In several instances it has been an ingested straight pin that found lodgment in the appendiccal lumen, and in one case it was a small piece of metal used to balance tires. Obviously, Amyand's hernia had been a difficult preoperative diagnosis in the days

S.R. Baker, *Notes of a Radiology Watcher*,
DOI 10.1007/978-3-319-01677-1_74, © Springer International Publishing Switzerland 2014

before CT, but with computed tomography now nearly ubiquitous, the radiologist can now make the finding which otherwise would have been a surprise at surgery.

We have now come to the inguinal canal where everything gets even more crowded. To refresh your memory, a direct inguinal hernia protrudes through the abdominal wall between the inferior epigastric artery and the edge of the rectus muscle, whereas an indirect inguinal hernia passes through the internal ring and then part of its same at least is in the inguinal canal. A femoral hernia, situated more posteriorly and medially, is so named because the hernial sac is situated in the femoral canal. One more anatomic point. Poupart's ligament is a fibrous band derived from the aponeurosis of the external oblique muscle, which extends from the anterior superior iliac spine to the pubic tubercle. Incidentally, Pascal Poupart was a French polymath who lived between 1616 and 1708. The seventeenth century in France was obviously a very fruitful time for anatomic discovery. Not only was Poupart a physician, he also made considerable discoveries in entomology. A particular type of inguinal hernia bears the eponym Holthouse in remembrance of its describer, an English surgeon of the nineteenth century. This designation, Holthouse hernia, applies to an extension of the inguinal hernia sac containing a loop of intestine along Poupart's ligament.

Kronlein's hernia is still another variant of inguinal hernia. Kronlein, a German surgeon of the nineteenth century, made his mark in the elucidation of surgery for appendicitis. He also described a complicated double sac protrusion with part of the inguinal canal and the other part projecting from the inguinal ring into the subperitoneal tissues. Thus, it is also known by its non-eponymic appellation as the properitoneal inguinal hernia. Joseph Francois Malgaigne, 1806–1864, best known for his description of a pelvic fracture which bears his name, concentrated his research predominately on the anatomy of the anterior pelvis. He was also a medical geographer and was a leader in mortality mapping to better understand the distribution of disease and from that gain an awareness of etiology

and spatial containment, especially of contagious conditions. Malgaigne's hernia occurs in the infant life in boys, with the sac presenting prior to the descent of the testes.

Femoral hernias are uncommon in men and nulliparous women, and appear predominantly in multiparas. Cooper's hernia, honoring the English surgeon Astley Cooper who was active in the eighteenth century, is a bilocular femoral hernia with one sac in the femoral canal and the other traversing a defect in the superficial fascia to appear immediately below the skin. The depiction of the appearance of this protrusion is ideally made by CT. Cooper's hernia also has the eponym "Hey hernia" in honor of William Hey, a near contempororary and a countryman of Cooper. Hey was a pioneer in the use of oxygen for antisepsis (he was a friend of Priestley).

Alfred-Armand Louis Marie Velpeau (1795–1867) was an illustrious surgeon, famous for his statement that has been found to be incorrect, thank God. He said, "the escape from pain in surgical operations is a chimera. Knife and pain in surgery are words which are always inseparable in the minds of patients". He was made to eat those words later in his career as he witnessed the development of anesthesia. Therefore, he later said on the subject of ether that it is a wonderful and terrible agent. His femoral hernia is a protrusion of the sac in women, passing in front of the femoral vessels to lie in the posterior aspect of the major labia. In contradistinction is the Cloquet hernia, in which the sac lies posterior to the femoral vessels as the hernia perforates the aponeurosis of the pectineus muscle. Cloquet was another nineteenth century French surgeon, more familiar perhaps for the lymph node that bears his name. Cloquet's node is a deep inguinal node located adjacent to the femoral canal which, when inflamed, sometimes can be mistaken for an incarcerated femoral hernia.

Our last eponymic hernia was described by Franz Caspar Hesselbach, who was the first to recognize the femoral hernia in 1798. He has also distinguished himself by being the first to differentiate a direct from an indirect inguinal hernia, an observation he made in 1810. Hesselbach's triangle is bounded by the inguinal ligament below, the rectus muscle medially and the inferior epigastric vessels laterally, the area where a direct inguinal hernia will protrude. The cribriform fascia is located immediately subjacent to it. Cribriforn means sieve-like. Therefore, Hesselbach's hernia (as distinguished from Hesselbach's triangle) occurs when the hernial sac has a lobular outline bulging the skin anterior to the femoral vessels. In effect, his hernia is located inferior to his triangle.

Reference

1. Souba WW. ACS surgery: principles and practice. New York: WebMD Professional Publishing; 2006.

In the proceeding essay, my theme was well-established misconceptions under the heading. "It ain't what you don't know it's what you do know that ain't so." If you are game, let's continue with some more examples.

Pills

Occasionally on plain films of the abdomen and on CT's, one or several discrete non-calcific opacities are recognized [1]. They are characteristically homogeneously dense and differ also from most stones by their smooth outline and by the fact that their density varies inversely with the extent of the "area" they present to the X-ray beam. That is, when the beam brings into view a larger "area" of the opacity it appears less bright than when a smaller area is presented, when it is correspondingly more radiodense. This is because these opacities are disc-shaped, unlike the more spherical configuration stones tend to assume. So by the characteristics of their conformation alone, one is apt to say that they are pills. Typically the radiologists report is limited just to that phrase. That is, pills are present.

I submit that such a brief interpretation is inadequate because we know more and should say so. I routinely ask senior medical students and residents—all of whom are at least 2 years beyond physiology class a simple question. Where is iron absorbed? Unless tipped off, almost all of them will say in the ileum and a few others will offer up the jejunum. Yet they have forgotten that iron is absorbed only in the twelve inches of the duodenum—not more distally.

How is that relevant? Well if we are to see a pill in the gut on X-ray, it must be intact and therefore it has resisted dissolution. Moreover beyond the duodenum it is of no value even if it could dissolve. And of course it must be opaque to begin with. Now, the only medications that satisfy both those criteria are Pepto Bismol tablets which are typically triangular in configuration and iron pills which have a range of shapes.

Besides being absorbed only in the duodenum, iron is irritating to the stomach. Hence solid iron-containing preparations are enteric-coated to bypass dissolution in the gastric lumen and therefore they are prepared to dissolve in the duodenum. This requires a pharmaceutical tour-de-force if you will. Enteric coats become more resistant the older the patient and the longer its shelf life before being ingested. Hence, often the pill is still intact as it enters the jejunum and thus it will not be absorbed.

The implication of this fact should not be avoided by the radiologist. The presence of a pill beyond the duodenum—and it is always an iron pill if it is rounded—is that the treatment of anemia for which the pill was administered is now recognized as being ineffective. The radiologists' report should mention this clinically relevant conclusion. Moreover, the referring physician should be specifically notified about this manifestation of a therapeutic failure. Merely to say pills are present should be regarded in this circumstance as inadequate reporting by a radiologist.

S.R. Baker, *Notes of a Radiology Watcher*,
DOI 10.1007/978-3-319-01677-1_75, © Springer International Publishing Switzerland 2014

Grading Pneumothorax

How do you grade a pneumothorax? Do you say it is 20 or 50 or 75 % with each of those percentages made by measuring the width of the lung from the midline horizontally to the edge of the displaced visceral pleura and comparing that figure to the corresponding width of the affected hemithorax? Yet is it correct to use a linear measurement to assess a volumetric phenomenon? Assume that a hemithorax is a sphere. Symmetric collapse of the lung by the pressure of air in the pleural space will decrease pulmonary volume by length, width, and height. Consequently a so-called 50 % pneumothorax is actually a decrease of volume of 87.5 %, a 50 % reduction side to side as well as a 50 % front to back reduction as well as a 50 % top to bottom decrease. According to this geometric simplification it is a (1/2) (1/2) (1/2) loss of volume. Thus it is a seven-eighths pneumothorax.

Therefore it is more accurate even if less precise to record the extent of a pneumothorax by semi-quantitative words that are readily and unequivocally appropriate. I use the 5M rule for this purpose. A pneumothorax can be minimal, mild, moderate, marked, or massive. A linear measurement, in contrast, is always an understatement.

The Chest X-Ray and Sickle Cell Disease

Sickle cell anemia is a terrible affliction affecting many people whose life is impaired by recurrent pain in the chest as assuredly as they impacted by the continuous ravages of a hemolytic anemia leading to heart failure, kidney failure, gallstones, and bone infarcts, to name just a few of sickle cell's other complications.

Chest pain is probably the most frequent manifestation of episodic discomfort in S-S disease. The acute chest syndrome is one adverse presentation, pneumonia is another, microinfarcts still another. The worry about the recognition and treatment of sickle related pulmonary changes that can be treated have led to the standard practice to obtain a chest X-ray at every one of a sickle cell sufferer's frequent visits to an emergency department. In our institution, we have studied the findings on those routine radiographic series. Unlike what has been reported in the literature, our true positive rate on X-ray was only 1 in 1,300 cases.

Yet there is more to the story, at least as it is germane to our experience at Newark. For many sicklers, who use our hospital E.R. exclusively, it is not uncommon for them to visit us according to a routinely chosen every 3 week schedule. They sometimes come in more often but mostly they return almost like clockwork every 21 days or so. Why? Well 3 weeks is the duration for completion of the course of pain medication they receive, assuming of course that they consume their daily doses. Now some *may* need to alter the medication protocol for pain control but others are actually giving or selling some of the pills to someone else. The dispensing E.R. physician therefore then becomes unwittingly complicit in the transfer of pain medication, first to the patient, and perhaps secondarily and illicitly to others. That the chest X-ray is almost always negative is irrelevant, because it is not used for diagnostic purposes, but instead serves only to legitimize the trip to the E.R. Perhaps, instead of persisting with this nonproductive exercise which continues to involve Radiology, another approach is required. There is a need for the establishment in a large institution of a sickle cell team of physicians which would function according to a defined structure and assignment regimen. The team members would get to know each recurring sickle cell visitor and come to realize if the reported chest pain was real, and whether at each time it is atypical and/or significant. They could then decide at each E.R. visit if radiographic evaluation was necessary for the patient in crisis. It would be likely that they could decide that a chest X-ray was not required for every painful episode and therefore its restriction could save time, cost and radiation.

Bowel Obstruction

Lastly let us come to that repertoire of you know but it ain't so—the assessment of bowel obstruction, particularly by plain films. Misconceptions, unverified but hardened notions, abound here,

I categorize them with the heading—No first name for obstruction please. Respect this serious condition. Some hallowed nostrums of obstruction—which is what I mean by "first names"—bring with them a measure of seeming familiarity with obstruction that are not borne out by careful consideration. Here are three.

1. Early obstruction

   Dilatation of gas-filled bowel presumably proximal to a luminal blockage is evidence of obstruction on plain films if clinical data are corroborative. When there is also flatus in a nondilated colon, the temptation is to label the overall appearance consistent with the diagnosis of early obstruction. Such a temporal assertion, however, is not justified from one image alone. The obstruction may just as well be recurrent or intermittent and prolonged as it can be early. Unless a series of sequential plain films is made available with the most recent one indicating obstruction, the distinction of early from persisting obstruction is not achievable.

2. Incomplete or partial obstruction

   In the setting of acute obstruction, a diagnosis of partial or incomplete luminal occlusion is often a consideration. The notion of less than total obstruction is compelling but cannot be validated by plain films. The appellations, partial or incomplete, are often given to radiographic presentations analogous to early obstruction. An example is dilation of gas containing bowel loops proximally with maintenance of lucency in nondistended intestinal loops beyond the site of occlusion. Longstanding stenosis of a bowel segment can be accompanied by specific signs and symptoms consequent to the persistent retardation of flow of intestinal contents. Yet acute partial or incomplete obstruction cannot be distinguished solely by plain radiologic observations, even in a patient whose bowel blockage is already suspected. It is best to say that an obstruction exists and resist the temptation to further specify its degree of completeness. That determination can be achieved by additional imaging studies, but not solely by the observation of the differential dilation of bowel loops.

Surprisingly, the surgical literature is conspicuously reticent on the issue of the "partialness" of an acute obstruction. Hence, in this regard, there is no good correlation between suppositions drawn from the plain film and operative facts. What is also possible is that so-called persistent partial or incomplete obstructions are really complete but intermittent. With each temporary respite, some gas is allowed to advance distally, simulating the expected distribution of intraluminal lucency in a partial or complete blockage. Yet this hypothesis, too, lacks proof and should not be included in a diagnostic impression of a plain film study. Thus, by plain films alone, the presence of an obstruction can be acknowledged but a recognition of its extent is more problematic.

3. Tube compression

   Decompression of the bowel proximal to an obstruction s often accomplished by the placement of nongastric tube. In some facilities, a long tube is inserted perorally and eventually progresses into the jejunum to foster the drainage of intestinal contents. A desired effect of tube placement is to relieve the pain and discomfort attendant upon bowel dilatation. Yet another effect is to remove the contrast material, that is, the swallowed air that helps characterize the plain film picture of obstruction. The patient may feel better, the X-ray looks better, but that does not mean that the obstruction is relieved. Such an encouraging development can only be appreciated when the patient resumes passing gas per rectum. Therefore, one should not presume that the reduction of dilatation during or after tube placement is a corollary of the resolution of the obstruction. Rather, it is a beneficial consequence of the treatment of symptoms, not necessarily a manifestation of cure. Yet surgeons love these terms and concepts about obstruction, even though they are wrong in fact and lack corroborative foundation.

Reference

1. Baker S, Cho K. Abdominal plain film with correlative imaging. 2nd ed. Radiology. 1999;212(3):724.

That witty aphorism of Will Rogers—It ain't what you don't know that'll hurt you. It's what you do know that ain't so—is often true in life. It is certainly frequently true in medicine, and radiology is no exception. Like many things accepted as correct in medical science and given the status of "law" by students and practitioners, it actually turns out to be "lore", which in many instances is really the product of bull times time. So often an official-sounding pronouncement is unquestioned but false. The job of an investigator and teacher in any discipline having at least a glimmer of scientific luster is twofold: the first is rare—it is discovery; the second is much more common—it is revision.

In this essay I endeavor to point out tried but not true notions, faithfully believed as being what you know but really they ain't so. I will confine my task of rectification to the chest and abdomen.

Example (1) If one is asked to list the causes of air in the biliary tree, the standard differential includes operations on the bile ducts, previous ERCP, gallstone ileus and cholangitis caused by a gas-forming organism. The first three are for sure, the fourth alleged cause, infection, does occur in the drainage ducts leading from the liver to the duodenum. Pneumobilia exclusively in the ducts but not the gallbladder, due to infection, has been recorded in books and reviews as a clinical observation, but the last time I searched several years ago it has never actually been reported. And I scanned the major radiology journals for 50 years to seek out a reference. It is perhaps reasonable to assume that it would occur but we deal with empirical information not logical deductions. How many other differentials can we recall in which not every possibility has actually been verified. Perhaps there are many like "phantom" pneumobilia.

Example (2) Association in time or space is not causality. Consider the implications of the porcelain gallbladder. A report from Argentina years ago concerned a group of patients, a very small group, in a large sample who had a calcified gallbladder and a carcinoma in it. This was the basis for the old adage that a porcelain or calcified gallbladder was a risk factor for cancer in that organ. But is it? One would have to know the clinical history of gallbladder wall calcification in a series of cases. Is it really a precursor? If so, what is the lag time? Are a few people apt to get cancer of the gallbladder independently developing calcification? Like the intersecting circles of a Venn diagram the diagnosis of gallbladder cancer and wall calcification are probably independent phenomena only occasionally coexisting. One uncontrolled retrospective report does not establish a causal link. Thus, a calcified gallbladder need not be removed, and most probably need not be closely watched. Without the presentation of evidence of a relationship so secure that the risks and costs of prophylactic cholecystectomy are justified, this putative relationship remains doubtful, and therapeutic intervention based on it would be no more than a surgical adventure not a prophylactic expedient.

Example (3) What is your preparation for CT studies of the abdomen to rule out intestinal

S.R. Baker, *Notes of a Radiology Watcher*,
DOI 10.1007/978-3-319-01677-1_76, © Springer International Publishing Switzerland 2014

obstruction? Do you give oral contrast material as part of your protocol? Remember many patients for whom obstruction is a concern are nauseated and have been vomiting. If they cannot keep food down why should you presume that oral contrast material, often Gastrografin, will not also be vomited? That is not a trivial issue. Because aspirated Gastrografin is extremely injurious to the lungs, it defies logic to give it automatically and thereby engender an unneeded risk. CT protocols especially for obstruction should be personalized. I am personally aware of two recent patients who died of aspiration pneumonitis from Gastrografin. Consider this recent malpractice scenario, 28 year old woman. Rule out small bowel blockage. Gastrografin administered by mouth. The patient vomited and aspirated the contrast material. Severe pneumonitis eventuated. The acute decrease in oxygenation became the precipitant cause of her myocardial infarction. And the abruptly decreased cardiac output resulted in a CVA for which she has made only a very partial recovery 6 months later.

Example (4) When a patient is admitted to the hospital with acute abdominal pain, does that automatically mean we must do immediate imaging? Well necessarily not, for most cases of acute pancreatitis. The surgical literature recently and from earlier references up to 20 years ago has affirmed that the treatment of acute pancreatitis is restriction of fluids by mouth, pain medication and rest. Imaging is not valuable if by other means including serum amylase and lipase, the diagnosis is established. One should not scan the abdomen unless the pancreatitis is severe and the initial course hectic. In the usual case, CT will often reveal extensive peripancreatic effusions which may look terrible but will resolve to at least some degree without intervention. The complication of pseudocyst will not develop in the first several days of an acute pancreatitis, and there is no gain in searching for it when the patient is uncomfortable during the initial manifestations of the acute attack. Moreover the search for gallstones, one or several of which may have occasioned the attack by the stone transversing the common bile duct and obstructing the main pancreatic duct, can be undertaken later

unless jaundice overwhelms the clinical situation. Ultrasonography in this setting is painful, intrusive and often non-contributory because of the presence of flatus overlying the pancreas in the transverse colon. Remember the predominant response of bowel to adjacent inflammation is distension and gas accumulation. And pressing the upper abdomen with a transducer hurts. So despite the urge to obtain pictures, the humane and the efficacious response to acute pancreatitis is to refrain from imaging at least early on in the typical hospital stay.

Example (5) The chest X-ray is a time hallowed maneuver for ER patients, almost irrespective of any presentation aside from minor extremity injury. In young and middle-aged adults, PA and lateral views encompass the routine set of images to assess the lungs, pleura, heart and mediastinum. But what about patients who are obtunded, unconscious, weak or ornery? Also what about those who cannot stand or those who are markedly obese? And what do we do for people who are loath to take a deep breath or for those who have ascites or cardiomegaly or a combination thereto? In all of these instances and many more, we get only an AP chest, sometimes as a portable view. The end result, too often, is an inadequate view; the lung bases are not clearly delineated. Especially the left lower lung field is obscured by the enlarged cardiac shadow. And if the patient is kyphotic, as are many elderly of both genders, then the heart and lower lung field are obscured by the projected higher than normal apparent position of both hemidiaphragms. In these circumstances the radiologist is apt to hedge because so much of the lung fields are obscured.

Yet that does not have to be the end of it. Without moving or inconveniencing the patient, we can often perceive the lung bases better by obtaining a second image, an AP film of the lower chest and upper abdomen, using the more penetrating abdominal technique to "burn" through the otherwise obscuring shadow of the heart and superior abdominal viscera. We have found this image so helpful that it has now become a standard radiographic procedure for our ER patients who meet the limitation criteria I just mentioned.

The result of this additional picture has been gratifying. It often eliminates the perceived presence of an infiltrate in some cases, and reveals it in others for which the standard AP chest view of the lower lungs was indistinct.

Example (6) And by the way, when do you get a chest-X-ray on a patient who may have CHF? The issues are CHF vs. no CHF or CHF and something else in the lung or no abnormal findings at all. The customary approach is to obtain a chest film promptly at presentation. But often, because the lungs have become opaque to varying degrees, one cannot distinguish between CHF and some other pathologic process. It is almost like trying to discern detail when a translucent screen is put between you and the object you are trying to identify, when what should be placed in front of you is a transparent screen. Thus, it is often more valuable to attempt to have the patient diurese first. Increased urine output among other indices documents fluid mobilization. That response will substantiate CHF and at the same clear the lungs of fluid, so that an appropriately-timed chest X-ray can clearly determine if other causes of lung opacities remain visible once the edema fluid has been drained away from the lungs.

The necessity of the immediate chest film with CHF is a rooted habit, but it is a handmaiden, if you will, of medical lore, an institutionalized maneuver often of less than optimal practice. You can change this practice if you want to. By so doing you will make better diagnoses and not hinder the initiation of therapy.

There are bound to be many more examples of procedures initiated long ago according to notion that just ain't so. A questing spirit will uncover them and lead to their abandonment if we have a mind to exercise our capability to revise and improve practice.

Illicit Drug Transport

One of the consequences of the ongoing global revolution in transportation and telecommunications is an increasingly uneven distribution of wealth both between rich and poor countries and within national borders in underdeveloped countries. New businesses stimulated by the enhanced demand created by these rapidly advancing technologies have made available a range of products and services, most of which are a boon to humankind, but others have created personal tragedies, social decay, and political instability. The transnational, even intercontinental, trade in illicit drugs is a prime example of the disruptive effects of high-speed travel and the instantaneous transfer of information. Today, the commerce in addictive substances such as marijuana, hashish, heroin, and cocaine in its various forms, including crack, has become a multibillion dollar worldwide industry. The fact that it is illegal in most jurisdictions heightens the risk but magnifies the profit for manufacturers, wholesalers, and retailers [1].

All of these providers must be constantly aware of changing terms of trade to stay one step ahead of the authorities. One of the job opportunities, generated by the widespread but clandestine delivery of drugs from source to market, involves the need for individuals to transport products not affixed to their person, but in their body. Known as mules, or body packers, these adventurous travelers have accustomed themselves to swallowing large quantities of packaged drugs, keeping them hidden in their gastrointestinal tracts as they cross international boundaries.

Some women have also utilized the vaginal vault as an auxiliary or prime storage site.

The most common points of entry for mules infiltrating the United States are the gateway airports in New York, Newark, Houston, Chicago, Miami, New Orleans, and Los Angeles. Radiologists are brought into the investigation after a suspect is detained, usually by U.S. Customs authorities. Plain films of the abdomen are obtained to confirm the presence of drug packets in the GI tract or vagina. Remember too, that many body packers may be initially successful but later seek medical care emergently because of signs and symptoms of bowel obstruction or drug overdose. Unless there is a high index of suspicion, the cause of their discomfort may be missed.

After September 11, 2001, increased security measures have increased the risk of conventional smuggling. Consequently, the frequency of body packing has also increased as evidenced by a higher frequency of interdiction at airports such as Kennedy in New York. Because of the real chance of perforation of the ingested drugs bags, intrusive diagnostic techniques such as endoscopy and barium enema are relatively contraindicated. Hence, the supine abdominal radiograph remains paramount for the detection of this condition. It is important to recognize the various plain film appearances of drug packets in the GI tract, in order to differentiate them from more innocuous conditions. Usually body packers undergo a period of training during which they learn how to secure and enclose their valuable cargo, how

S.R. Baker, *Notes of a Radiology Watcher*,
DOI 10.1007/978-3-319-01677-1_77, © Springer International Publishing Switzerland 2014

to ingest it, and how to retain it for delivery or possible reingestion. Typically, between 20 and 100 packets are swallowed in preparation for one flight.

Besides the risk of discovery, a body packer must be concerned with obstruction and drug perforation. In most cases, if a single packet passes through the esophagus, it will make its way unimpeded through the anus. However, two or more packets can become entangled, allowing obstruction to ensue in either the stomach or more distally.

For cocaine the LD 50 dose is approximately 500 mg, but much smaller absorptions can also lead to a rapid death. Obviously, it is crucial that the packets do not leak. Care should be exercised by these individuals to guarantee that the narcotics are enclosed in such a way that they remain intact. Yet with prolonged retention in the GI tract, drug powder or paste may become contaminated, or the balloon or condom in which it is housed may rupture or leak more insidiously. In the past, individuals who made the mistake of using a natural skin condom ran a great risk for seepage of drug into the stomach or bowel, a complication that is often fatal.

Today, toy balloons have been employed, especially in the European trade, but these can be associated with a heightened risk of obstruction. For the most part, latex condoms are preferred and the drug, be it in powder or paste form, is encased in two to five condom skins. If this cladding fits tightly, the overall density on plain films is a smooth, round or ovoid mass outlined by flatus in the colon or air in the stomach and small bowel. The bags are often tied at both ends, so they may present a projection reminiscent of a rosette or bowtie, extending beyond the contour of the packet.

Most condom bags appear as egg-shaped or round densities about the size of a ping-pong ball. They characteristically have a homogeneous density, similar to feces or soft tissue. Some may be fastened with tape as further prophylaxis from rupture or leakage. If the tape contains enough aluminum to be detected on plain films, each condom bag may have a marginal radiodense accentuation.

In the 1970s, a radiopaque material had been interposed within the substance of cocaine or heroin to render them diffusely radiodense on plain films. This distinctive finding is rarely noted today. Occasionally, a lucent halo, separate from colonic flatus, can be seen. It is introduced during the wrapping process and a residue of air remains between concentric condom layers. This encircling lucency is a pathognomonic finding, readily identifiable and often multiple, situated along the course of the large bowel. Even carefully waxed and wrapped condoms are potentially liable to rupture, especially when cocaine is introduced as a powder. In the form of a paste, cocaine in condoms is less resistant to seepage or perforation, especially if carefully packaged. Today, drug packets are more standardized, suggesting an industrial process of formulation, rather than them being artisanal products. The condom or balloon is usually sealed with a wax cladding.

A finding of extensive feces in the colon is an unusual one in a young adult, the typical age of most body packers. Neurologic injury and obtundation can lead to fecal accumulation. So, too, can mechanical obstruction in the distal large bowel. A further cause is persistent use of constipating narcotic medications. However, body packers are not always addicts themselves and should be considered to be neurologically intact. Hence, the appearance of rounded, scybalous-type "feces" in the large bowel of a young adult recently entering a country from abroad, should be a warning signal. Mention must be made of a simulating condition. Some psychiatric patients who swallow Vicks inhalers or other cylindrical nonmetallic objects have X-ray findings very similar to the illicit ingestion of drug-filled balloons.

One should not confuse body packing with another form of illegal drug ingestion visible on plain films. Cocaine or crack for street use is delivered in small, closed, tube-like containers, which may have a plastic or thin glass-like envelope. The latter is radiodense to a slight degree. To avoid detection emergently, drug users have been known to quickly swallow crack containers. These can be identified on plain films of the abdomen, not as rounded soft-tissue densities but as smaller, oblong structures in the stomach or small bowel, some of which are marginally opaque. It is important to be aware of both types of illicit drug ingestion so that the apprehended individual can be placed under continuous surveillance for his or her own good in the event of inadvertent rupture of the container and entry of the substance into the circulation. Also, radiologic recognition is crucial so that appropriate police action can be taken against these individuals who have broken the law.

As mentioned before, the plain film of the abdomen is the mainstay of imaging diagnosis, having a reported sensitivity of 85–90 %, at least among those interpreters familiar with the appearance of drug packets. Ultrasonography and CT have been proposed as adjunctive tests but, in my opinion, their adoption for this condition is problematic. Ultrasound is operator specific and thus the suspect most likely will be transported to a sonography unit away from the airport. This transference raises questions of cost and risk. Who will care for the patient if he or she gets sick at the U.S. facility especially if it is an outpatient center? Moreover, since the plain film is 90 % sensitive, only a few individuals need ultrasound diagnosis or corroboration. CT poses additional issues. For one, if the plain film is negative, how can the additional radiation dose be justified, especially to young adults? Also, a pregnancy test must be administered to a female in the child bearing age. And most important is the civil liberties issue of a suspected mule who has a negative plain film and then is forced to undergo a procedure for which, as of yet, there are no studies of its efficacy.

Reference

1. Baker S, Cho K. Abdominal plain film with correlative imaging. 2nd ed. Radiology. 1999;212(3):724.

The Spleen: The Forgotten Organ, Is There Anything To Say?

78

By my last counting I have identified 74 specialty organizations in Radiology. They cover a wide spectrum of narrow interests. There are specialty groups devoted to VA radiologists and women radiologists. Others are directed to a focus in the hospital like the American Society of Emergency Radiology. Yet for the most part the specialty societies are devoted to separate organ systems or specific organs as their focus of attention. So there are neuroradiologic societies, societies of head and neck radiology and societies for chest, GU, Gyn, Pediatrics etc. Yet a major solid organ of the abdomen is an orphan because no society is dedicated to it. I refer of course to the spleen. Sure, there is the Society of Gastrointestinal Radiology, but very little consideration is given to splenic abnormalities in GI Radiology journals or in national meetings of the SGR.

Perhaps this is wise, because not that much happens in the spleen. It gets large, it can have calcifications and lucencies, but they are caused by only a few conditions. My purpose here is not to provide a revisionist notion that the spleen has the same importance as the liver or the kidney, but rather to point out some unusual entities that you might like to know about despite their rarity and their location in the obscure reaches of the left upper quadrant [1]. So the following will be a potpourri of interesting entities, at least to me.

Wandering Spleen

The wandering spleen can remain asymptomatic throughout life. If it twists on its pedicle, however, it can become infracted because its blood supply is compromised. Plain film findings include a mobile left abdominal mass as demonstrated by successive views, a medially and posteriorly displaced splenic flexure, an elevated left kidney that lacks a splenic hump, and a laterally deviated stomach.

Splenic Calcification

Splenic calcifications can be divided into multiple discrete nodular densities, cysts and solid calcifications or opacifications. The most common entities with multiple discrete calcifications are tuberculosis and histoplasmosis. In recent decades, with the AIDS epidemic, Pnuemocysitis carinii infestation can sometimes involve the splenic substance producing diffuse multifocal opacities. There has also been a report of small ring-like opacities in this condition. But if you are looking for distinctive calcifications separate from TB or histoplasmosis, another bacterial infection should come to mind.

S.R. Baker, *Notes of a Radiology Watcher*,
DOI 10.1007/978-3-319-01677-1_78, © Springer International Publishing Switzerland 2014

Brucellosis is an infectious disease with a predilection for splenic calcifications. Untreated patients have repeated episodes of fever and malaise, alternating with asymptomatic intervals. The disease is caused by one of three species of *Brucella*, but, as in the liver, only B. suis engenders calcification. Interestingly, the calcifications are often so characteristic in brucellosis that a plain film diagnosis can be made with assurance. Granulomas contain a flocculent central nidus averaging 5–10 mm in diameter.

Emanating from the central focus are irregular linear densities and a separate encircling margin of calcification. In some cases, the calcification resembles a snowflake or a target. Calcified granulomas are multiple, never confluent, and usually associated with splenomegaly.

Tumors of the Spleen

The spleen contains numerous small veins. These can proliferate, forming a hemangioma. Hemangiomas elsewhere in the body in certain locations can develop phlebolithic-like calcifications. For example, opaque venous stones are found in the soft tissues, in the stomach and in the pancreas, but peculiarly almost never in the liver, despite the frequency of hemangiomas in the liver. In the spleen, hemangiomas are not rare, but phlebolithic calcifications are exceedingly uncommon. What is the explanation for the absence of calcified phleboliths in the liver and the spleen, despite their frequency of hemangiomas of soft tissue and in other solid organs and in the stomach? This is one of the many mysteries for which theorists have no convincing answer.

Other primary tumors of the spleen are seldom encountered. In this category one should include hamartomas, which occasionally calcify, but generally appear as a non-calcified solid mass. With cystic lesions in the spleen the list of entities is long including epidermoid cysts and cystic hemangiomas. Worldwide, two thirds of all reported calcified cysts are caused by *Echinococcus granulosus*, but they are very rare outside the geographic distribution of the parasite. In the United States, by far the most common cystic lesions of the spleen are really false cysts related to trauma.

Eighty percent of these are hemorrhagic cysts. Their formation is probably a result of the liquefaction of hematomas. It is not known why some traumatized spleens rupture and others form cysts. Surprisingly, cystic degeneration is a rare event, considering the large number of cases of splenic trauma. Serous cysts, which make up approximately 20 % of all nonechinococcal, acquired cysts of the spleen, also have a traumatic etiology. Like hemorrhagic cysts, they have a fibrous lining. Most probably, serous cysts are hemorrhagic cysts from which the blood has been totally resorbed, leaving only a fibrous wall and clear fluid. Hemorrhagic and serous cysts are found most often in women of childbearing age, for reasons which remain obscure.

A small percentage of cystic lesions are true cysts with epithelial or endothelial linings. Epithelial cysts are probably due to squamous metaplasia in a preexisting mesothelial cyst and are congenital. They appear sporadically, but a familial epidermoid cyst is a known hereditary entity. Calcified epidermoid cysts and cystic hemangiomas have been observed on occasion but are much less common than radiodense pseudocysts. Splenic cysts are either asymptomatic or cause vague sensations of discomfort or fullness in the left upper quadrant. Thus, they can grow to a large size before detection. Sometimes plain films of the abdomen, obtained for other reasons, demonstrate calcified cysts that were completely unexpected clinically.

A recent review of nonparasitic splenic cysts revealed that true cysts are usually first noted in adolescence, whereas false cysts come to attention somewhat later. Both enlarge the spleen and sometimes produce a localized bulge in the splenic contour. Less than 5 % of true cysts have radiodense walls on plain films, but almost 30 % of false cysts calcify. Hence, in an area not endemic for *E. granulosus*, the finding of a single large annular calcification within the spleen is most likely a "false" cyst related to previous trauma.

Lucencies in the Spleen

The most common condition with scattered lucencies in the spleen is a splenic abscess. The most frequent cause is embolization of the splenic tissue from a primary site elsewhere in the vascular system in patients with a history of drug abuse. Generally, the abscess bubbles are small and regular in size, but occasionally a very large lucency can appear. Recently a case was presented in which the splenic abscess led to a generalized pneumoperitoneum, providing one more entry into the ever expanding list of causes of free air.

Embolization of the spleen is often done for therapeutic purposes. Two situations may occur post embolization. One, there may be the immediate accumulation of gas in the splenic substance. Just as in the liver or kidney, non-suppurative intrasplenic gas can be found after transcatheter splenic infarction. A benign condition, unassociated with clinical symptoms, it first appears 3–4 days after the procedure and persists for several weeks. The gas is arrayed as small bubbles diffusely distributed throughout the area of infarction.

On the other hand, embolization can induce an abscess which may appear rapidly or be delayed. Thus, the presence of lucencies after transcatheter splenic embolization must be evaluated in the clinical context to distinguish between the expected accumulation of bubbles in noninfected spleen and the superimposition of infections by a gas forming organism.

Reference

1. Baker S, Cho K. Abdominal plain film with correlative imaging. 2nd ed. Radiology. 1999;212(3):724.

Acute Pancreatitis: What and When Is There Room for Imaging in the Diagnosis and Followup of Patients with Acute Inflammation of the Pancreatic Gland?

79

This is a fundamentally important question because appropriate care of this disease requires careful monitoring of the patient and sometimes judicious but intrusive interventions. Certain presentations provide an impetus for pictorial representation of the presence and extent of the disease. In many institutions CT has become by force of use routine in the initial assessment of patients presenting with signs and symptoms suggestive of acute inflammation of the pancreas. As we move from the exploitative phase of imaging to a more conservationist role, every imaging protocol should be assessed for appropriateness. The purpose of this review is to consider why imaging, particularly CT, has become part and parcel of the initial workup of patients with this disease, and to examine if such a notion has been established beyond doubt or is open to question. If one were to go back to the literature of 10 or 15 years ago, one would see articles advocating sonography in acute pancreatitis. It should be gratifying to all of us that this examination really has no place in the acute assessment of patients with pancreatitis. One study revealed that the ability to visualize the pancreas by ultrasonography was less than 15 % in patients with acute inflammation of that organ. Thus, most of the results of ultrasound evaluation upon entry to emergency suite were that the studies were equivocal, occasioned by the presence of gas in the stomach and transverse colon, which obscured visualization of the solid pancreatic mass beneath it and below it. Moreover, sonography in this setting should be regarded as an invasive procedure because the pressure of the transducer on a patient with acute upper abdominal pain makes the discomfort worse. The only role for sonography in acute pancreatitis is to help to determine whether the etiology is related to the presence of gallstones, one of which may have passed from the gallbladder into the common bile duct and along the way blocked the pancreatic duct, causing acute pancreatic inflammation. However, this need not be done initially as the main function of treatment in the early phase is to prevent serious complications and to be supportive in mild and moderate cases.

CT has been advocated to demonstrate the complications of pancreatitis. What are they? One complication of pancreatic inflammation is the development of a pseudocyst. However, almost always a pseudocyst does not appear in the initial period but occurs after the patient for the large part has recovered from the acute inflammation. Thus, the chance that upon entry one would see a pseudocyst on CT is remote, and by itself not a justification for CT evaluation. A more important reason advocated for CT is the demonstration of a pancreatic abscess. This terrible complication may be occasioned on CT by the appearance of a large area of liquifaction, poorly delimited but nonetheless clearly fluid-containing or (and perhaps and) by the presence of gas bubbles generated by bacterial suppuration. In most cases the demonstration of an abscess is not a finding seen initially but will develop after several days in a patient who is almost always hectically ill.

S.R. Baker, *Notes of a Radiology Watcher*,
DOI 10.1007/978-3-319-01677-1_79, © Springer International Publishing Switzerland 2014

Some surgeons and radiologists maintain that lack of perfusion of the pancreatic gland which has become inflamed is an indication of necrosis. Hence that there is a rating system for CT to assess if this complication has occurred. It has been suggested that if necrosis has developed, as evidenced by lack of perfusion, then the patient will not recover in the absence of surgical removal of the necrotic area. Acceptance of this putative relationship has further substantiated the need for CT. However, the idea that the lack of perfusion is equivalent to necrosis and the subsidiary belief that necrosis must be treated aggressively are open to question. What may appear to be lack of necrosis may in fact be lack of perfusion due to edema alone. The persistence of that area of decreased perfusion need not result in drastic consequences if untreated surgically. Most patients with mild to moderate pancreatitis will get better with supportive therapy, without any further intervention or sophisticated diagnostic imaging tests to help monitor the patient condition. The issue of the value of CT pertains primarily to patients who come in with serious and severe pancreatitis as manifested by score values either using the APACHE or Ranson scores. The APACHE scores are primarily a measure of systemic problems with acute pancreatitis. They do not correlate well with evidence of local manifestation of severe pancreatitis. Thus the correlation between APACHE scores and CT use has yet to be established.

In sum, acute pancreatitis is the model disease that lends itself to prompt, uncritical deployment of an expensive cross-sectional imaging modality according to the fallacy of the vivid example. Because CT can demonstrate dramatic findings, it is tempting to use it to reveal those dramatic findings primarily because they are dramatic. They tempt us with their vividness, but for mild and moderate presentations of acute pancreatitis, they do not demonstrate their usefulness. They engender rewards for the radiologist but not usually for the patients. This disease and its customary workup clearly illustrate the disconnect between the lure of technology and service of the satisfaction of imaging physicians, and the lack of relevance to the immediate care of patients, rare exceptions notwithstanding.

Index

41289041R00194

Made in the USA
Middletown, DE
08 March 2017